T0275639

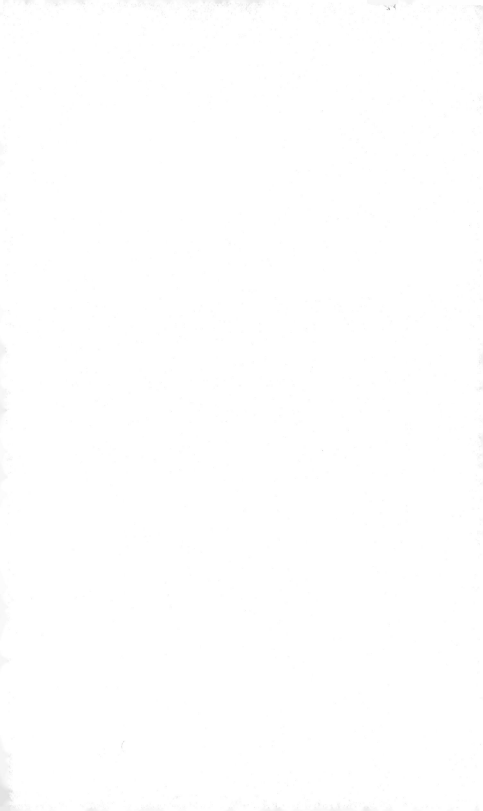

CAMBRIDGE LIBRARY COLLECTION

Books of enduring scholarly value

History of Medicine

It is sobering to realise that as recently as the year in which On the Origin of Species was published, learned opinion was that diseases such as typhus and cholera were spread by a 'miasma', and suggestions that doctors should wash their hands before examining patients were greeted with mockery by the profession. The Cambridge Library Collection reissues milestone publications in the history of Western medicine as well as studies of other medical traditions. Its coverage ranges from Galen on anatomical procedures to Florence Nightingale's common-sense advice to nurses, and includes early research into genetics and mental health, colonial reports on tropical diseases, documents on public health and military medicine, and publications on spa culture and medicinal plants.

A Treatise of the Scurvy, in Three Parts

Born in Edinburgh, with family connections to the local medical profession, James Lind (1716–94) went on to spend nine years at sea as a surgeon for the Royal Navy. His service made him familiar with one of the most common and debilitating ailments of the eighteenth century. Scurvy posed a particular problem for Britain, an island nation seeking to assert itself overseas through its navy. The symptoms of the disease had been recognised for centuries, but the causes remained elusive. First published in 1753, Lind's treatise explores the topic thoroughly, weighing the evidence and presenting a theory of the disease's aetiology, suggesting methods of prevention and treatment, and also discussing previous work on the subject, including ancient texts. Lind provided the groundwork for later investigations, his research lending support to the later practice of including the juice of citrus fruit in a sailor's diet, even though vitamin deficiency was not yet understood.

Cambridge University Press has long been a pioneer in the reissuing of out-of-print titles from its own backlist, producing digital reprints of books that are still sought after by scholars and students but could not be reprinted economically using traditional technology. The Cambridge Library Collection extends this activity to a wider range of books which are still of importance to researchers and professionals, either for the source material they contain, or as landmarks in the history of their academic discipline.

Drawing from the world-renowned collections in the Cambridge University Library and other partner libraries, and guided by the advice of experts in each subject area, Cambridge University Press is using state-of-the-art scanning machines in its own Printing House to capture the content of each book selected for inclusion. The files are processed to give a consistently clear, crisp image, and the books finished to the high quality standard for which the Press is recognised around the world. The latest print-on-demand technology ensures that the books will remain available indefinitely, and that orders for single or multiple copies can quickly be supplied.

The Cambridge Library Collection brings back to life books of enduring scholarly value (including out-of-copyright works originally issued by other publishers) across a wide range of disciplines in the humanities and social sciences and in science and technology.

A Treatise of the Scurvy, in Three Parts

Containing an Inquiry into the Nature, Causes, and Cure, of that Disease

JAMES LIND

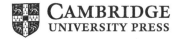

CAMBRIDGE
UNIVERSITY PRESS

University Printing House, Cambridge, CB2 8BS, United Kingdom

Cambridge University Press is part of the University of Cambridge.

It furthers the University's mission by disseminating knowledge in the pursuit of
education, learning and research at the highest international levels of excellence.

www.cambridge.org
Information on this title: www.cambridge.org/9781108069984

© in this compilation Cambridge University Press 2014

This edition first published 1753
This digitally printed version 2014

ISBN 978-1-108-06998-4 Paperback

A

TREATISE

OF THE

SCURVY.

IN THREE PARTS.

CONTAINING

An inquiry into the Nature, Caufes, and Cure, of that Difeafe.

Together with

A Critical and Chronological View of what has been publifhed on the fubject.

By *JAMES LIND*, M. D.

Fellow of the Royal College of Phyficians in *Edinburgh*.

EDINBURGH:

Printed by SANDS, MURRAY, and COCHRAN.
For A. MILLAR, in the Strand, *London*
MDCCLIII.

T O

The RIGHT HONOURABLE,

GEORGE Lord ANSON,

&c.   &c.   &c.

Who, as a juft reward for the great
and fignal fervices done to the BRI-
TISH NATION, does now prefide
over her NAVAL AFFAIRS,

The following TREATISE

IS INSCRIBED,

With the greateft refpect,

By his LORDSHIP's

Moft devoted, and

Moft obedient

humble fervant,

JAMES LIND

P R E F A C E.

THE *subject of the following sheets is of great importance to this nation; the most powerful in her fleets, and the most flourishing in her commerce, of any in the world. Armies have been supposed to lose more of their men by sickness, than by the sword. But this observation has been much more verified in our fleets and squadrons; where the scurvy alone, during the last war, proved a more destructive enemy, and cut off more valuable lives, than the united efforts of the* French *and* Spanish *arms. It has not only occasionally committed surprising ravages in ships and fleets, but almost always affects the constitution of sailors; and where it does not rise to any visible calamity, yet it often makes a powerful addition to the malignity of other diseases. It is now above* 150 *years since that great sea-officer,* Sir Peter Hawkins, *in his observations made in a voyage to the South sea, remarked it to be the pestilence of that element. He was able, in the course of twenty years, in which he had been employed at sea, to give an account of* 10,000 *ma-*
riners

riners *deftroyed by it. But I flatter myfelf, that
it will appear from the following treatife, that
the calamity may be prevented, and the danger of
this deftruftive evil obviated: nor is there any
queftion, but every attempt to put a ftop to fo
confuming a plague, will meet with a favourable
reception from the public.*

*It is a fubjeft in which all praftitioners of
phyfic are highly interefted. For it will be found,
that the mifchief is not confined to the fea, but is
extended particularly to armies at land; and is an
endemic evil in many parts of the world. This
difeafe, for above a century, has been the fuppofed
fcourge of* Europe. *But how much even the
learned world ftands in need of farther light in
fo dark a region of phyfic, may appear from the
late mournful ftory of the* German *troops in*
Hungary, *the difafter in* Thorn, *and from many
other relations in this treatife.*

*What gave occafion to my attempting this work,
is briefly as follows.*

*After the publication of the Right Honourable
Lord* Anfon's *voyage, by the Reverend Mr* Walter, *the lively and elegant pifture there exhibited*

of

*of the diftrefs occafioned by this difeafe, which
afflicted the crews of that noble, brave, and experienced Commander, in his paffage round the
world, excited the curiofity of many to inquire into
the nature of a malady accompanied with fuch
extraordinary appearances. It was acknowledged,
that the beft defcriptions of it are met with in the accounts of voyages: but it was regretted, that thofe
were the productions only of feamen; and that no
phyfician converfant with this difeafe at fea, had
undertaken to throw light upon the fubject, and
clear it from the obfcurity under which it has lain
in the works of phyficians who practifed only at
land. Some time afterwards, the fociety of furgeons of the Royal navy publifhed their laudable
plan for improving medical knowledge, by the labours of its feveral members; who have opportunities of infpecting Nature, and examining difeafes, under the varied influence of different climates, feafons, and foils. I then wrote a paper
on the fcurvy, with a defign of having it publifhed
by them. It appeared to me a fubject worthy of
the ftricteft inquiry: and I was led upon this occafion to confult feveral authors who had treated of
the difeafe; where I perceived miftakes which
have been attended, in practice, with dangerous
and fatal confequences. There appeared to me an*

evident

*evident neceſſity of rectifying thoſe errors, on ac-
count of the pernicious effects they have already
viſibly produced.   But as it is no eaſy matter to
root out old prejudices, or to overturn opinions
which have acquired an eſtabliſhment by time,
cuſtom, and great authorities; it became therefore requiſite for this purpoſe, to exhibit a full
and impartial view of what has hitherto been publiſhed on the ſcurvy; and that in a chronological
order, by which the ſources of thoſe miſtakes may
be detected. Indeed, before this ſubject could be
ſet in a clear and proper light, it was neceſſary
to remove a great deal of rubbiſh. Thus, what
was firſt intended as a ſhort paper to be publiſhed
in the memoirs of our medical navy-ſociety, has
now ſwelled to a volume, not altogether ſuitable
to the plan and inſtitution of that laudable and
learned body.*

*I cannot, however, upon this occaſion, omit
acknowledging with gratitude the many excellent
practical obſervations I have been favoured with
by ſome of its moſt worthy members; eſpecially by
the ingenious Mr Ives of Goſport; and Mr John
Murray, an eminent ſurgeon at Wells, in Nor-
folk. Notwithſtanding which advantages, I am
ſenſible of many inaccuracies and imperfections in*
this

this performance. They are perhaps the more numerous, as it has been sent to the press sooner than was at first intended. There are, however, two things that may appear exceptionable, which I ought here particularly to mention.

The first is the plan of the work.

I am sorry to find myself under a necessity of offering what some of my readers may think very indifferent entertainment, and that at their setting out, in the critical chapters of the first part. But it was not easy to fall upon a method equally adapted to all readers: nor indeed is the arrangement of the several chapters a matter of any great importance. The order here followed, is that in which it ought to be perused by physicians and men of learning, who have made this disease their study, and are previously acquainted with former writings upon it. It was necessary, in order to prevail with some of these gentlemen to peruse the second part with less prejudice against me, to endeavour first to remove such objections as might arise from doctrines imbibed in younger years, in schools and universities. Others, who are not so well acquainted with the subject, I would advise to begin with the second part; which

b   *will*

will enable them to form a better judgment of the first. The Bibliotheca fcorbutica, *or the col-lection of authors on the fcurvy, is placed at the latter end of the book, as proper to be confulted in the dictionary-way.* And it is to be remark-ed, that when, to avoid repetitions in the firft and fecond parts, an author's name is barely mentioned, recourfe muft be had to the Alpha-betical Index; which points out the page where the title of the book referred to, or its abridgment in part 3. is to be found.

In the order of the chapters, the prevention of the difeafe precedes its cure: and the firft being the moft material, I have thrown great part of the latter into it; this method of treating the fcurvy fuiting it better than perhaps any other. It will appear, that in the plan I have purfued, I had in view an author whofe book has met with a ge-neral good reception, Aftruc de morbis venereis; *and were other difeafes treated in like manner, it would greatly abridge the enormous, and ftill increafing number of books in our fcience.*

What may be deemed by critics equally excep-tionable with the order of the chapters, are fome few repetitions. But in certain cafes they were neceffary, neceſſary, in order to obviate prejudices at the time they might naturally ariſe, and to inforce the argument.

As to the contents of the book in general :

In the firſt part, I have endeavoured, by a connected courſe of reaſoning in the ſeveral chapters, to eſtabliſh what is there advanced, upon the cleareſt evidence, confirmed by ſome of the beſt authorities ; and have laid aſide all ſyſtems and theories of this malady which were found to be diſavowed by nature and facts. Where I have been neceſſarily led, in this diſagreeable part of the work, to criticiſe the ſentiments of eminent and learned authors, I have not done it with a malignant view of depreciating their labours, or their names ; but from a regard to truth, and to the good of mankind. I hope ſuch motives will, to the candid, and to the moſt judicious, be a ſufficient apology for the liberties I have aſſumed.

Dies diem docet.

The principal chapters of the ſecond part, containing a deſcription of this diſeaſe, its cauſes, the means of preventing and curing it, are alſo

founded

founded upon attested facts and observations, with-
out suffering the illusions of theory to influence and
pervert the judgment. For, that things certain
may precede what is uncertain, the theory, and the
inferences from it, are placed at the latter end.

In the third part, where I have given an a-
bridgment of what has been written upon the sub-
ject by the most celebrated medical authors, and
others, I have always endeavoured to express
their sentiments with as much clearness and con-
ciseness as I could. I have indeed through the
whole aimed at perspicuity rather than elegance of
diction, as most proper in a book of science. To
know a disease, and to cure it, being the two
things most essential to be learned; I have there-
fore transcribed the symptoms and cure of the scur-
vy from those authors, where they do not entirely
copy from each other.

CONTENTS.

PART I.

CHAP. I.

PART

P A R T   II.

C H A P.   I.

C H A P.

E R-

A

TREATISE

OF THE

SCURVY.

PART I.

CHAP. I.

A critical history of the different accounts of this disease.

IN the first accounts given us of this disease, by *Ronsseus*, *Echthius*, and *Wierus* (a), it is surprising to find, not only an accurate description of it, but an enumeration of almost all the truly antiscorbutic medicines that are known to the world even at this day.

(a) The first authors on the scurvy. *Ronsseus* and *Echthius*, though cotemporary, wrote separately, without having the benefit of seeing each others works.

Ronsseus,

Rouffeus, who believed it to be the fame difeafe that is defcribed by *Pliny (b)*, and is faid
to have afflicted the *Roman* army under the
command of *Cæfar Germanicus,* obferved, that
in his time it was to be met with only in *Holland, Friefland,* and *Denmark*; though he had
heard of its appearing in *Flanders, Brabant,*
and fome parts of *Germany.* From feeing
fome of thofe countries entirely free from this
diftemper, he was induced to afcribe its frequency in other places to their foil, climate,
and diet. In order to prove which, he wrote
his firft epiftle *(c)*.

Echthius feems to be the firft who gave rife
to the opinion of its being a contagious or infectious *lues.* He was led into that miftake, by
obferving whole monafteries who lived on the
fame diet, and in the fame air, at once affected with it, efpecially after fevers; which no
doubt might become infectious in clofe and
confined apartments. He imagined, therefore,
that a fcurvy might in a manner be the *crifis*
of a fever, which as fuch he deemed contagious.

(b) Vid. part 3. chap. 1.

(c) Intitled, *Quare apud Amfterodamum, Alecmariam, atque
alia vicina loca, frequentiffime infeftet fcorbutus ?*

But

But where *Wierus* tranſcribes the ſymptoms from this laſt author, (which he does almoſt *verbatim*), upon this occaſion he very juſtly differs from him. He obſerves, that the ſcurvy is not properly the *criſis* of a fever; but, like many other diſeaſes, may be occaſioned after it by unſound viſcera, and a vitiated ſtate of blood. He imagines people were induced to believe it a contagious malady, by ſeeing many whole families alike affected; but this he aſcribed to the *ſameneſs* of their diet. He was however deceived (probably by the authority of *Echthius*) in thinking, that where the gums were putrid, the diſeaſe might be infectious: and accordingly makes it a doubt, whether in ſome parts of the *Lower Germany*, where it had lately appeared, it was owing to their diet, or to infection. But it ſhall be fully proved hereafter, that the ſcurvy is not contagious or infectious *(d)*.

It may be proper to obſerve further, that *Wierus* had deſcribed the various and extraordinary ſymptoms of this malady, in ſo accurate a manner, that the ſucceeding authors for a long time did nothing more than copy him. It was a conſiderable time afterwards, when

(d) Chap. 4.

Solomon

Solomon Albertus wrote a large treatiſe on this ſubjeƈt, wherein he aſſumes great merit to himſelf in diſcovering a ſymptom not taken notice of by any author, and which he had once or twice obſerved in this diſeaſe, *viz.* a *rigor* or ſtiffneſs of the lower jaw. However, *Wierus* ſtill continued in the greateſt eſteem and reputation; and his book was deemed the ſtandard on this ſubjeƈt, even till the time of *Eugalenus*, who gives it that juſt charaƈter, and refers to it almoſt entirely for the cure. He muſt be allowed therefore to have been a good judge of this diſtemper: and as he was a perſon of eminent learning, as well as probity, (which his writings on this and many other ſubjeƈts ſufficiently ſhew), his word may be relied upon, when he tells us, that in his time this diſeaſe was peculiar to the inhabitants of the countries upon the north ſeas: he had never met with it in *Spain*, *France*, nor in *Italy;* nor was it to be ſeen in the large traƈt of *Upper Germany:* and as to *Aſia* and *Africa*, if ever it appeared there, it would no doubt be in ſuch places as lay adjacent to the ſea; where ſuch a ſituation, and a groſs diet, with the uſe of putrid water, might give riſe to it, in the ſame manner as they do in the countries where

it

it was endemic.   Thefe were not conjectures in our author; for he was a great traveller, and had vifited all the places he talks of *(e)*.   A book wrote in thofe times by him, *De præftigiis dæmonum*, adds much to his reputation; as it fhews he was neither fo weak, nor credulous, as fome later writers on the fcurvy.

Brunnerus, who may be deemed the next judicious author after him on this fubject, obferved, that in his time, when the ufe of wine was become more common, the fcurvy was not fo frequent as formerly, even in thofe countries where it had been endemic.

Notwithftanding which, in a very fhort time after, we are furprifed with accounts of this fuppofed contagious *lues* having fpread far and wide.   In lefs than thirty years after *Wierus*, *Solomon Albertus*, in his dedication to the Duke of *Brunfwick*, after fome very pathetic declamations on the vices of the times, obferves, that he had met with the fcurvy every where; and that it prevailed in *Mifnia*, *Lufatia*, on the borders of *Bohemia* and *Silefia*, *&c.*

However, the difeafe as yet ftill retained the fame face; the fymptoms and appearances in it the fame.   For though this author (who

(e) Vid. Melchior Adam in vita Wieri.

practifed

practifed in a place where *Wierus* fays the fcurvy was uncommon) had difcovered one extraordinary fymptom, before mentioned, fometimes accompanying it; and which certainly was but rarely to be feen, as it efcaped the obfervation of every one but himfelf: yet in other refpects, he, as well as his contemporary writers, gives us the fame account of it as *Wierus* had done before; and particularly, that the putrid gums and fwelled legs were the moft certain and only characteriftic figns of it *(f)*.

But in eleven years after him, we are likewife acquainted by *Eugalenus*, with the furprifing rapidity with which this contagious *lues* had made its progrefs over almoft the whole world. And what is ftill more remarkable, the face of the difeafe was in a few years fo much changed, that the putrid gums and fwelled legs were no longer characteriftical figns of it, as it often killed the patient before thefe fymptoms appeared *(g)*. And it is highly probable from

(f) Signa mali hujus charaƈteriftica non alia funt, præter duo illa (quorum fuprà meminimus) gemina, fymptomata pathognomica appellata, indubia morbi indicia, viz. ftomacace et fceletyrbe. Cætera fymptomata ancipitia funt et vaga. Alberti hiftoria fcorbuti, p. 546.

(g) P. 10. and 211. The *Amfterdam* edition of *Eugalenus*, publifhed in the year 1720, is here quoted.

the

the hiftories of above 200 cafes of patients delivered in his book, wherein mention is made
of the gums being affected in one perfon only,
that fuch fymptoms did now but rarely, if at
all, occur.

This malady was alfo greatly increafed in
virulence, as he gives us to underftand in different parts of his performance: all which he
would perfuade us to have proceeded from a
very fingular caufe *(h)*.

Its effects and fymptoms were now various
and innumerable *(i)*: and it was alfo become
a much more frequent calamity than it appears
to have ever been formerly; at leaft, if we
may take this author's word for it, who upon

(h) P. 250. where talking of the pox and fcurvy as both
modern difeafes, *Utrique etiam peculiare hoc noftro feculo fuit, ut
quàm longiffimè latiffimèque fua pomæria dilatent et diffundant, atque
procul à generationis fuæ locis et terminis, ad incognita et remota loca excurrant evagenturque, atque fub diametrali linea, quâ fibi in-
vicem, fub polorum oppofitione, oppofita funt, fe mutuò quafi comple-
ctantur, et inter fe virus ac venenum fuum communicent. Ita fit ut
hodie etiam Germaniæ, Angliæ, Galliæ, hic morbus innotefcat;* a-
pud quos antea ne quidem auditum ejus momen fuit. He fays the
fame thing in the dedication of his book to the Count of *Naffau.*
Some of his editors have taken care to have this dedication fuppreffed in the later editions. It is indeed a moft curious piece.

*(i) Tam varii funt effectus quos hic morbus edit, ut minimas o-
mnium differentias numero comprehendere non magis ferè poffibile fit,
quàm arenam maris numerare,* p. 217.

this

this occafion expreffes himfelf in very hyper-
bolical terms. And we muft indeed allow
him to have had a very extenfive practice, fince
he informs us that he had feen almoft innumerable patients afflicted with only one particular fymptom of the malady *(k)*.

But befides the natural reafons which he affigns, he is likewife pleafed to introduce fome
moral confiderations, to account for the great
frequency and virulence of this diftemper, and
the extraordinary fymptoms which he afcribes
to it. In one place *(l)* he attributes its irregular appearances to the operation of the de-
vil. But in another, he thinks this new and
furprifing calamity fent, by divine permiffion,
as a chaftifement for the fins of the world.
And as he really thought himfelf (as appears
through the whole treatife) the moft fagacious
detector of this *Proteus*-like mifchief, lurking
under various and furprifing appearances, he

(k) Thus in a fcorbutic quotidian, *Plures mendaci quotidianæ
febris typo ab hoc morbo ægrotarunt, quàm ut numero hîc comprehendi
queant,* p. 231. Talking of fcorbutic pains in various parts of
the body, *Defcribendis nominibus eorum qui ab his doloribus variè
exercitati elapfis hifce annis fuere, vix fufficeret præfens charta,*
p. 51. Thofe patients, he again repeats, were almoft innumerable, p. 258.

(l) P. 81.

very

very religiouſly thanks Heaven for the important diſcovery *(m)*.

Now, as this book has been often reprinted in different parts of *Europe*, has been recommended by the greateſt authority, by *Boerhaave* to his pupils, by *Hoffman*, *&c.* and is looked upon at this day as the ſtandard author on our ſubject *(n)*; it may be worth while to inquire into the contents of it, as well as the merit of its author. And we ſhall begin with obſerving wherein he differs in his account and deſcription of this diſeaſe, from all preceeding authors. For as to thoſe who ſucceeded, they did little more than copy him. So that I ſhall have few remarks to make upon theſe, till we come to Dr *Willis*, who gives us a ſomewhat different account of its ſymptoms.

(m) Quod ideò permittere Deus videtur, ut hoc modo iram ſuam adverſus peccata oſtendat, dum novis et inuſitatis morbis et ægritudinibus, nunquam priùs cognitis ac viſis, mortale genus in ira ſua viſitat et caſtigat; ut etiam vulgus noſtras, morborum novitate admonitum, intelligat differentes hujus temporis febres ac morbos eſſe, ab iis qui ante aliquot annos homines afflixerunt. Agamus igitur Deo gratias, quòd pro ſua infinita miſericordia ac clementia tam benignè eos nobis revelare dignatus ſit, p. 222.

(n) It is ſaid very lately by *Haller*, to be univerſally eſteemed the beſt book written on the ſcurvy. *Vid. Boerhaave methodus ſtudii medici.*

B   *Eugalenus*

Eugalenus differs from all preceeding authors.

1*ſt*, In ſuppoſing the malady may be far advanced, before (what they judged) the moſt equivocal and uncertain ſigns appeared in it. " Thus, (ſays he), after a long continuance " of the diſtemper, the patient has a conſtant " *languor*, a numbneſs, a ſenſe of heavy pain " in his legs, or an acute pain in any part *(o)*." But ſuch ſymptoms are by *Echthius* claſſed in a ſeparate chapter, under the denomination of *the remote ſigns common to this diſeaſe with others*. And *Forreſtus*, who had the greateſt opportunity of being converſant with ſcorbutic caſes, by living in a ſea-port town, mentions them as the ſymptoms only of the approaching evil. He ſays, that upon their appearance he heſitated for ſome time, till the proper and peculiar ſymptoms of this diſeaſe appeared, *viz.* the putrid gums, *&c.* which put the matter out of all doubt. But *Eugalenus* ſuppoſes the ſcurvy often to deſtroy the patient before the appearance of theſe latter *(p)*.

2*dly*, On the contrary, he ſuppoſes, that thoſe ſymptoms which, according to all others, ap-

(o) P. 14.   *(p)* P. 10. et 211.

pear

pear only in the laft and moft advanced ftage of this malady, often occur in the very beginning, and without any other previous fcorbutic fign; fuch as, frequent fainting-fits, atrophies, dropfies, *&c.*; which laft are mentioned by *Brucæus* and others, as the confequences of the moft inveterate and confirmed fcurvy.

So that whereas formerly the malady had a regular progreffion of fymptoms in its different ftages, accurately related by *Wierus* and many others, it became in *Eugalenus's* time the moft irregular and deceitful evil that we can well imagine.

3*dly*, *Eugalenus* differs from all preceeding authors in his defcription of many fymptoms peculiar to this difeafe. Thus, fcorbutic ulcers, according to him, are dry *(q)*: whereas thefe ulcers are defcribed formerly in this difeafe, as having quite a contrary appearance, *viz.* fungous, fœtid, *&c.* Alfo the *dyfpnœa* in fcorbutic perfons, formerly moft troublefome upon u- fing exercife or motion, is defcribed by *Euga- lenus* with very different marks; as is the *di- arrhœa*, and almoft all the other fymptoms.

(*q*) Sect. 49. In the firft pages of his book, which are copied from *Wierus*, he defcribes the ulcers more truly.

4*thly*, He has afcribed to this difeafe many
new fymptoms, feemingly oppofite to the genius
of it; at leaft never taken notice of by any
before him: though *Dodonæus*, *Wierus*, and
many other writers, may be fuppofed to have
had an opportunity of feeing it in its utmoft
virulence, when epidemic in the year 1556, in
the places where they then lived; and where in
all probability it has never finee raged in fuch a
degree.   The fymptoms he mentions, are cancers, buboes, ulcers of the *penis*, lofs of memory, fymptoms of the plague, &c.

Now, thefe different accounts and defcriptions of the fame difeafe, can be accounted for
but in two ways.

This diftemper muft, in a very fhort time after the firft accounts of it were publifhed, have
made an incredible progrefs, become an univerfal
calamity, and affumed quite a new appearance
and different fymptoms.   This was the opinion of *Eugalenus*; who, although he has given
fuch a new and different relation of it, yet tells
us exprefsly, it was the *ftomacacia* of *Pliny*, the
difeafe defcribed by all other authors under the
name of *fcurvy*; with whom he agrees in affigning the fame caufes and cure.   For which laft,
in particular, he refers us to thefe authors.

Or

Or we may ſuppoſe, that this author might be miſtaken, in thinking the diſeaſe he has deſcribed, to be preciſely the ſame that was formerly known by that appellation: yet perhaps there may be found ſome analogy or reſemblance betwixt what he deemed ſuch, and the former accounts we had of the ſcurvy; ſo that they may be ſaid to border on each other. Or at leaſt he has given this denomination to a complication of various ſymptoms firſt deſcribed by himſelf; and thus has characteriſed under the name of *ſcurvy*, a particular diſeaſe, or claſs of diſeaſes; in which he has been followed by ſucceeding authors.

Upon the firſt ſuppoſition, before we can give entire credit to him, and believe ſo great an alteration to have happened in this diſtemper, it is neceſſary we ſhould know what grounds he had for his opinion, and what reaſons induced him to believe, that ſo many diſeaſes, various and oppoſite in their appearances, were nothing more than the ſcurvy lurking under theſe different forms. It is at leaſt required, that there ſhould have been in the effects or appearances of the diſeaſes, ſome diſtant analogy or reſemblance left; otherwiſe there will

be

be a ftrong prefumption that here he might be miftaken.

But inftead of pointing out to us any fuch fimilarity or refemblance betwixt the difeafes he has defcribed, and the real fcurvy as defcribed by all others before him; he has fallen upon a moft extraordinary method of proving their identity, by *affuming for pathognomic and demonftrative fcorbutic figns, fuch fymptoms as had never been obferved in the difeafe before*; *viz.* fuch a ftate of urine and pulfe as is entirely different from the defcription given of them by the moft accurate writers *(r)*.

Now,

(r) Vid. part 3. chap. 2. *Forreftus* tells us, that in this malady the ftate of the urine deferves no regard ; and wrote three books to prove it fallacious. Although *Reufnerus* does not in this agree with *Forreftus*; yet he, as well as *Wierus*, differs widely from *Eugalenus* in the defcription of the urines in this difeafe. As to the ftate of pulfe defcribed by *Eugalenus*, which he afferts to be the moft conftant concomitant of this diftemper, p. 30. it is remarkable, he is the firft author who mentions fuch a condition of pulfe to have ever been obferved in the fcurvy. *Reufnerus* fays, the pulfe is here inordinate ; in which he likewife differs from all other authors : but it is plain by his book, this was a fuppofition made from theory, and not from obfervation. (Vid. *Reufner.* p. 382.). He makes it at the fame time flow.

Notwithftanding all which, the pulfe and urine, or either of them, convince *Eugalenus* of the exiftence of the fcurvy, though in other refpeəts the fymptoms fhould differ from it as much as

the

Now, upon a fuppofition that the pulfe and urine, like the reft of the fymptoms, had alfo varied in this diftemper from their former appearances, it was then incumbent upon him to prove the identity of thefe difeafes by other marks, and not by thofe fymptoms wherein the difeafe differed from itfelf.

Befides the pulfe and urine, which were to him the moft demonftrative figns, he often mentions fome other marks or diagnoftics; upon which, however, he does not depend fo much as on the former; though he often in-

the plague does from a dropfy. *Sufficiant ad denotandam mali caufam quæ ab urina et pulfu indicia fumuntur,* p. 120. *De his o-mnibus, certum à pulfu & urina, vel ab horum alterutro, indicium eft, minimèque fallax,* p. 89. *Citra alia indicia, non femel ad morbi cognitionem nos fola urina deduxit,* p. 23.

Our author could not perhaps well have fallen upon two more uncertain diagnoftics than thofe of the pulfe and urine, by which alone he charaƈterifes fo many various difeafes, acute and chronic. The mighty faith he had in urine, the moft fallacious of all medical figns, one would have thought fufficient to have deftroyed his credit with the judicious. As to the pulfe, it varies fo much in old and young, and in the different fexes; the conftitution of the body, the fituation, and other circumftances of the artery, all what phyficians call *the nonnaturals,* have fo remarkable an influence upon it, as to make the diagnoftics taken from it fingly, to be very fallacious in any difeafe.

There is indeed the utmoft abfurdity in his accounts of both; and, what is very remarkable, moft of the cafes at the latter end of his book, are manifeft contradiƈtions to the diagnoftics delivered in the firft part of it.

troduces

troduces them to confirm the judgment he had formed of ſuch diſeaſes. And it may be proper, in juſtice to him, to take notice of them all; which I think may be properly referred to theſe two claſſes.

1ſt, Such ſymptoms as the before mentioned conditions of pulſe and urine, that never were remarked in the ſcurvy by any but himſelf; and ſeem indeed more peculiar to other diſtempers; *viz.* recurring anxieties at the region of the ſtomach, under the diaphragm *(ſ)*; — a ball in the throat *(t)*; — a tumor moving from one part of the body to another *(u)*; — retchings to vomit in the beginning of a fever *(x)*.

2dly, Such as are common to this diſeaſe with many others; and which the authors who preceeded him, call the remote and doubtful ſymptoms; *viz.* an obtuſe or dull pain of the legs, which he often mentions as a convincing proof of the ſcurvy *(y)*; — dejection of mind *(z)*;

(ſ) P. 142. and in many other places.
(t) P. 154.
(u) Diag. 23. p. 212.
(x) P. 235.
(y) P. 145. 201. 206. 216. 235. and particularly p. 50.
(z) Obſ. 15.

— being

— being worſe after purgatives *(a)*; — a *languor*, rather than ſickneſs; — a ſlow diſeaſe without any evident cauſe; — ſometimes a vomiting, faintings, and a change of colour in the face; — an eruption on the face and breaſt in a fever *(b)*; — nay, an eruption on the body after death, and not till then, he makes a demonſtrative ſign of the ſcurvy *(c)*, or juſt at the approach of it *(d)*.

But theſe diagnoſtics he ſeems to rely upon no further, than to corroborate the proofs he had from the pulſe and urine.

Now, as theſe are the principal marks and diagnoſtics of the diſeaſes deſcribed by *Eugalenus*; among which there are not to be found any of thoſe ſymptoms which the authors preceeding him thought abſolutely neceſſary to demonſtrate the exiſtence of the diſeaſe which they had deſcribed under the name of *ſcurvy*; and as *Eugalenus* aſſumed for demonſtrative and conſtant ſigns of this diſeaſe, ſuch as were never before obſerved in the true ſcurvy, nor are ever ſeen to occur in it at this day, as afterwards will be more fully proved: we muſt neceſſarily conclude, that he has deſcribed a

(a) P. 152.   *(c)* P. 124.
(b) Diag. 25. p. 236.   *(d)* P. 187. et 189.

different

different difeafe; which appears from his whole treatife, and will be further confirmed by what follows.

It is indeed furprifing, in fo extenfive a practice as he pretends to have had, that in his book, containing 72 obfervations, and above 200 cafes of different patients, given us by him or his editor, there is not mention made of one truly fcorbutical cafe wherein the gums were affected, except in a very extraordinary and dubious relation of a clergyman *(e)*; who contracted his indifpofition by a coftive-nefs, being accuftomed when in health to have ten or twelve natural ftools a-day; whom he cured by bleeding, and fome antifcorbutics which he does not mention; and by reftoring his belly to its ufual lax ftate.

It is true, he maintains, that the fcurvy often kills before it affects the gums or the legs *(f)*. But is it credible, among fuch a number of patients as he treated in this difeafe, which in many places he tells us were almoft innumerable, that in the before mentioned cafe alone the putrid gums were obferved; which formerly, during the moft virulent rage of this evil, and at this day, as fhall be afterwards proved,

(e) Obf. 72.   *(f)* P. 10.

is

is the moſt conſtant, chief, and characteriſtic ſymptom of it?

For a ſpecimen of the queſtions he aſked his patients, ſee *p*. 32. & 98. where he reca-pitulates all his diagnoſtics of ſcorbutic diſeaſes; and it does not appear he ever looked for ſuch ſigns.

He gives but one inſtance of the teeth being looſe *(g)*; where he obſerves there were much more demonſtrative ſigns of the ſcurvy, *viz.* the pulſe, urine, oppreſſion on the *præcordia*, and faintings; adding it in the laſt place, as a ſymp-tom of the leaſt moment *(h)*.

He takes notice of ſpots as a ſign of this diſ-eaſe, only in the ſcorbutic atrophy; though he produces but one very doubtful ſcorbutic atro-phical caſe *(i)* wherein they appeared.

We ſhall compare him in this reſpect once more with the authors who preceeded him. *Reuſnerus* wrote but four years before him, and has collected into a volume of conſiderable bulk, almoſt all that had been written upon

(g) Obſ. 47.

(h) Ultimo, et dentium laxatio. Sed quia hæc primùm ſub morbi finem incidit, minus ad monſtrandum morbum hunc ponderis habuit; quòd priùs ægrota ab hoc morbo interfici potuit, quàm ab hoc ſigno morbus cognoſci.

(i) Obſ. 34.

C 2   the

the ſcurvy. After deſcribing the putrid gums
and ſpots, he expreſſes himſelf thus. " Theſe
" are the pathognomic ſigns of the ſcurvy,
" without whoſe appearance the diſeaſe can-
" not ſubſiſt *(k)*."

IT may be ſaid, that though the diſeaſes were
not preciſely the ſame, yet *Eugalenus* under
the ſame name has charaċteriſed a certain diſeaſe, or ſpecies of diſeaſes, in which he has
been followed by all other authors; and his
ſuccesful cures, to which he ſo often appeals,
ſeem to confirm it. This leads me to the only diagnoſtic which I have omitted to mention;
being reſerved for this place, as the moſt diſtinguiſhing charaċteriſtic of all the diſeaſes deſcribed in his book, and which is to be met with
almoſt in every page *(l)*. It is there called
Regula diagnoſtica generaliſſima (m), *viz.* its
                                        being

(k) *Et hæ ſigna ſunt ſcorbuti pathognomica, quæ ſine rei in qua
ſita ſunt interitu abeſſe nequeunt.* Reuſneri exercitat. de ſcorbuto,
p. 328.

(l) P. 27. 127. &c.

*(m) Viz. Nam ſi quis nobis in his regionibus morbus occurrat rarus,
vel etiam aliquis veteribus cognitus, ſub aliis, et diverſis, atque plurimum
ab eorum deſcriptione diſcedentibus ſignis, ſtatim mendacem ejus ſpe-
ciem ſuſpeċtam habere oportet, et huc atque ad hunc morbum cogitati-
ones dirigere, diligenterque cum morbi mores, et cauſas ejus antecedentes,*
                                                              tum

*being a diſeaſe not properly deſcribed by the an-
cients :* to which he often adds, its not ſubmit-
ting to the cure preſcribed for it by theſe old
authors.

He recommends the peruſal of his book to
ſuch only as are converſant in the writings of
the ancient *Greek* and *Roman* phyſicians *(n)*;
otherwiſe he obſerves they will never be able
to diſtinguiſh old diſeaſes from the new. The
laſt of which, or what he imagined to be ſuch,
he has promiſcuouſly claſſed, without any o-
ther diſtinction, under the general name of
ſcurvy.

To give the reader the true idea the author
had of the ſcurvy, by which he may be enabled to judge what particular diſeaſe, or ſpecies
of diſeaſes, he has characteriſed; it is preciſely
this.

He ſeems to have been of opinion, with an e-
minent phyſician of that age, who takes occaſion
from *Solomon's* ſaying, there was nothing new
under the ſun, to aſſert, that all diſtempers were

tum pulſum et urinam explorare, taliane ſint quæ huic morbo conve-
niant, eumque quadam ſuâ proprietate exprimant et demonſtrent.
Soon after adding, *Non video quis præterea dubitationi locus eſſe
poſſit, niſi perpetuo cogitationibus noſtris oberrare et incertum vagari
velimus,* p. 179.

(n) P. 227.

the

the fame formerly as at prefent. To this our
author, however, makes two exceptions, in the
pox and fcurvy, *(p. 250.)*; where he imagines
that the one travels from the north, the other
from the fouth ; and that, upon their meeting,
they communicate and intermingle their poifon
with each other. But he was entirely unacquainted with hyfteric and hypochondriac ailments, and a train of others now going under
the name of *nervous*. He knew very little of
the rheumatifm, rickets, and many others;
which, if at all, have been very imperfectly
defcribed by the ancients. Hence, whenever
fuch cafes occurred, with this peculiarity, of
not being defcribed in ancient authors, he
directly pronounced them fcorbutic.

Thus, he imagined, that the fcurvy might af-
fume the form of almoft all difeafes, acute or
chronic, incident to the human body: or, in
other words, that the numerous and various
diftempers defcribed in his book, from the
plague to a fimple intermitting fever, might be
produced by this one fcorbutic caufe;   and
that each of thefe manifold difeafes might fubfift fingly and feparately, without the appearance of any fymptom formerly obferved in the
fcurvy defcribed by others; or even any one
                              fymptom

symptom common to thofe defcribed by himfelf, except the appearances in the urine and
ftate of the pulfe. The firft of which, he tells
us himfelf, is often fallacious; and though he
mentions the pulfe as the only fymptom *(o)*
in which all fuch difeafes agree, yet, from
many other parts of his book, it appears, that
the pulfe alfo was, and certainly muft be very
various in fo many different cafes *(p)*.

But as difference of climates muft needs
have a great influence, even on the fame difeafe; accordingly we find the crifes and types
of fevers and other diftempers, to vary in thefe
cold climates, from the defcription given of

(o) P. 30.
(p) If the criticifm on *Eugalenus* appears too tedious, it muft
be confidered, that it is the bafis of all the reafoning in this firft
part of the work. Nor muft the reader imagine, that although
he be found to have publifhed very great abfurdities, yet he is
but one author only, and feems not to deferve fo ferious a confutation. Such as are ignorant of the hiftory of the difeafe,
and have not taken the pains to look into the *Bibliotheca,*
part 3. muft be informed, that his whole book almoft is tranfcribed by *Sennertus* and *Martini*; and its greateft abfurdities by
Horftius, Lifter, and many others. Had thefe authors confirmed what he advances, by faꞔts and obfervations, *Eugalenus* had
juftly merited the compliment they pay him. But, on the contrary, they affert moft things in their writings entirely upon the
faith of *Eugalenus*; fo that, according to his fate, the credit of
many authors muft ftand or fall.

                                                    them

them in more ſouthern countries, where the
ancients practiſed. Theſe and other incidental
circumſtances, muſt needs vary the juſt indications of regimen and cure. This our author
makes no allowance for: but when the moſt
common and uſual malady deviated in the leaſt
from the graphical account given of it by thoſe
accurate authors, eſpecially when it did not
yield to the method of cure directed by them;
all ſuch irregular and untoward ſymptoms he
likewiſe referred to the ſcorbutic taint.

Now, whether the diſeaſe was altogether
and purely ſcorbutic, or the ſcurvy was joined
or complicated with another malady, no cure
could poſſibly be made in either caſe, without
the common and ſpecific antiſcorbutic medicines; which, upon the laſt ſuppoſition, were
to be compounded with others proper for theſe
diſeaſes, and which, according to his own account, proved always ſuccefsful *(q)*.

But here we have reaſon to ſuſpect ſomewhat worſe than ignorance, by which it would

(q) In his omnibus, cum, propter multiplicem ſymptomatum va-
rietatem raritatemque, cauſam ſubeſſe raram, et veteribus incogni-
tam, conſiderarem; poſt varias habitas mecum deliberationes, et di-
ligentem pulſuum urinarumque examinationem, tandem ſcorbuto ad-
ſcribendam inveni, conjecturam meam ac σοχασμὸν de his, compro-
bante felici curationis eventu, p. 30.

ſeem

ſeem he has chiefly impoſed upon the world. He informs us, that if the diſeaſe was but known, it was very eaſily cured *(r)*; and re-fers us to *Wierus,* who had wrote moſt learn-edly on this ſubjeƈt before him; the inten-tion of his book being only to deteƈt this *Proteus*-like malady, lurking under ſo many various and fallacious appearances *(ſ)*. He has indeed furniſhed us with no other antiſcor-butic remedies, than what were recommended before him; as may be ſeen by his *Therapeutic canons (t)*. His principal antiſcorbutic medi-cine was ſcurvy-graſs, and next to it, water-creſſes and brook-lime. He however fancied ſome of theſe to have a more ſingular and pe-culiar virtue in particular ſymptoms of this diſ-eaſe, than others of them. For a *coma* (or *carus* as he terms it) in the ſcorbutic fever, he particularly recommends *naſturtium aquat. (u)*, and gives what may be called a miraculous in-ſtance of its good effeƈts *(x)*: whereas in con-vulſions attending ſcorbutic fevers, he prefers

(r) P. 140.
(ſ) Ibid.
(t) P. 26. 42. 43.
(u) P. 44. Canon. ther. 11. Item, p. 124. 125.
(x) Obſ. 54.

ſuc. cochlear. (y), and gives an equally ſurpriſing
hiſtory of its good effects *(z)*.

But what idea can any perſon entertain of
this author's veracity, when he relates ſuch numerous and extraordinary cures, in the moſt
tedious and obſtinate diſeaſes, performed by
ſuch ſimple medicines; and in ſo ſhort a time
as exceeds all manner of belief? Such was then
the efficacy of thoſe herbs, that they reſcued
many long-unhappy patients from the jaws of
death. They removed diſeaſes which had re-
ſiſted all other methods of cure, and had baf-
fled the ſkill of the beſt phyſicians. With ſuch
aſſertions this book every where abounds.
" Many who had laboured under this calami-
" ty, confined to bed for weeks, months,
" nay, years, (as, at the time he was writing,
" was the caſe of a widow, owing to the ig-
" norance of her phyſician), were in a few
" days, by theſe powerful antiſcorbutic juices,
" cured of the moſt obſtinate and inveterate
" ailments *(a)*."

In a ſeemingly very bad caſe of a childbed-
woman *(b)*, the ſcorbutic *deliquium* and *anxiety* were put off for ſeveral hours when ap-

(y) Canon. ther. 13. p. 44.   *(a)* P. 129. 147.
(z) Obſ. 53.   *(b)* Obſ. 69.

proaching,

proaching, by thefe antifcorbutic medicines; which upon this account were repeated eight or nine times a-day.   Any one who perufes this relation, will find as extraordinary cafes, *viz.* ulcers gaping and fhutting, *&c.* as are to be met with in the records, or perhaps the legends of phyfic *(c)*.

He performed feveral cures, even in apparently dangerous cafes in fevers, by an infufion of a little fcurvy-grafs in goat-whey *(d)*.   He removed a malignant fever, chiefly by the addition of *fuc. cochlear. dr.* ii./s. to an aperient potion; which, upon taking four or five times, abated the fever with all its untoward fymptoms; but upon difcontinuing the medicine for two days, it returned *(e)*.

The vanity and prefumption of this author are indeed intolerable, when he affures us, that he would cure beginning confumptions in fourteen days *(f)*; palfies in five days *(g)*, in four days often, but in fourteen at moft *(h)*;

(c) P. 264. 265.   Vid. Obf. 33. et 50.
(d) Obf. 32.
(e) Obf. 59.
(f) P. 192.
(g) Obf. 16. et 23.
(h) P. 63.

violent

violent toothachs in a few hours *(i)*; several
quartan agues in ten days, otherwise not cu-
rable in a year *(k)*.   In short, according to
him, no disease is any longer incurable; and
by his means the art of physic is restored to
credit and reputation *(l)*.

Sometimes indeed the patient expired before
the antiscorbutic medicines could be got ready;
as was the case of a young girl to whom this
fatal accident happened.   Here he offered to
prove the wonderful effects of his remedies, to
the conviction of the whole family, in the el-
dest son, who laboured also under this affliction.   But after a fruitless trial of eighteen days
he was dismissed; the father being informed,

(i) P. 52.
(k) P. 40.
(l) *Futurum enim est, ut in morbi notitiam deductus, paucis die-
bus gravissimas quasque febres sit curaturus, quibus nulla prius veterum profuit curatio.*   Soon after adding, *Quæ, quia à nemine
hactenus satis animadversa sunt, quod sciam, hinc factum esse ar-
bitror, quòd tantopere vilescere apud nos et in his regionibus medicina cæperit, utpote quæ nullius febris curationem certò promitteret.*
p. 36.
And repeating the same remark in another place, *Hoc sine
arrogantia dicere possum, me certam harum febrium curationem pro-
mittere omnibus audere, qui nostris præceptis ac monitis obtemperare,
et in assumendis hisce medicamentis consilium nostrum sequi non detre-
ctant: siquidem (absit arrogantia dicto) non minùs certò harum
febrium curatio mihi nota est, atque digitorum numerus.* Obs. 56.

that

that ſuch medicines were hurtful and improper for ſo tender an age *(m)*.

His extreme ignorance in phyſic, appears,
among many other inſtances, from his taking
a proneneſs to faint in childbed-women for a
demonſtrative ſign of the ſcurvy *(n)*. In a man
of ſeventy years, he judged a mortification of
the foot to be ſcorbutic, by the black and
purple ſpots which appeared upon the mortified part; and the ſmall, weak, and unequal
pulſe, naturally to be expected in ſuch a ſituation *(o)*.

He ſeems to have known no other diſtinction betwixt the *lues venerea* and ſcurvy, but
the pulſe *(p)*, and ſometimes the urine *(q)*.

ALL the ſucceeding authors, for a conſiderable time after *Eugalenus*, follow him moſt religiouſly and minutely in their deſcription of
this diſeaſe. So great a compliment is paid
him by *Martini, Horſtius*, and *Sennertus*, that
they copy out of him with a ſcrupulous exact-

(m) Obſ. 59.
(n) P. 194. 197. Item, Obſ. 11.
(o) P. 108.
(p) P. 51.
(q) P. 263. Vid. p. 60. 126. 137.

ness, not only the many symptoms he describes
peculiar to the malady; (and especially his great
dependence on the pulse and urine, for ascer-
taining its existence); but where he or his editors, in their extraordinary relations of scorbutic cases, mention some very uncommon and
singular appearances, these are likewise added
by them to the diagnostics of the scurvy.

What additional observations they themselves
made, may be seen in the proper place *(r)*.
They even exceed him in absurdities. Their
merit seems chiefly to have consisted in furnish-
ing us with cures, or at least with many medicines for the different diseases described by
Eugalenus. However, as an apology for *Sennertus,* he informs us, that he transcribed
chiefly from this last author, because the scurvy was not a disease so frequent or common
in his own country *(s)*.

Eugalenus

(r) Part 3.
(s) Tractatus de scorbuto, p. 140.
To give the reader some idea of the consequence of such
writings, and the high esteem these authors gained by their
works; we find *Moellenbroek,* who pretended likewise to write
upon this disease, or at least a species of it, setting out in his
introduction thus. *Immo nullus ferè jam morbus est, cui se non ad-
jungat scorbutus; unde nisi antiscorbutica interdum reliquis admisceat
medicamenta, vix eos curabit medicus. Quod in praxi mea exper-
tus sum non raro. Et novi aliquos, qui scorbutum ejusque antidota
negligentes,*

Eugalenus had not talents fufficient to form any fort of theory for illuftrating the nature of the many difeafes referred by him to the fcorbutic taint. The principles he affumes upon particular occafions, of obftructions in the liver and fpleen, overflowing of the *atra bilis*, and corruption of the humours, are all borrowed from other authors, lamely explained by him, and often contradicted in his book. *Sennertus*'s hypothefis confutes itfelf. So it

negligentes, in morborum curatione, fuum non potuerunt obtinere fcopum: ac propterea meo exemplo edocti, maximo cum ægrorum fuorum emolumento, eadem poftea exhibuere. Quamvis autem valdè frequens fit fcorbutus, fymptomatibus tamen variis oculatiffimos fæpe medicos illudit et decipit; immo ex mille medicis (ut fcribit Frentag. cent. 1. obferv 99.) ne ternos quidem invenias fcorbuti fat gnaros, ut ut fe fingant Æfculapios. Hinc tantæ ægrotorum ftrages, tanta mortalitas, tanta archiatrorum, necdum gregariorum errata; ut ftatuas mereantur Fracoftoriana fplendidiores, ære perenniores, viri clariffimi Sennertus et Martinus, (adderem ego Gregorium Horftium), qui, penicillo plus quam Apelleo, medicorum opprobrium nobis depinxerunt. Meruiffet pyramidem Eugalenus, ni curationem fubticuiffet.

This laft is certainly a falfe imputation on *Eugalenus.* He feems to have concealed no part of the cure that he knew. Befides referring to *Wierus*, he gives twenty-one general therapeutic canons, and twenty-nine fpecial ones; under moft of which he mentions antifcorbutic herbs, adapted to the feveral intentions of cure If it was found, that in parallel cafes thefe herbs did not fucceed, it does not follow he concealed the cure; the contrary of which appears through his whole book.

Four years after *Moellenbroek* wrote, and had publifhed the fame of the preceeding authors, the world was obliged with Dr *Willis*'s treatife.

was

was left to Dr *Willis*, with the affiftance of
Dr *Lower*, to clear up a fubject that lay under
very great obfcurity, by reducing the whole
into an ingenious fyftem, which continues eftablifhed and adopted even at this day.

It may be worth while to take notice, that
until *Eugalenus*'s time, as before mentioned,
putrid gums and fwelled legs were the pathognomic figns of the fcurvy. This laft author
made them to be a fmall, quick, and unequal
pulfe, together with a peculiar ftate of urine *(t)*.
But fuch a condition of pulfe is not mentioned
by *Willis* to have been obferved in any of the
cafes he gives to illuftrate his account of this
difeafe; nor is it fo much as mentioned in his
book, except under the title of the *Pulfus in-
ordinatus (u)*; where it is put down with fifty
other fymptoms; and has no preference given
it as a characteriftic of the fcurvy, more than
palfies, convulfions, and the reft of the fymptoms which he there enumerates, from the
crown of the head to the fole of the foot. It
is explained by him afterwards *(x)*, when he
tells us, that this inordinate pulfe, being une-

(t) Vid. part 3.
(u) P. 228. Amfterdam edition.
(x) P. 254.

qual

qual and intermitting, attended with frequent faintings, occurs only in the moft inveterate fcurvy; but he no where gives any ftate of pulfe as peculiar, or an index to the difeafe. And although he lays great ftrefs on the appearances in the urine *(y)*; yet here he in fome refpect likewife differs from *Eugalenus (z)*.

There is another very material difference in their accounts of this difeafe. *Eugalenus*, who, if we take his own word for it, had many more patients than ever fell to Dr *Willis*'s fhare, found it in his time very eafy to remove *(a)*. Accordingly, his book abounds with fome very fpeedy and miraculous cures. But now the fcurvy is become much more obftinate, proceeds from various and oppofite caufes, requiring very different methods of cure; and the fimple antifcorbutics fo much extolled by *Eugalenus*, are by no means fufficient to remove it.

Willis has alfo given a different account of this difeafe from all others; as will appear by comparing the fymptoms defcribed by each *(b)*. It is very natural then to in-

(y) P. 256.
(z) P. 229.
(a) *Cognito morbo, facilè curatur.* Eugalen. p. 140.
(b) Vid. Part 3.

quire.

quire, what fingular and diftinguifhing marks
and characteriftics he has given of fuch a variety of diftempers, in order to their being with
any manner of propriety claffed under one denomination, and referred to the difeafe we are
now treating of. And they are as follows.

" The figns of the fcurvy are: Firft, Certain
" outward marks and circumftances, which
" give a fufpicion of it, until the more certain
" fymptoms appear. Thus, if one is born of
" fcorbutic parents, has been converfant with
" a fcorbutic wife, or other fcorbutic compa-
" ny; lives near the fea, or in an unwholfome
" marfhy place; has had a long fever, or o-
" ther tedious chronic difeafes; or if he finds
" benefit from antifcorbutic remedies; fuch
" a perfon, difpofed to be valetudinary, with-
" out having a fever, or certain figns of any
" other diftemper, we may juftly fuppofe to
" have contracted the fcorbutic taint *(c)*."

But it fhall be proved in another place *(d)*,
that the fcurvy does not feem to be properly a hereditary malady, and that it certainly never is
contagious or infectious. People living near
the fea, in unwholfome damp fituations, as well
as thofe who are recovering from fevers and

(c) Cap. 3. p. 247.   *(d)* Chap. 4.

other

other ailments, are fubject to many other difeafes befides this: the former, (as in *Holland*), to
anomalous agues, with very deceitful appearances. His argument, of their finding relief
from antifcorbutics, fhall be examined afterwards. But what he adds next, *viz.* their being free from a fever, is pretty extraordinary.
Eugalenus, Sennertus,· and moft other authors,
had included fevers in a fpecial manner as fymptoms of this difeafe, though *Willis* hardly makes
mention of them. So that the marks he has
given us as yet, are at beft but doubtful and
precarious, if not moftly falfe. He indeed
hints a little at what others had fpoke out more
freely, when he concludes with *not having the
figns of any other diftemper (e).*

He proceeds *(f).* " Secondly, The other
" figns of this diftemper, are its immediate
" fymptoms and effects. As thefe are mani-
" fold, they are commonly differently divided,
" and reduced into certain claffes, *viz.* as they
" are proper to the fcurvy, or common to it
" with other difeafes ; — or according as they
" ocour in the beginning, increafe, or ftate of
" the malady;—as they are external, or inter-
" nal ;— or they may be diftributed according

(e) *Abfque alterius morbi certis indiciis.*   (f) Cap. 3. p. 247.

" to

" to the different parts of the body affected,
" *viz.* the head, breaſt, *abdomen*, or the mem-
" bers, and habit. And in this laſt manner
" we have deſcribed them."

Had he taken the firſt method he mentions,
and deſcribed the ſymptoms proper and peculiar to this diſeaſe alone, as *Echthius* has done;
— or the ſecond method, that of deſcribing it
in its beginning, progreſs, and different ſtages,
as the firſt and pureſt writers have all done; he
might have given us ſome light into the matter. Whereas in his manner of delivering a detail of almoſt all diſtempers incident to the human body, in a progreſſion from the head to
the foot, without any diſtinguiſhing marks to
know when they proceeded from the ſcurvy,
and when from other cauſes, he has acted
much more irrationally than *Eugalenus*; who,
although he aſcribes as many diſeaſes to the
ſcorbutic taint, yet gives the peculiar character-
iſtics of pulſe and urine proper almoſt to each;
by which they may be known to proceed from
that, and no other cauſe. But this Dr *Willis*
no where does.

It may be aſked then, What idea this author
had of the ſcurvy? This we can only gueſs at
from

from one paffage of his book *(g)*, where he pretends to deliver the difcriminating marks of fome particular fcorbutic difeafes, *viz.* palfies, convulfions, *vertigo*, dropfies, tumors, and ulcers; and which conveys to us the only notion he feems to have had himfelf of this difeafe, if we lay afide his theory; which can never be admitted, until we know what he wants to account for by fuch a new and extraordinary hypothefis as he there advances.

He makes the principal diagnoftics of thefe fcorbutic difeafes to be the two following.

Firft, Their yielding chiefly and principally to antifcorbutic medicines.   If he hereby means only the fimple and moft approved antifcorbutic herbs, fcurvy-grafs, brook-lime, and creffes; in this cafe he will gain as little credit as *Eugalenus*, who afferts, that in palfies, convulfions, lethargies, dropfies, *&c.* they have extraordinary virtues.   The daily experience of practitioners convinces us of the contrary. But this author cannot mean only the fimple and common antifcorbutics.   There is here a greater abfurdity than may appear at firft fight.   His book abounds with the moft various indications of cure, and with a great num-

(g) Cap. 5. p. 274.

ber

ber of antifcorbutic remedies of the moft oppofite virtues. He defires, that when one of
thefe does not fucceed, we fhould try another,
and another, until fuch time as we luckily fall
upon fomething which may give relief *(h)*.
For this purpofe, he furnifhes us with as many
different receipts as are fufficient to compofe a
pharmacopœia. Yet, after all, makes the cure
a proof of the difeafe. It is furely lefs fo of
the fcurvy, as he has defcribed it, than of any
other difeafe he could have well mentioned;
and is, without fome other figns, an indication
of no particular one whatever.

He is pleafed, however, to give us but one
other mark of diftinction, which he places in
the formal caufe, as he terms it *(i)*. And his
meaning feems to be, that in the fcurvy, the
blood and other juices are principally affected
and vitiated, without any fixed difeafe, defect,
or obftruction in the folids. So that here
he would fay there is no topical difeafe in
any part of the body, efpecially the *vifcera*;
but a fcorbutic dyfcrafy of different forts, fometimes in the blood, and at other times in the
animal fpirits.

It muft be owned, this is a diftinction extremely nice and ſubtile.   One would willingly be informed, how it is known, when in palſies, dropſics, and ſuch diſeaſes as he there mentions, the cauſe is only in the fluids.   Is it not abſurd to characteriſe ſcorbutic ulcers and tumors in that manner *(k)?*   But he ſaves the trouble of going farther on this head, by contradicting himſelf immediately after, or at leaſt making this diſtinction hold only betwixt a beginning, and confirmed (or, as he calls it, a deplorable) ſcurvy *(l).*

Towards the cloſe of his book, he opens a little the myſtery to us, in the relation of the caſe of a nobleman, which ſeems to have been as different from the ſcurvy as from the pox. " As this caſe cannot properly be referred to " any other diſeaſe, it may juſtly be deemed " ſcorbutic *(m)*."

Dr *Willis* is copied by moſt of the ſucceeding authors, eſpecially by *Charleton*; by *Hoffman*, in the diſtribution of the ſymptoms; and by *Boerhaave*, in the grand diſtinction into a hot and cold ſcurvy, in the proceſs of cure, as alſo in the medicines preſcribed for it.   But theſe already mentioned, having been

(k) P. 274.   *(m)* P. 334
(l) P. 275.

deemed

deemed the standard and original writers on this subject, I shall not trouble the reader with any farther animadversions upon them or their followers. I am persuaded, that many observations will naturally occur to those who peruse Part III. of this treatise with attention.

What were the sentiments of a most judicious physician, may be there seen by looking into *Sydenham;* what were the dreadful consequence of such writings, will appear by looking into *Kramer:* but how many unhappy patients must have suffered in this disease, before the slaughter of thousands at a time *(n)* began to open the eyes of mankind, is too melancholy a subject to dwell upon!

We are now arrived to a period of time, when many distinctions and divisions were introduced and made in the scurvy. An inquiry into the propriety of these, we shall make the subject of the following chapter.

(n) Vid. *Kramer.*

CHAP.

C H A P. II.

Of the several divisions of this disease, viz. *into scurvies cold and hot, acid and alcaline, &c.*

AUthors had now gone on for near seventy years *(a)*, by collecting from each other, and adding something themselves, to make up a very extraordinary number of scorbutic symptoms. They had ascribed to this modern calamity, almost every distemper or frailty *(b)* incident to the human body; so that no room was here left for farther invention. It became afterwards absolutely necessary, and was a sufficient task for their ingenuity, to make distinctions and divisions of it.

The daily experience of practitioners, and their observations in physic, must soon have convinced them of the inefficacy of one uniform method of cure. The simple antiscorbutics, how much soever extolled by *Eugalenus,* failed to remove the many various and complicated disorders that were classed under

(a) From *an.* 1604, when *Eugalenus* wrote.
(b) *Omnes qui ex senio moriuntur, moriuntur etiam ex scorbuto.* Dolæus.

F   the

the name of *scurvy*. Thus they found themselves under a consequent neceffity of having
recourse to different diftinctions at firft, divifions and fubdivifions afterwards, of the malady.
And as the *Materia medica* abounded with antifcorbutics of different and oppofite virtues,
taken from all parts of the animal, mineral,
and vegetable kingdoms, it was proper to diftinguifh for what particular fymptoms, difeafes, or ftages of the difeafe, each was peculiarly adapted.

But it may be afked, In what difeafe did
fuch diftinctions become fo neceffary? And it
evidently appears, in that alone *which was
firft defcribed by Eugalenus, and from him tranfcribed by Horftius and Sennertus; and has been
defcribed by Willis, and his copier Charleton;*
who have always been efteemed the principal
and ftandard authors on the fcurvy. But if
the critical remarks that have been made upon
thefe original authors be found true, the diftinctions made here are founded in abfurdity;
and the former chapter is a fufficient confutation of them.

Thefe indeed, when firft introduced by
Willis, were not univerfally received. *Cha-
meau*, with great ftrength of reafon, confutes
Willis's

Willis's hypothefis; as many others have done. *Maynwaringe* upon this occafion obferves, that there is no effential difference in fcurvies; but that the fcurvy *(quafi genus morborum)* hath a latitude and extent more than any fpecific difference.

However, after all, thofe who have made the moft diftinctions of thefe difeafes, feem to have acted moft rationally. In which *Gideon Harvey*, phyfician to King *Charles* II. has exceeded all others. He obferves, that here the exacteft diftinctions are requifite. Thefe (he fays) are to be taken, " 1*ft*, From its growth " or different ftages; in which cafe, it is ei-" ther a *preliminary, liminary, recent, invete-* " *rate*, or *terminative fcurvy*; the laft of which " is the difeafe into which it paffes, and " puts a termination to the diftemper, or life " of the patient.

" 2*dly*, From its origin; in which refpect it " is either *hereditary* and *connate*, when deri-" ved from the parents; or *adventitious*, when " got fome time after being born: and this " laft is either *contagioufly adventitious*, when " got by infection; or *non-naturally adventi-* " *tious*, when contracted by fome error in the " non-naturals.

" 3*dly*,

" 3*dly*, From the part chiefly affected, this
" difeafe may be named an *hepatic*, *fplenetic*,
" or *ftomachic fcurvy*.

" 4*thly*, From the internal caufe, it may be
" termed either an *acid*, or *lixivial fcurvy*.

" 5*thly*, From the parts where the fymp-
" toms concentrate, or from fome predomi-
" nating fymptom, it often takes a particular
" name; as, a *mouth fcurvy*, *leg fcurvy*, *joint*
" *fcurvy*, an *afthmatic fcurvy*, a *rheumatic fcur-*
" *vy*, a *griping fcurvy*, a *diarrhæous fcurvy*, an
" *emetic* or *vomiting fcurvy*, a *flatulent hypo-*
" *chondriac fcurvy*, a *cutaneous fcurvy*, an *ul-*
" *cerous fcurvy*, a *painful fcurvy*," &*c*. To
which a *face fcurvy*, and many others, may be
added.

" 6*thly*, It may be diftinguifhed into a *la-*
" *tent* and *manifeft fcurvy*. The firft is made
" known by no external or manifeft fymp-
" toms; only a neutrality is obfervable in point
" of health, a defect of appetite, lazinefs, dul-
" nefs, &*c*.

" 7*thly*, It is either a *mild* or *malignant*
" *fcurvy*, an *Englifh* or *Dutch fcurvy*, a *fea*
" or a *land fcurvy*, &*c*."

This writer and *Charleton* are almoft the only authors who deliver the fymptoms peculiar

to the different kinds of ſcurvies, by which they may be known and diſtinguiſhed from each other. Whereas others found this a taſk too difficult for them; and that it was much eaſier to give a long detail of ſymptoms and diſeaſes; leaving it to the ſagacity of their readers to apply fewer, more, or all of them, to the different ſpecies of ſcurvies conſtituted by them. For this purpoſe, it was alone ſufficient that their theories were rightly underſtood; as when the ſulphurs abounded in the blood, and when they were depreſſed; when this vital fluid was too hot or cold, or inclined to an acid, alcaline, and briny acrimony, or an oleous rancidity.

The firſt and beſt authors *(c)*, whoſe method of cure was ſimple, uniform, and for the moſt part ſuccesſful, having conſequently no occaſion for ſuch various diſtinctions, univerſally aſcribed the malady to a fault in the ſpleen. They miſtook this diſeaſe for a very different one deſcribed by *Hippocrates (d).* But it being ſuppoſed, that the ſcurvy ſince

(c) Ronſſeus, Wierus, Echthius, Albertus, Brucæus, Brunnerus, &c.

(d) Vid. part 3. chap. 1.

their

their days, had by contagion *(e)* diffufed itfelf over the whole world, infeƈted the child
unborn *(f)*, and that few efcaped this modern
calamity *(g)*; (as a pimple appearing on the
fkin, was thought to indicate this mifchief
lurking in the blood); to fupport thefe ill-
grounded conceits, theories were invented, galenical, chymical, and mechanical, according
to the whim of each author, and the philofo-
phy then in fafhion.

Firft, The galenical qualities of heat and
cold, which *Willis* defines *a fulphureo-faline,
and a falino-fulphureous ftate of humours ;* and
which the more modern writers have diftinguifhed by the appellation of *alcaline* and *acid
fcurvies,* were introduced; and the diftinƈtion
continues to this day. By which they mean,
that the fcurvy occurs in different habits and
conftitutions, or at different times; proceeding
from as oppofite caufes as can well be imagined; as from heat and cold, or the hoftile and

*(e) Tacitè ferpit infidiofum virus ab hofpite in hofpitem, fpiri-
tûs, lecti, menfæ, poculorum communione.* Charleton, p. 17.
Contagium celere. Boerhaave.
*(f) Fuere qui liberis fuis fcorbutum legarent jure poffidendum
hereditario.* Charleton, p. 17. Vid. Willis, p. 242.
(g) Nemo ferè hodie ab eo planè immunis exiftit. Dolæi Ency-
clopædia. See chap. 1. p. 30.

repugnant

repugnant qualities of an acid and alcali: and accordingly the different kinds of it require the moſt different methods of cure; what proves ſalutary in one ſpecies, being experienced hurtful, nay, poiſonous in another. This was the conſequence of *Eugalenus's* book, and other like writings.

It muſt be owned, the general name of a diſeaſe does not always lead us to the true nature of it. The habit of the body, and many other circumſtances, are carefully to be examined; as alſo, the different degrees and ſtages of it, together with whatever other ſpecialties may occur, in order to furniſh juſt prognoſtics, proper indications, and a rational method of cure. But the diviſions and diſtinctions that have been made here, are not only altogether unneceſſary and perplexing, but have a pernicious tendency to confound it with other diſeaſes, between which there is not the leaſt analogy to be found.

The term *cold* or *acid ſcurvy*, is often met with in converſation, and frequently in the writings of very great phyſicians. Now I take it for granted, that they who uſe this term, do it in the ſame ſenſe as the moſt eminent writers on the ſcurvy who firſt introduced it, and have

                                                    explained

explained its meaning. It will therefore be fufficient for our purpofe, to fhew in what fenfe it was underftood by *them*, and indeed by all who have attempted to explain it.

Soon after *Eugalenus*'s book was publifhed, it was found he had defcribed in it many fymp-toms of the hypochondriac difeafe. Accord-ingly, *Sennertus*, in the preface to his fo much efteemed treatife, which has been reputed the beft on the fcurvy, tells us, as an apology for having tranfcribed this author, that if we live in a country where the fcurvy is not very com-mon, we fhould at leaft learn from his book many fymptoms of the hypochondriac difeafe. Yet what is furprifing, this author, as well as all other fyftematic writers, has defcribed the latter, in other parts of his works, as altogether different from the fcurvy.

Thefe authors, by confounding the two difeafes, occafioned the utmoft perplexity to fucceeding writers on the fubject. *Willis*, and all the followers of *Eugalenus*, maintain that the fcurvy was nearly allied to the hypo-chondriac difeafe. But to fet limits to both, and determine wherein they differed, puzzled authors not a little. Some thought they were fo clofely connected as not to be defcribed fe-

parately

parately *(h)*.   The excellent *Riverius*, who knew little of this diftemper but from books, conjectured it to be the hypochondriac difeafe, complicated with a certain malignity.   Some were of opinion it was this laft when beginning.   But the more general notion of thefe miftaken authors *(i)* was, that the melancholic malady often terminated in the fcurvy, as being the laft and moft exalted degree of it. The moft judicious, fuch as Drs *Pitcairn* and *Cockburn*, (the laft of whom efpecially had great opportunities of being acquainted with the fcurvy), tell us plainly, that if any thing is meant by the term of a *cold fcurvy*, it is nothing elfe but the hypochondriac difeafe. And any perfon will be convinced, that this is truly the cafe, by looking into *Charleton*; who muft mean that, if he means any thing; and is the only writer of character who has diftinguifhed the acid fcurvy by its fymptoms and cure *(k)*.

But it is certainly paying too great a compliment to *Eugalenus*, to extend this denomina-

---

(*h*) *Ettmullerus, Dolæus, &c.*

(*i*) *Moellenbroek, Barbette, Deckers, &c.*

(*k*) P. 40. He fays, it is fo nearly allied to the *melancholia hypochondriaca*, as to differ from it only in certain degrees.

tion

tion to the hypochondriac difeafe, or any fpecies of it; to peftilential fevers, cancers, buboes, &c. as he has done. Nor is it fufficient
to alledge, that time and cuftom have given a
fanction to fuch terms; as this is paying a de-
ference to ignorance and cuftom, no ways
confiftent with the improvement of arts and
fciences.

The hypochondriac diftemper, according to
Sydenham (l), is the fame in men, that hyfteric diforders are in women. In this, with
fome little variation, moft phyficians agree
with him. But fuch difeafes have no manner
of connection with the fcurvy: their feat and
caufe in the human body, and efpecially their
fymptoms, are widely different; fo that there
is hardly to be found one conftant fymptom
in either, which is common to both.

It is indeed furprifing, that fome very eminent authors fhould have endeavoured to perfuade us, that from fuch oppofite caufes, as
heat and cold, or alcaline and acid falts abounding in the body, not only the fame feries of
fymptoms fhould arife, (for if they do not,
they fhould certainly have noted which were

(l) Vid. Differ. epiftol. ad Gul. Cole.

peculiar

peculiar to each), but that then likewife the fame ftate of the blood fhould alfo exift. Thus, the learned *Boerhaave* and *Hoffman*, after giving a regular detail of fymptoms, wherein they widely differ from each other, both agree in affigning one only immediate caufe of all fcurvies; which they fuppofe to be an extraordinary feparation of the ferous part of the blood from the *craffamentum*; the former being diffolved, thin, and acrid; whilft the latter, or the grumous part, is too thick and vifcid. From the predominancy of different acrimonious falts, or oils *(m)*, in this ferum, the fcurvy was to be denominated, according to *Boerhaave*, either *muriatic, acido-auftere, foetid-alcaline, rancid-oily, &c. (n)*

It

(m) *Vix equidem plura fulphurum faliumque genera in hermeticorum ergafteriis, quàm in fanguine fcorbuticorum eft reperire.* Charleton, p. 58.

(n) *Boerhaave* having defcribed the fymptoms peculiar to the beginning, progrefs, and end of the malady, it may be afked, To which of the different fcurvies are the fymptoms (*Aph.* 1151.), and their fo regular progreffion, to be applied? It would appear, to all of them, not only by his defcription in this manner, but by the prefcriptions in his *Materia medica*; where, for example, putrid gums, the pathognomic fign of the malady, as will afterwards be fhewn, are fuppofed to occur both in the hot and cold fcurvy, which are the moft oppofite fpecies of the difeafe. Vid. *Aph.* 1163.

It were to be wished, after having laid down as the sole immediate cause of all scurvies whatever, however different in other respects they might be from each other, such a broken

The whole indeed consists of scraps taken from different authors. He has picked the symptoms out of one book, *Sennertus*'s collection, as he acquainted the pupils in his lectures; the cure out of another, *viz. Willis*. But it will appear to any person who peruses the authors from whom he has borrowed the description of the symptoms, *viz. Echthius, Wierus, &c.* that they described a very different disease from what *Willis* did. Dr *Willis*'s method of cure may perhaps be rationally applied to the diseases he described; but is by no means adapted to the disease characterised by the first writers on the scurvy.

I have been told, that *Boerhaave* has described a *cacochymia* under the appellation of *scurvy*. But if any thing else is meant besides a scorbutic *cacochymia*, which must be the same thing as the disease called *scurvy*, why misapply and confound terms? This must occasion a confusion of the things themselves; and hath produced very dreadful consequences, of which I will give but one instance. Mercury may be reputed a poison in the scurvy; *Kramer* gives an account of 400 men destroyed by it, (See Dr *Grainger*'s letter, part 2. cap. 2.): yet *Boerhaave* recommends it; and in such a state of the malady (*Aph.* 1151.*n.* 4.) where it must certainly become a very deadly one. This fatal mistake has been copied from him, and even inforced by his authority. See *Heucher*.

It is true, he says, what is proper for one scurvy, is a poison in another. But this is not easily reconciled with the causes he assigns of the disease; all which (except the *cort. Peruv.* which is a good antiscorbutic) would seem, either separately or jointly, to produce similar effects. Let us suppose, for a moment, they produced very different effects; what criterion have we to distinguish, by his aphorisms on this disease, a poisonous from a salutary medicine? As I have before observed, he delivers

broken texture in the blood, and a remarkable separation of the serum from the grumous part, with so great an acrimony in the first alone, that those learned authors had furnished us with some better reasons for this opinion. Here we must have recourse to the first author of this hypothesis, *Moellenbroek*, in his book *De varis, seu arthritide vaga scorbutica.*

But it may be proper, before we go farther, to remark, that this writer has taken upon him to describe a disease as scorbutic, which *Wierus*, the first who mentions it, had described as

livers the most regular uniformity of appearances; and the pathognomic signs seem to be the same in every species of scurvy.

To so great an authority, which, as far as is consistent with truth and the good of mankind, I shall always respect, may be opposed a much greater, *viz.* the experience of a physician who had the greatest opportunity perhaps any one ever had, of being conversant with scorbutic patients; woful experience gained by being witness to the death of many thousands, when *Boerhaave's Aphorisms* on this subject were of no use to him! *Non nisi unica species veri scorbuti datur, eaque foetida, putrida, &c. Gravissimus est error, quamlibet cacochymiam, imo etiam cachexiam, &c. scorbutum putare, quum verus scorbutus species cacochymiæ singularis sit.* Kramer epistol. p. 27. 28. Such indefinite terms are indeed but a subterfuge for ignorance, and have been long a reproach to the art of medicine. *Antiquorum cacochymia, et modernorum scorbutus, æqualia habent fata; nam nomen suum in omnibus illis affectibus dare debent, ubi causæ morborum et symptomatum nullo alio vocabulo exprimi possunt. Et sic tanquam asylum ignorantiæ hæc nomina consideranda veniunt.* Junckeri conspectus medicinæ, tab. 69.

a

a very different one, in a treatife *De morbis a-
liquot hactenus incognitis*; in which he tells us,
the one was peculiar to the people of *Wcft-
phalia,* the other to *Holland, &c. Forreftus,*
upon receiving an account of the *die varen,*
from *Henricus a Bra,* ingenuoufly owns, that
in fifty years practice it had never occurred to
him. He thinks it a new difeafe, and very
different from the fcurvy *(o).*

Now it is this author, in his account of
what he calls *the fcorbutic wandering gout,*
who *(p)* makes the immediate caufe of the
fcurvy to be a volatile fcorbutic falt. He obferves, that this falt muft needs be volatile, o-
therwife it would too tenacioufly adhere to
the parts, as in the true gout; and the
pains would not move or fhift fo fuddenly as
they do in the fcorbutic gout *(q):* and for
the fame reafon it muft refide in the ferum a-
lone, as the moft proper vehicle to circulate it
fo quickly. This the other vifcid humours
with which fcorbutic habits abound, as is plain
from the blood taken from their veins, cannot
be fuppofed to do. He afterwards affigns thefe

(o) Vid. Obf. medicinal. lib. 20.
(p) P. 11.
(q) P. 12.

vifcid

vifcid humours as the caufe of the putrid gums
and fome other fymptoms *(r)*.

The celebrated Profeffor *Hoffman (f)* makes
ufe of pretty much the fame arguments. He
judges the falivation, flying pains, and hæmorrhages ufual in this difeafe, to proceed from the
thinnefs and acrimony of the *ferum,* and its
feparation from what he calls the folid parts of
the blood; and the more fixed pains, tumours,
&c. to arife from the vifcidity or *lentor* of the
latter.

But the truth is, there is no fuch ftate of
blood in this difeafe. It is indeed contrary to
reafon, to fuppofe, in fo high a degree of putrefaction as appears in fcorbutic cafes, that
the *craffamentum* of the blood fhould continue thus thick and vifcid; which, by all experiments made on putrified blood, appears
quickly to be diffolved and thinned by corruption *(t)*. It certainly is fo in all putrid dif-

(r) P. 18.

(f) Medicin. fyftematic. tom. 4. part. 5. cap. 1.

(t) By Dr *Pringle's* experiments, not only the *craffamentum*
of the blood is the firft refolved by putrefaction, which the *ferum* refifts for a much longer time; but the feptic or putrid particles feem principally to be intangled in the grume: fo that fuch
acrimony would appear to refide chiefly there, by experiment
42. Vid. Appendix to Obfervations on the difeafes of the
army.

eafes. This is further made evident to a demonſtration, by the diſſections afterwards to
be related *(u)*; or, if theſe be liable to objections, from the appearance of the blood in
Lord *Anſon*'s ſcorbutic crew while alive *(x)*;
which in every ſtage of the diſeaſe, and from
whatever part of the body it was diſcharged,
was always found in a different condition:
the *craſſamentum* was altogether diſſolved and
broken; and there was not ſo much as any regular ſeparation *(y)*, much leſs ſuch an extraordinary one, as has been by ſome made the
only immediate cauſe of the ſcurvy, the baſis
of a theory, and of a practice founded upon it.

The aſſuming likewiſe the chymical principles of acid and alcaline ſalts, as the foundation of a method of cure, from a preſumption
of the predominancy of ſuch ſalts, or of an
acid or alcaline tendency in the blood in this
diſeaſe, is exceptionable on many accounts.

We may allow the predominancy of ſuch
ſalts, or the exiſtence of ſuch an humour in
the *primæ viæ*, as may be ſuppoſed to have the

(u) Part 2. chap. 7.
(x) Ibid.
(y) This is confirmed by *Kramer*.   See Part 3. and Dr
Grainger's obſervations, chap. 5. part 2.

phyfical marks and properties of what is faid
to be acid or alcaline. But as the blood of no
living animal was ever found to be either acid
or acaline *(z)*, it is hard to grant the exiftence
of fuch qualities, latent and occult there, when
they do not manifeft themfelves by any figns
in the body, from which we can be affured of
their exiftence. Thefe, according to all the
authors of fuch theories, ought principally to
be in the firft paffages. But, in the higheft
degree of the hot, putrid, and what is called
the *alcalefcent fcurvy*, there is generally neither lofs of appetite, putrid belchings, nor any
other marks, delivered by thofe authors, as
proofs of an alcalefcent tendency in the ftomach and inteftines ; nor is there commonly
any præternatural thirft, or heat of the body,
fuppofed always to accompany an alcalefcent
ftate in the blood. On the contrary, fuch

(z) Although the recent urine of thofe who took Mrs *Ste-*
phens's medicine was found to effervefce with acids, yet this experiment by no means authorifes us to conclude that the blood
of fuch people was alcaline, for very obvious reafons. It however furnifhes one of the ftrongeft arguments againft the opinion of putrid fcurvies being of an alcalefcent nature ; as pills
made of foap, garlic, and fquills, was the common medicine
given by our moft experienced navy-furgeons, and ufed at feveral hofpitals, particularly at *Gibraltar,* for recovery of many
thoufand feamen half-rotten in this difeafe.

people have for moſt part a good appetite,
without any heat or drought, even till their
death.

One would naturally have expeȼted here, e-
ſpecially in the *muriatic ſcurvy*, as it is denominated, (which in another place ſhall be proved altogether a chimerical diſtinȼtion), a violent thirſt, a vehement deſire of aqueous and
diluting liquors. Theſe alſo would ſeem the
moſt rational and effeȼtual remedies, in ſuch
a ſaline ſtate of blood, at leaſt upon chymical principles. Accordingly, a great chy-
miſt, *Hoffman (a)*, though he admits different ſalts in the blood as the cauſe of ſcurvies,
obſerves, that nothing can be ſo ridiculous as
the laboured and anxious pains taken to correȼt
theſe by oppoſite ſalts. " For (ſays he) I will
" prove it to a demonſtration, there is but one
" way, and it is the moſt effeȼtual and ſafeſt,
" to correȼt morbid ſalts of any kind ; that is,
" by diluting them ſufficiently with water."
His reaſoning is at leaſt plauſible, it being certain water is the proper menſtruum and ſolvent
of all ſalts.

The terms of *acid* and *alcaline*, have not indeed been ſufficiently defined and reſtriȼted, ſo

(a) Medicin. ration. ſyſtem. tom. 4. part. 5. cap. 1.

as

as to be a very solid foundation for any theory of diseases *(b)*, beyond those of the *primæ viæ*. For even such as are generally deemed of either class, though obtained in their utmost purity, are found to differ extremely from each other in their properties, more especially in their effects upon the human body *(c)*; as unfermented and fermented, vegetable and fossil acids do; some coagulating, others attenuating the blood. Thus likewise, volatile and fixed alcalies differ extremely, though pure. But this purity being seldom attainable, their virtues and properties are still infinitely more varied, according to the manner of their preparation, and their different and various combinations with other substances.

But to bring this matter to a conclusion: Such theories are entirely overthrown, upon having recourse to experience, the only test by which they must stand or fall. We find in practice, that in such hot, putrid sea-scurvies, as have

(b) Frustra quærimus limites quibus utralibet species contineri debeat. Hinc quàm rectè ii faciant, non difficilis est conjectura, qui theorias, non chymicas modò, sed et medicas, ex acidorum alkaliumque doctrina confingunt, dum ne vocabulorum quidem vim intelligunt. Jo. Freind prælect. chymic. p. 12.

(c) Vid. Hoffman. observ. physic. chymic. lib. 2. obs. 29. et 30.

been

been referred to the alcaline clafs, the hot alcalefcent plants, *viz.* creffes, onions, muftard, and
radifhes, prove ferviceable. Thefe, from fuch
theories, have been condemned by authors, as
noxious and pernicious in the higheft degree.
But the contrary is demonftratively evinced, by
the deplorable cafe of the failor left behind at
Greenland, related by *Bachftrom* and others,
who was cured by fcurvy-grafs alone *(d)*;
and by the experience of all our naval hofpitals, where the moft high and putrid fcurvies
are daily removed by frefh flefh broths; wherein are put great quantities of celery, cabbage,
colewort, leeks, onions, and other alcalefcent
plants. In fuch cafes all acid fruits and herbs
are likewife experienced to be of great benefit.
So that the uncertainty of fuch theories plainly
appears. And they ought the more now to be
difregarded, as putrid fubftances and alcalines
are proved by experiments to be different *(e)*.
Yet it was upon a fuppofition of their bearing

(d) Though it is not fo acrid as our fcurvy-grafs, yet it has a
tendency that way. See Mr *Maude*'s letter concerning the
Greenland fcurvy-grafs, part 2. chap. 5.; which is a fufficient
confutation of the vulgar error, that acids alone are proper in
putrid fcurvies.

(e) See Dr *Pringle*'s experiments read before the Royal Society.

a

a great similitude to each other, or being properly different degrees of the same thing, that
this theory was first devised. Upon the faith
of which, many improper chymical preparations, and especially opposite salts highly extolled in such cases, have been recommended
and administered in the scurvy, to the manifest
detriment of the patient. Be it remembered,
*Chymia egregia ancilla medicinæ, non alia pejor
domina.*

C H A P. III.

*Of the distinction commonly made into a land and
sea scurvy.*

THis disease has been always most common at sea. It is well known there in
the present age, by reason of the frequent voyages to the most distant parts of the world.
The symptoms, though numerous, are yet observed to be regular and constant; so that the
most ignorant sailor, in the first long voyage,
becomes well acquainted with it. But as many
were supposed to die at land of the scurvy,
though none of the most equivocal and uncertain,

tain, much lefs the ufual fymptoms of the marine difeafe, appeared; it became neceffary, in
order to fave the credit of the phyfician, and
to juftify his opinion of the difeafe, to pronounce it *the land-fcurvy*, or a fpecies of fcurvy different from that at fea.

This is a diftinction often made in converfa-
tion, and fometimes in books. In order to
judge of the juftnefs and propriety of it, we
fhall here confider, what certainty we have
that this diftemper is the fame on both elements; and what particular proof can be
brought at any time, to afcertain the identity
of two difeafes, afflicting different perfons, in
different climates, and at different times.

The phænomena or appearances in any difeafe, which are obvious to our fenfes, or by
their affiftance may be made evident to our
reafon, are the fymptoms or diagnoftics of it.
Whether they be the immediate caufes or effects of the malady, they are properly called
fymptoms; a fymptom being part of the difeafe;
and the whole fymptoms taken together con-
ftituting the whole difeafe; from the aggregate
or affemblage of which we draw conclufions.

Such appearances or fymptoms, then, as are
peculiar to the nature of the malady, and are
more

more conftantly experienced to accompany it, are called *pathognomonic* or *demonftrative figns*; and thefe conftitute the greateft medical evidence which can be obtained of the exiftence and identity of difeafes. Befides which, it is a corroborating proof of their identity, if they proceed from fimilar caufes: And, laftly, if they are removed by the like medicines or method of cure.

1*ft*, As to the pathognomonic figns of this difeafe: If we compare its fymptoms as defcribed by *Echthius*, *Wierus*, and all other authors till the time of *Eugalenus (a)*, with the accounts given of them in books of voyages, particularly the extraordinary narrative of what happened to the great Lord *Anfon*'s crews in their paffage round the world *(b)*, we fhall perceive an entire agreement in the effential figns of the diftemper, (making a proper allowance for the different defcriptions that may be expected from feamen and phyficians), and appearances fo fingular as are not to be met with in any other. Thus, putrid gums, fwelled legs, and fpots, accompanying each other, and in their progrefs ufually attended with rigid tendons in the ham, are obferved in no other diftemper.

(*a*) Vid. Part 3.   (*b*) Ibid.

It

It is alſo peculiar to it, that perſons thus afflicted, though otherwiſe apparently healthful, are
upon the leaſt motion, or exertion of ſtrength,
apt to faint, and do often ſuddenly drop down
dead.

This evil the medical writers have deſcribed
as peculiar to certain countries.   They tell us
of its being epidemic one year over all *Brabant (c)*; ſome years in *Holland (d)*.   *Forreſtus,* though he had frequent opportunities
of ſeeing it in ſailors, yet in all his hiſtories
gives us but one caſe of a mariner. His moſt
faithful accounts of this malady, are illuſtrated
by patients who had always lived at land; ſome
of whom muſt have been infected in a very
high degree, when they dropped down dead
ſuddenly, to the ſurpriſe of their relations; of
which he gives an inſtance.   *Dodonæus (e),*
a very accurate writer on the ſcurvy, relates no
caſes of it in ſailors, but in people on ſhore,
particularly in a perſon who contracted it in
priſon *(f)*.

(c) *Dodonæus, Forreſtus.*   (d) *Ronſſeus.*

(e) *Praxis medic. et obſervationes.*

(f) Yet elſewhere, *Angli maritimis commerciis dediti, et nau.
tæ potiſſimum, ſtomacace affliguntur.   Sive id fit. cereviſiæ potu ex
paluſtribus aquis coctæ, ſive ex aëris putredine, cælique nebulis aut
vaporibus, hujus noſtri inſtituti explicare non eſt.* Hiſtoria ſtirpium.

It

It is indeed remarkable, that the first just description published of this disorder in *Europe*, was in an account of its raging in besieged towns, by the historian *Olaus Magnus (g)*, where it was attended with such symptoms as occur always at sea.   We have likewise about the same time a very elegant picture of it drawn by *Adrian Junius*, a physician and historian in *Holland*, cotemporary with *Ronsseus (h)*.

Moreover, the sea-scurvy is called by several authors *the Dutch distemper*; especially by the celebrated *Francis Gemelli Careri*, who has wrote the best voyages in the *Italian* language. And indeed the symptoms of the malady are at this day uniform and the same, both at sea and land; in *Holland (i)*, *Greenland (k)*, *Hungary (l)*, *Cronstadt (m)*, *Wiburg (n)*, *Scot-*

(g) Vid. Part 3. chap. 1.

(h) Hollandiæ itaque peculiari dono Natura dedit proventum lætum Britannicæ herbæ, (which he afterwards calls *cochlearia*), *quam præsentanei remedii vim præbere in profliganda sceletyrbe et stomacace experiuntur, cum incolis, exteri quoque: quibus malis dentes labuntur, genuum compages solvitur, artus invalidi fiunt, gingivæ putrescunt, color genuinus et vividus in facie disperit, livescunt crura, ac in tumorem laxum abeunt.* Histor. Bataviæ, cap. 15.

(i) Vid. Dr *Pringle*'s observations on the diseases of the army, p. 10.

(k) Act. Haffnien. vol. 3. obs. 75.   *(m) Sinopæus.*

(l) Kramer.   *(n) Nitzsch.*

I   *land*

land (o), &c.: which ſufficiently evinces the abſurdity of the aſſertion advanced by ſeveral authors, that ſince the firſt accounts of it were publiſhed, the face and appearances of the calamity have been greatly changed.

2*dly*, As to the cauſes of this diſeaſe; they are the ſame on both elements: for it will be fully proved *(p)*, that there is not to be found any one cauſe productive of it at ſea, which is not alſo to be met with at land; though ſuch cauſes, by ſubſiſting longer and in a higher degree, uſually give riſe to its greater virulence in that element.

It is indeed a ſufficient and juſt confutation of many writers on the ſcurvy, that they pretend to deſcribe a malady to which ſeamen are peculiarly ſubject, and which they ſay proceeds from the *nauticus victus*, putrid water, and ſea-air. Yet their aſſertion, That the diſeaſe deſcribed by them, *(viz. Eugalenus (q), Willis*, and their

(*o*) Vid. Dr *Grainger's* account of the ſcurvy at *Fort-William*, part 2. chap. 2.

(*p*) Part 2. chap. 1.

(*q*) *Eugalenus* practiſed at *Embden*, and other places of *Eaſt-Frieſland*; where the cold, thick, and moiſt air, the raw unwholſome waters uſed by the inhabitants along that tract of the ſea-coaſt, and the *craſſus et nauticus victus*, (as he terms it), occaſioned the ſcurvy to be a univerſal diſeaſe. But it muſt be granted,

their followers), is properly a marine disease, is refuted by the observation of all practitioners at sea.   And the same may be said of the different species of scurvies alledged by *Boerhaave* to proceed from the causes above mentioned.

But a heavier charge lies against them.   When granted, that the scurvy never was so epidemic or fatal there as in ships and fleets.   All the causes he assigns as productive of it, do subsist at times in a much higher degree at sea than at land.   I have had 80 patients out of the number of 350 men afflicted with it ; and have seen a thousand scorbutic persons together in an hospital, but never observed one of them to have the diseases described by *Eugalenus*.   Nor did I ever hear of a practitioner at sea, where it would have been most allowable, who assumed his principles ; and supposed, that almost all diseases there must be complicated with the scorbutic *virus* ; that the most extraordinary and uncommon which occurred at sea, (as was supposed at *Embden* and *Hamburg*), were, this mischief lurking under deceitful appearances ; and that such diseases could not be cured without a mixture of antiscorbutics, which seldom failed to remove them.   This last, surely, could never have escaped the observation of our many ingenious navy-surgeons, and of our physicians and surgeons to naval hospitals ; some of whom had seldom less than a thousand patients from the sea.   Mr *Ives*'s ingenious journal, (placed at the end of chap. 1. part 2.), is a proof of the variety of diseases which occur there, without the least connection with the scurvy.   If it often killed the patient (as it would seem always to have done in *Friesland*) before the gums and legs were affected, or the spots appeared ; this likewise must have escaped our observation.   But though *Eugalenus* may be justly condemned as the parent of these absurdities, greater mischief, however, has been done by succeeding authors, from their digesting them into a system.   Such remedies and cures have been directed, as are not only altogether unserviceable, but for the most part highly pernicious.

the

the true ſcurvy does really occur, their writings, ſo far from being uſeful, are rather hurtful to practitioners; which I think needs no farther proof, than *Kramer*'s letter to the college of phyſicians at *Vienna*. Their doctrines have perverted the judgment of even ſome of the beſt writers. I ſhall inſtance only in *Sinopæus*. That author has taken his deſcription of the diſeaſe from nature and obſervation; but, unluckily, his medicines from thoſe authors; otherwiſe I am morally certain, the calamity would not have ariſen to the height it did at *Cronſtadt*, and uſually does every ſpring; where it ſeems to be abated annually more by change of weather, than the ſkill of phyſicians.

3*dly*, The cure of ſcorbutic diſeaſes contracted either at land or ſea, is entirely the ſame. This will appear to any perſon who peruſes *Backſtrom*'s and *Kramer*'s obſervations, and ſeveral other hiſtories related in this treatiſe. And every practitioner who has treated ſuch caſes, muſt be further convinced of it; as the firſt remedies which were caſually found out by the vulgar, and are recommended by the firſt and purer writers on the ſubject, have preſerved their reputation and eſteemed virtues even to this day.

Laſtly,

Laftly, If to fuch convincing proofs it may be neceffary to add authority, I fhall beg leave to quote a very great one.   The learned Dr *Mead (r)* informs us, that incited by the extraordinary events publifhed in Lord *Anfon's* voyage, to make a full inquiry into this whole affair, he had not only the honour of difcourfing with his Lordfhip upon it, but had alfo been favoured with the original obfervations of his ingenious and fkilful furgeons; and, upon the whole, he found, that this difeafe at fea was the fame with the fcurvy at land; the difference being only in the degree of malignity.

IF objectors fhould reply, 'That tho' the feafcurvy often occurs at land, and, as has been demonftratively proved, is the only difeafe that was defcribed by the firft writers on the fubject, as a malady peculiar to the marfhy and cold countries which they inhabited; yet that they, neverthelefs, underftand by what may be termed, in contradiftinction to the other, a *land-fcurvy*, a difeafe, or clafs of difeafes, different from the appearance of the marfh or marine fcurvy: then it is incumbent upon them, and would be much for the benefit of mankind, to define,

(r) Difcourfe upon the fcurvy, p. 97.

defcribe,

describe, and characterise this singular species, and distinguish it from the appearances of the said disease, either at land or sea. This they must know has not been attempted by any author in physic. The greatest modern writers, *viz. Boerhaave, Hoffman,* and *Pitcairn,* have made no such distinction, either in the causes or diagnostics of the disease, nor indeed in any part of their description of it. And I mention these last, as having had a very extensive practice, besides the advantage of perusing all books wrote before them on the subject.

It may be said, That there are certain disorders, *viz.* many cutaneous eruptions, ulcers, a species of toothach, *&c.* which, for a considerable time, have passed under the character and denomination of *scorbutic*; a term introduced by our predecessors in the science, and which most practitioners have agreed to make use of at this day, and which there may perhaps be a necessity of retaining, as it is not easy to assign a proper appellation to every disease, or case of a patient.

This reason is commonly urged. In answer to which I shall, *first,* inquire, how or when this term came first to be so generally applied; or whence such ulcers, the itch, *&c.* were denominated

minated *fcorbutic?* I think it will admit of no
doubt, that it was firſt applied to ſuch ulcers
and eruptions on the ſkin as did not readily
yield to the ſkill of the praƈtitioner *(ſ)*. Dr
Muſgrave (t) informs us, that all *Europe* was
ſo much alarmed with the apprehenſions of this
evil in the laſt century, as appears from the
Recipe's of praƈtitioners in thoſe times, that
the whole art of phyſic ſeems to have been
employed in grappling with this univerſal calamity, which was ſuppoſed to mingle its malignity with all other diſeaſes whatever *(u·)*.
Thus the term was originally impoſed through
ignorance, and a miſtaken opinion of the pre-
valence of the ſcurvy. There would indeed
be ſome difficulty in conceiving how men of
ſuch wild fancies, as were they who have been
deemed the principal authors on the ſcurvy,
and to whom we are indebted for this general
name, could ever get into poſſeſſion of that degree of fame which they have acquired, did
we not experience how much the world is diſ-
poſed to admire whatever ſurpriſes; as if we
were endued with faculties to ſee through or-

(ſ) *Vid.* Sydenham.
(t) De arthritide ſymptomatica, p. 98.
(u) Vid. note, p. 30.

dinary follies, while great abfurdities ftrike with an aftonifhment which overcomes the powers of reafon, and makes improbability even an additional motive to belief. There are few now who fet fo fmall a value upon their time, as to read thefe authors; and by that means their merit is little examined into, and is admitted upon the credit of others.

2*dly*, If it be urged, That the denomination of fuch difeafes ought ftill to be retained, as being now generally adopted; I anfwer, That, upon the fame principles, the moft ridiculous terms in any art may be vindicated. Lord *Verulam*, and the firft reformers of learning in *Europe*, met with this very objection. The learned ignorance of that age lay concealed under a veil of unmeaning, unintelligible jargon. But, in order to make way for the reftoration of folid learning, it was found neceffary to expunge all fuch terms as were contrived to give an air of wifdom to the imperfections of knowledge.

It may be believed, that there are few people who have had opportunities of reading more upon this fubject than I have done; and that there are few books or obfervations publifhed upon the difeafe, that have not fallen under

my

my infpection. If I could, with any manner
of propriety, have characterifed any other fpecies of fcurvy than that which is the fubject of
this treatife, I fhould have confulted the fecurity of my character more, than in advancing
an uncommon doctrine, as all novelties are
expofed to oppofition. But, in attempting a
thing of that fort, I did not find two authors
agree who founded their doctrine upon facts
and obfervations. I obferved, that ten different practitioners pronounced ten cafes to be
fcorbutic, which, upon examination, did not
bear the leaft refemblance or analogy to each
other. Upon this occafion, I might have followed the example of fome writers; and, dif-
liking the former diftinctions made, might have
introduced others, accommodated either to
the opinion of the country, and thus, by adopt-
ing vulgar errors, have endeavoured to eftablifh
and confirm them; or to fome new principles;
and fo might have multiplied abfurdities, in like
manner as every private practitioner does, who
thinks he has a right to term what he plea-
fes a *fcurvy*; though the propriety of the appellation cannot be juftified from the accepta-
tion of it, by the moft authentic authors of

K   facts

facts and obfervations, nor has any foundation in the genuine principles of phyfic.

It may be faid, That the world would reap great advantage by having a compleat treatife of the caufes, cure, *&c.* of the many difeafes which commonly go under the denomination of the *fcurvy*. But this is not an eafy tafk: and it might as well be expected, that an author, who lived in a country, or at a time, when the moft obftinate and uncommon appearances were afcribed to witchcraft, and had taken pains to banifh fuch ignorant conceits, fhould be able to account for the various diftempers and *phænomena* afcribed to that imaginary evil. It has been ufual for ignorant and indolent practitioners, to refer fuch cafes as they did not underftand, or could not explain, to one or other of thefe caufes; according to the obfervation of a very learned and late practitioner *(x)*.

With regard to the neceffity of retaining the name, as if an unmeaning term was as re-

---

(x) *Mos adeò invaluit, ut hodie medici imperitiores, fi quando ex certis fignis neque morbum nec caufam ejus ritè poffunt cognofcere, ftatim fcorbutum prætendant, et pro caufa fcorbuticam acrimoniam accufent. Deinceps non rarò accidit, ut adfectus quidam fæpe planè fingularis, cui portentofa fpaftico-convulfiva junguntur fymptomata, in artis exercitio occurrat; et tum ufu receptum eft, ut illam vel ad fafcinum vel ad malum fcorbuticum rejiciant.* Fred. Hoffman. med. fyftemat. tom 4. p. 369.

quifite in phyfic as pious frauds in certain religions: *Si vulgus vult decipi, decipiatur.* If
the good of mankind will have no effect upon
thefe gentlemen, I am afraid no other argument will.   We fhall however lay before them
a view of the fatal effects produced by the ufe
of fuch vague and indefinite terms.

1*ft*, On young practitioners and ftudents in
phyfic; who being provided with fuch a general
name as that of the *fcurvy,* comprehending almoft all difeafes, think themfelves at once acquainted with the whole art of medicine; as they
may be furnifhed with numerous cures for it
from the many Pharmacopœias with which
the prefent age abounds.

2*dly*, Older practitioners, by referring many various and uncommon difeafes to fuch imaginary caufes *(y)*, deprive the world of the true
improvement of their art: which can only be expected from accurate hiftories of different cafes,
faithfully and honeftly ftated; and diftinguifhed
from each other, with the fame accuracy that
botanical writers have obferved in defcribing
different plants. The ancients have been at great

<hr>

(y) *Notandum eft, quòd quando multa fymptomata numerantur, tunc*
effe cogitandum de nomine congeriem morborum indicante, ut fcor-
butus.   Waldfchmid praxis medicinæ rationalis.

pains

pains to diſtinguiſh the diſeaſes of the ſkin,
which at this day make up a very numerous
and conſiderable claſs, and have indeed treated
that ſubject with prolixity. But the moderns
have claſſed almoſt all of them under that one
very improper denomination of the *ſcurvy (z),*
even from the higheſt degree of the leprous e-
vil, to the itch and common tetters; and with
theſe have confounded the pimpled face, ſcall
head, moſt cutaneous eruptions uſual in the
ſpring, the eryſipelas, *&c.*; nay dyſepulotic
ulcers, eſpecially on the legs, and various o-
ther ailments of the moſt oppoſite genius to
the true ſcurvy, have been ſuppoſed to proceed
from it. The different cauſes of which various
diſtempers cannot be with propriety reduced

(*z*) Dr *Pringle* very juſtly obſerves the impropriety of the
appellation of *ſcurvy* generally given to the itch, various kinds
of *impetigo, &c.*; and remarks, that in the marſhy parts of
the *Low Countries,* where the true ſcurvy is moſt frequent, and
of the worſt kind, the itch is a diſtemper unknown. A real
ſcurvy (ſays he) imports a ſlow, but general reſolution or putrefaction of the whole frame; whereas the *ſcabies, impetigo,* or le-
proſy, will be found to affect thoſe of a very different conſtitution.
The true ſcorbutic ſpots are of a livid colour, not commonly ſcur-
fy, or raiſed above the ſkin, *&c.* Vid. chapter on the itch, in
Obſervations on the diſeaſes of the army.

In his Appendix he obſerves, that the muriatic and putrid
ſcurvy are properly the ſame thing, and that the ſuppoſed ſpecies of acid ſcurvy is at leaſt very improperly denominated.

under

under any divifion of the fcurvy as yet made, nor from thence the peculiar and diftinct genius of each known and afcertained; which, however, is abfolutely neceffary towards undertaking their cure.

3*dly*, and *laftly*, It has a moft fatal influence on the practice. Thus the original and real difeafe has been loft and confounded amidft fuch indefinite diftinctions and divifions of it, that it is fometimes not known by the beft practitioners, when it really occurs. *To this was owing the lofs of fo many thoufand Germans in Hungary (a), not many years ago; where the phyfician to that army, together with the whole learned college of phyficians at Vienna, affifted by all the books extant on the fubject, were at a lofs how to remedy this dreadful calamity.* And for this reafon many unhappy people are daily injudicioufly treated at land, as muft have been obferved by every one acquainted with the diftemper. Thence likewife pernicious methods have been recommended at fea, and too often put in practice.

(a) Vid. *Krameri epiftola de fcorbuto.*

C H A P.

C H A P. IV.

Of the scurvy being connate, hereditary, and infectious.

VArious have been the opinions concerning the causes and propagation of this evil. Some believed it to be connate, and the direful seeds of it transmitted from scorbutic parents, and that sometimes it was derived from a scorbutic nurse.

Horstius (a) had so very accurate a discernment, as to find, that the grandfather might infect a grandchild, though his own son escaped the infection. He ascribes the spreading of the contagion in *Holland* to the custom of salutation by kissing; and pities the poor infants, whom every person must salute, to avoid giving offence to the family. He is not at all surprised, that the calamity was so frequent in the *Hanse Towns*, and in the *Lower Saxony*, as they used but one cup at table; where there was rarely wanting some scorbutic person with rotten gums, who with his *saliva* might infect the whole company. *Sennertus* asserts

(a) *Tractatus de scorbuto.*

it

it to be infectious from venereal embraces, and
mentions an inftance of its being communicated even from a dead body. *Boerhaave*, *Hoffman*, and almoft all authors, make it a very
infectious poifon; and *Charleton* was of opinion, that more got it in this way than in any
other.

Several of thefe chimerical opinions deferve
no ferious confutation. It is indeed far from
being probable, that this is what may properly
be called a hereditary or connate difeafe; as
we feldom in practice fee it rife to a great height,
without the influence of fome obvious external caufes; and experience fhews, that when
the taint is but flight and beginning, it may
for the moft part be quickly and eafily fubdued.

It is a matter of more confequence, to be
rightly informed whether it is really contagious, as hath been confidently afferted by moft
authors. The effect of contagious poifons
can only be known *à posteriori*, and by no reafoning deduced *à priori*. So that thefe authors
fhould have given us attefted hiftories of perfons infected in this manner, where the other
caufes that always produce the difeafe had no
influence. But no fuch hiftories are to be
found.

found. On the contrary, where-ever the calamity has been general, it was known to proceed from ftrong and univerfal caufes; and, in the times of its moft epidemical ravage, perfons properly guarded againft the influence of thefe caufes, were not infected with it. Thus, when it lately raged with fuch a remarkable devaftation among the *Germans* in *Hungary*, the phyfician to that army *(b)* was furprifed to find, that not one officer, even the moft fubaltern, received the infection.

At fea likewife, where the frequency of the diftemper gives the greateft opportunities of determining this point, it never has been deemed infectious. If it had been fo, it could not there have efcaped obfervation. Taught by fatal experience the fpeedy progrefs and great havock that all contagious diftempers, *viz.* fevers, dyfenterics, *&c.* make among a number of men fo clofely confined, it is common to ufe many precautions to prevent their fpreading. They feparate the difeafed from the reft of the crew, deftroy the bedding and cloaths of thofe who die, fend immediately on fhore patients afflicted with fuch difeafes upon coming into port, and afterwards fmoke and clean the fhip.

(b) Kramer.

But

But long and conftant experience having fufficiently convinced them, that fcorbutic ailments
are not infectious, no fuch precautions are ever
taken. In flight cafes, and even where the
gums are very putrid, the men are often kept
on board, and cured; there being no inftance
of fuch perfons ever infecting the reft of the
crew, or of thofe who are fent on fhore carrying the infection into the hofpitals; though,
upon many other occafions, the patients in
thefe hofpitals fuffer extremely by contagious
difeafes introduced amongft them.

In an epidemic fcurvy at fea, the indifpofition attacks, in a regular order, fuch people as
are predifpofed to it by manifeft caufes. It is
for a long time confined at firft to the common
feamen: and though the officers fervants are at
fuch times often afflicted with it, while ufing
the fame cups and difhes with their mafters;
yet it is but rare to fee this difeafe in an officer, nay even a petty officer.

I could produce many inftances, and well-
attefted facts, which prove beyond all doubt,
that drinking out of the fame cup, lying in the
fame bed, and the clofeft contact, does not
communicate this diftemper. But to multiply
proofs of a thing fo univerfally known, is

needlefs. Perhaps the following may fuffice.
A *French* prifoner was taken on board his Majefty's fhip the *Salifbury* from a prize-veffel,
with the moft putrid fcorbutic gums that I ever
obferved. The ftench and putrefaction of his
mouth were indeed intolerable, even at fome
diftance. Yet though he eat and drank out of
the fame difh and cup with five of his companions for a fortnight, he did not infect one of
them: they all arrived in harbour in perfect
health.

Nor is this difeafe communicated by infection from thofe that die: for the diffections made
at *Paris (c)*, of the moft putrid fcorbutic bodies, do not appear to have produced any fuch
effect.

From whence we may judge how much authors have been miftaken, when they imagined
this dreadful calamity to have diffufed itfelf by
contagion over the whole world, after it had
quitted its native feat in the cold northern
climates.

(c) Vid. *Memoires de l' academie des fciences* 1699, *p.* 237.

A

A

T R E A T I S E

O F   T H E

S C U R V Y.

P A R T   II.

C H A P.   I.

The true caufes of the difeafe, from obfervations made upon it, both at fea and land.

THE fcorbutic taint is induced chiefly by the agency of certain external and remote caufes; which, according as their exiftence is permanent or cafual, and in proportion to the different degrees of violence with which they act, give rife to a difeafe more or lefs epidemic, and of various degrees of malignity.

Thus, where the caufes productive of it are general, and violent in a high degree, it becomes an epidemic or univerfal calamity, and rages

L 2   with

with great and diffusive virulence: as happens
often to feamen in long voyages; sometimes to
armies *(a)*, very lately to the *German* foldiers
in *Hungary (b)*; frequently to troops when
closely befieged, as to the *Saxon* garrison in
Thorn (c), the befieged in *Rochelle*, as also
Stetin (d): and at other times to whole countries; as in *Brabant*, in the year 1556 *(e)*;
and in *Holland, ann.* 1562. *(f)*.

2*dly*, Where these causes are fixed and permanent, or almost always subfifting, it may be
there said to be an endemic or conftant difeafe;
as in *Iceland, Groenland (g), Cronftadt (h)*,
the northern parts of *Ruffia (i)*, and in most
northern countries as yet difcovered in *Europe*,
from the latitude of 60 to the north pole.
It was also formerly in a peculiar manner endemic in several parts of the *Low Countries*, in
Holland and *Friefland*; in *Brabant, Pomera-
nia*, and the *Lower Saxony (k)*; and in some

(a) Vid. *Nitzfch.*   *(b)* Vid. *Kramer.*
(c) Bachftrom.   *(d) Krameri epiftol. p.* 23,
(e) Dedonæus, & Forreftus. *(f) Ronffeus.*
(g) Herman. Nicolai. Vid. act. Haffn.
(h) Sinopæus.
(i) Vid. *Commerc. literar. Norimb. an.* 1734, *p.* 162.
(k) Wierus, Ronffeus, &c.

places

places of *Denmark (l)*, *Sweden*, and *Nor-way (m)*, chiefly upon the fea-coafts.

Laftly, Where thefe caufes prevail lefs fre-quently, and are more peculiar to the circum-ftances of a few, it may be there faid to be fpo-radic, or a difeafe only here and there to be met with; as in *Great Britain (n)* and *Ireland*, feveral parts of *Germany*, &c.

Now, by confidering the peculiarity of the circumftances, fituation, and way of life of thefe people; and by attentively obferving, what at any time gives rife to this difeafe, what is feen to remove it, and what to increafe or mitigate its malignity, we fhall be able to form a judgment, not only of the principal caufes productive of it, but likewife of the fubordi-nate, or thofe that in a lefs degree may con-tribute their influence. It is indeed a matter of the utmoft confequence, to inveftigate the true fources of this evil; as, upon the removing or correcting of thefe, the prefervation of the body from its firft attacks, as well as its confe-quences, in a great meafure depends. And

(l) Vid. *Concilium facultatis medicæ Haffn. de fcorbuto.*

(m) *Brucæus.*

(n) Vid. Dr *Grainger*'s account of the fcurvy at *Fort-Wil-liam*

we

we fhall begin with confidering the fituation of thofe at fea, among whom it is faid to be fo often an epidemic calamity.

In the proof of the identity of this difeafe on both elements *(o)*, I obferved, that the caufes productive of it at fea, were to be found alfo at land, in a fmaller degree: but before determining what are the true caufes of its being fo often epidemic at fea, it may not be amifs to remark what they are not, although commonly accufed.

Many have afcribed this difeafe to the great quantity of fea-falt *(p)*, neceffarily made ufe of by feamen in their diet: and it has been therefore denominated a *muriatic fcurvy.*

Whether this falt, inftead of producing the fcurvy, may not, on the contrary, from its antifeptic quality, become the means of preventing it for fome time, I fhall not take upon me to determine, as my experiments do not authorife this conclufion; though they plainly prove, that it neither caufes the diftemper, nor adds to its malignity. For in the cruifes after mentioned, where the fcurvy raged with great violence, it was then a fafhionable cuftom to

(o) Part 1. chap. 3.
(p) *Lifteri exercitatio de fcorbuto.*

drink

drink the falt water, by way of gentle phyfic. I have been told, that Admiral *Martin*, and feveral officers in his fleet, continued the ufe of it during a whole cruife.   I had at that time feveral patients under a purging courfe of this water, for the itch, and obftinate ulcers on their legs; and have experienced very good effects from it, efpecially in the laft cafe: yet none of thefe people, after continuing this courfe for a month, had the leaft fcorbutic complaint.

But to put it beyond all doubt, that fea-falt is not the occafion of the fcurvy, I took two patients, (in order to make trial of the effects of different medicines in this difeafe, to be more fully related afterwards), with very putrid gums, fwelled legs, and contracted knees, to whom I gave half a pint of falt water, and fometimes more, every day for a fortnight: at the expiration of which time, I was not fenfible of their being in the leaft worfe; but found them in the fame condition as thofe who had taken no medicine whatever *(q)*.   From which I am convinced, that fea-falt, at leaft

(q) This experiment, of giving fcorbutic people falt water, has been often tried; and fome have thought they received benefit from it. See chap. 4.

the

the drinking of falt water, by no means dif-
pofes the conftitution to this difeafe.

But I would not be underftood here to mean,
nor does it follow from what has been faid,
that although fea-water, which is a compofition in which this falt is a principal ingredient,
has no bad influence upon the fcurvy, that a
diet of falt flefh and fifh is equally innocent.
The contrary of which will appear in the fe-
quel. The brine of meats, in particular, is of a
different quality from either purified fea-falt or
falt water; for we find that this falt may be fo
intangled by the animal oils, efpecially in falt
pork, that it is with great difficulty difen-
gaged from them after many wafhings, and the
moft plentiful dilution So that as this faline
quality is inextricable from fuch food, it is rendered improper in many cafes to afford that
foft, mild nourifhment, which is required to
repair the body. It is remarkable, that the
powers of the human machine can animalife o-
ther falts; that is, convert them into the ammoniacal fort, or that of its own nature: while
this fea-falt feems to elude the force of our folids and fluids; and retaining its own unchange-
able nature in the body, is to be recovered un-
altered from the urine of thofe who have taken

it.

it. Thus, fea-falt has no effect in producing this difeafe; whatever meats hardened and preferved by it may have, by being rendered of hard and difficult digeftion, and improper for nourifhment. And this is farther confirmed by the daily experience of feamen; who, upon the firft fcorbutical complaint, are generally debarred the ufe of every thing that is the leaft falted: notwithftanding which, the difeafe increafes with great violence: While at other times, it breaks out when there is plenty of frefh flefh-provifions on board; as was the cafe in Lord *Anfon*'s fhips, on their leaving the coaft of *Mexico* (*r*).

Others, again, have fuppofed fuch to be the conftitution of the human body, that health and life cannot be preferved long, without the ufe of green herbage, vegetables, and fruits;

(*r*) Vid. Part 3. chap. 2. Dr *Mead*, who was thoroughly acquainted with their fituation, obferves, that, upon that occafion, frefh flefh-provifions, and plenty of wholfome rain-water, did not avail them. *Difcourfe on the fcurvy, p.* 100.

That falt flefh-meats have fometimes no fhare in occafioning this difeafe, is demonftrable from the many *Germans* in *Hungary* deftroyed by it, who eat neither falt beef nor pork; on the contrary, they had frefh beef at a very low price. *Vid. Krameri epift. p.* 33.

The foldiers in the *Ruffian* armies alfo had no falt provifions. *Vid. Nitzfch.*

and

and that a long abftinence from thefe, is alone the caufe of the difeafe *(f)*.

But if this were truly the cafe, we muft have had the fcurvy very accurately defcribed by the ancients; whofe chief ftudy feems to have been the art of war; and whofe manner of befieging towns was generally by a blockade, till they had forced a furrender by famine. Now, as they held out many months, fometimes years, without a fupply of vegetables; we fhould, no doubt, have heard of many dying of the fcurvy, long before the magazines of dry provifions were exhaufted. The continuance of thofe fieges far exceeded moft of our modern ones; even the five months blockade of *Thorn*, upon which *Bachftrom* has founded this fuppofition. It would likewife be a much more quent difeafe in every country, than it really is: for there are perfons every where, who, from choice, eat few or no green vegetables; and fome countries are deprived of the ufe of them for five or fix months of the year; as is the cafe of many parts in the highlands of *Scotland*, *Newfoundland*, &c.; where, however, the fcurvy is not a ufual malady.

It would be tedious to give many inftances,

(f)· Obfervationes circa fcorbutum ; auctore Fre. Bachftrom.

they

they being notorious, of fhips crews continuing feveral months at fea, upon their ordinary
diet, without any approach of the fcurvy. I
have been three months on a cruife, during
which time none of the feamen tafted vegetables or greens of any fort; and although for
a great part of that time, from want of frefh
water, their beef and pork were boiled in the
fea-water, yet we returned into port without
one fcorbutical complaint. I have known meffes, as they are called, of feamen, who have
lived, during a whole voyage of three years, on
the fhip's provifions, for want of money to
purchafe better fare, efpecially greens; and
who were fo regardlefs of health, as to expend
what little money they could procure, in brandy and fpirits: fo that a few onions, or the
like, was their whole fea-ftore; and a meal
with vegetables was feldom eat by them, above
twice or thrice in a month, during the whole
voyage. Notwithftanding which, they have
kept free from the fcurvy.

But it was remarkable, in the two cruifes
afterwards to be mentioned, in his Majefty's
fhip the *Salifbury*, where I had an opportunity
of making obfervations on this difeafe, that it
began to rage on board that fhip, and indeed

M 2   all

all the *Channel* fquadron, upon being lefs than
fix weeks at fea; and after having left *Plymouth*,
where plenty of all forts of greens were to be
had ; by which, as one would have thought,
the failors had fufficiently prepared their bodies
againft the attack of this malady. Yet here, in
fo fhort a time as two months, out of 4000 men
in that fleet, 400 at leaft became more highly
fcorbutic *(t)*, than could reafonably have been
expected, had they all been debarred the ufe
of vegetables for fix months on fhore, like our
highlanders, and many others. And what
puts it beyond all doubt, that the difeafe was
not occafioned folely by the want of vegetables
for fo fhort a time, is, that the fame fhip's
company of the *Salifbury*, in much longer crui-

(t) Upon the return of the fleet to *Plymouth*, Dr *Huxham*
makes the following remark in the month of *July* 1746. *Ter-*
ribilis jam fævit fcorbutus inter nautas, præcipue quos fecum reduxit
Martin, claffis occidentalis præfectus. Excruciantur perplurimi ulceri-
bus fædis, lividis, fordidis, ac valde fungofis: mirum eft profecto et
infolitum, quàm brevi tempore fpongiofa caro, fungi ad inftar, his ulceri-
bus fuccrefcit, etfi paulò antè fcalpello derafa, eaque interdum ad ma-
gnitudinem enormem. Non folùm miferis his, at verè utilibus homini-
bus, per fe infenfa eft maximè fcorbutica lues, fed et illos etiam omni
penè morbo, qui ab humorum corruptione pendet, obnoxios admodum
reddit ; febribus nempe putridis, malignis, petechialibus, peffimo va-
riolarum generi, dyfenteriæ cruentæ, hæmorrhagiis, &c. Multo
magis adeò bonis his fuit exitio quàm bellicum fulmen! Obfervationes de aëre et morbis epidemicis.

fes,

fes, kept quite free from the diftemper, where their circumftances as to want of frefh vegetables were fimilar. It was obfervable, that in the longeft cruife fhe performed, while I was furgeon, there was but one fcorbutical patient on board, who fell into the difeafe after having had an intermitting fever. We were out at that time from the 10th of *Auguft* to the 28th of *October* ; which was a twelve weeks continuance at fea, and confequently as long an abftinence from vegetables.

So that although it is a certain and experienced truth, that the ufe of greens and vegetables is effectual in preventing the difeafe, and extremely beneficial in the cure; and thus we fhall fay, that abftinence from them, in certain circumftances, proves the *occafional caufe* of the evil : yet there are unqueftionably to be found at fea, other ftrong fources of it; which, with refpect to the former, (or want of vegetables), we fhall hereafter diftinguifh by the name of the *predifpofing caufes* to it. The influences of which latter, at times, muft be extremely great, as in the cafe of Lord *Anfon*'s fquadron in paffing round *Cape Horn (u)*, to induce fo univerfal a calamity; from which hardly any

(u) Vid. Part 3. chap. 2.

one

one of them feems to have been exempted, attended with the mortality of above one half of them, when they had been but little more than three months at fea: while whole countries are obferved to live on the fame, nay, even a lefs wholfome diet; and many people for years abftain from vegetables, without almoft any inconveniency.

Some have alledged this to proceed from fomething peculiar in the confined and polluted air of a fhip; and the ftagnation of the bilge-water in the hold has been accufed as a main caufe of the diftrefs. But had this laft the effects prefumed, they would be moft fenfibly fel by thofe who are moft expofed to it, *viz.* the carpenters; who at fea are often obliged to meafure, every four hours, the quantity of bilge-water; and do then, and at other times in mending the pumps, fuffer very great inconveniencies, being almoft fuffocated by it: nay inftances are not wanting where they have been killed at once with this noxious vapour, to which they lie the nearceft when in bed. Yet it does not appear from my own experience, nor from the accounts which I have been able to collect. that they are more liable to the fcurvy than others on board.

As

As to any other inconveniencies from filth, or want of cleanlinefs, in a clofe place, and where the cutaneous and pulmonary perfpiration of a multitude is pent up and confined; they are not peculiar to fhips, but common to all crouded jails, hofpitals, &c.: and whatever bad effects fuch a vitiated air may have on this difeafe, yet it is certain the fcurvy is not the ufual and natural confequence of it. This is the more particularly to be noted, in order to determine the genuine effects of this peculiar evil difpofition of air; which are at all times, and in all places, a malignant, highly-contagious fever, known by the name of *the jail-diftemper*. This is almoft the only difeafe obferved in the tranfport-fhips which daily carry over numbers of people to *Virginia*, few or none of whom become fcorbutic; as likewife in fhips that have been crouded with foldiers. And, univerfally, whenever many perfons are confined together long under clofe-fhut hatches, they will at length contract this fever, without any approach of the fcurvy amongft them; unlefs, as may fometimes be the cafe, the body, weakened and exhaufted by the preceeding ficknefs, is afterwards rendered more fufceptible of the fcorbutic taint, where

other

other fcorbutic caufes prevail.   Though I have oftentimes had occafion to fee this contagion bred by putrid air, yet I never obferved any fcurvies, either at the time, or after it.

In the latter end of the year 1750, the government contracted with a *Dutch* mafter of a veffel to carry over 200 *Palatines* to our colony in *Nova Scotia.* The brutal *Dutchman,* contrary to exprefs orders, confined thefe poor people below, and would not permit them to come fo often upon deck as was requifite for their health; by which means they contracted this malignant fever, which killed one half of them.   And here it was remarkable, there was not one of thefe people who, after recovering at fea, or upon land, became fcorbutic; nor had they any fuch diftemper in the fhip (*x*).

The

(*x*) Communicated by Mr *Ives.* This contagious petechial fever was as a plague to the fhip *Dragon,* of 60 guns, and 400 men, for the fpace of fix months. During which time I feldom or never had in my lift lefs than fixty or feventy patients. Many of them relapfed to the third and fourth time. It was a dreadful, painful fcene! Not a fifth part of our people efcaped. My firft mate, Mr *Blincow,* foon died in it. Another gentleman, whom our neceffities obliged the Commodore to warrant as mate from another fhip, died alfo. My other mate, Mr *Thomas Peck,* (prefent furgeon to the fick and wounded at *Deal),* narrowly efcaped

The truth really is, a putrid air, though never obferved folely to be productive of this difeafe, has a pernicious influence in aggravating its feveral fymptoms: and where an epidemic fcorbutical conftitution at the fame time fubfifts, they give rife to a complicated, fcorbutical and malignant fever; which I fhall have occafion to mention among the fymptoms of this malady.

But the fcurvy by itfelf is often experienced to make great ravage, where the air has been properly renewed and ventilated, and the whole fhip kept clean and fweet. I have been told, that the *Namur's* crew, in their expedition to the *Eaft Indies*, though very healthy at the Cape of *Good Hope*, became fcorbutic at the time they arrived at *Fort St David's*, notwithftanding the ufe of that truly noble

efcaped with life. To thefe loffes I muft add my own dear brother, who commanded the foldiers on board, feveral gentlemen of the quarter-deck, and fixty of our ftouteft and beft failors. Yet, amidft all this danger, through the providence of God, I efcaped untouched, to the furprife of all who knew our circumftances, and the fatigue I underwent, when for moft part deftitute of all affiftance. But I have not feen one inftance of this illnefs having been complicated with the fcurvy, or of the fcurvy feizing a man recovered from that fever for at leaft fix months afterwards; which was indeed one of the longeft intervals we ever enjoyed freedom from it.

N   invention,

invention, *Sutton*'s machine *(y)*. And though Lord *Anfon*'s fhip was kept uncommonly clean and fweet after they left the coaft of *Mexico*; yet the progrefs of their mifery was not at all retarded by it. And, what is further pretty remarkable, we know, that the fcurvy may be perfectly cured in the impure air of a fhip; of which the following is a memorable inftance.

His Majefty's fhip the *Guernfey* brought into *Lifbon*, after a cruife off *Cadiz*, 70 of her crew afflicted with this difeafe. Many of them were far advanced, even in the laft ftages of it. The plague at this time raging at *Meffina*, it was with great difficulty our fhips could obtain

(y) When accounts were received from that great and experienced officer Admiral *Bofcawen*, of the general healthfulnefs of his fquadron at the Cape, it was with great reafon afcribed to the benefit derived from thefe ufeful pipes; though their prefervation from the fcurvy in particular feems to have been owing chiefly to their having had a good paffage, and touching at different places, where proper refrefhments were procured them by their brave and wife commander. Upon their arrival at *Fort St David's*, the furgeon to that hofpital acquaints me, that the men of wars crews became as highly fcorbutic, as any of the others, whofe fhips were not provided with the machine.

The cafe of our annual *Greenland* fhips, who are fo well fitted, large, and convenient, and carry no more men than are juft fufficient to navigate them, puts it beyond all doubt, that confined putrid air, bad provifions and water, have often no fhare in producing this difeafe. For confirmation of which, fee Mr *Maude*'s account of them, part 2. chap. 5.

pratique

pratique in any port: fo that it was found impracticable to land them. There was another very troublefome circumftance. For, in order to conceal fo great a number of fick from the vifit of the officers of health, they were under a neceffity of fhutting them up for fome time together in a clofe place. For this purpofe they were with great difficulty removed into the Captain's ftore-room; where there is generally worfe air than in any other part of the fhip. This was performed with imminent danger to many of their lives. Several of them, though moved with extreme caution, fell into the fcorbutic *deliquium*; whofe prefervation was owing to the judgment of their ingenious furgeon, and to the liberality of the Captain, who, upon this occafion, ordered them to be plentifully fupplied with his richeft cordial wines. But every one of thefe men recovered on board before they left that place, without being landed. The fhip lay ftrict quarantaine a fortnight. After that they were obliged to be extremely circumfpect in allowing even thofe who were pretty well recovered, to go on fhore; as their ill looks might have betrayed their fituation to the *Portuguefe.* This fhip had no ventilators: and it is natural to fuppofe there might be fome remiffnefs in the article of cleanlinefs, where there was fuch a number of fick; who, notwithftanding, all recovered.

The learned writer *(z)* of the great Lord *Anfon*'s voyage, after clearly evincing the falfity of many fpeculations concerning this difeafe, and juftly exploding fome opinions which ufually pafs current about its nature and caufe, is pleafed modeftly to offer a very plaufible and ingenious conjecture, well deferving confideration. " Perhaps a diftinct and adequate know-
" ledge of the fource of this difeafe may never
" be difcovered. But, in general, there is no
" difficulty in conceiving, that as a continued
" fupply of frefh air is neceffary to all animal
" life, and as this air is fo particular a fluid,
" that without lofing its elafticity, or any of
" its obvious properties, it may be rendered
" unfit for this purpofe, by the mixing with
" it fome very fubtile, and otherwife imper-
" ceptible effluvia; it may be conceived, I fay,
" that the fteams arifing from the ocean may
" have a tendency to render the air they are
" fpread through, lefs properly adapted to the
" fupport of the life of terreftrial animals,

(z) The Reverend Mr *Walter.*

" unlefs

" unlefs thefe fteams are corrected by effluvia
" of another kind, and which perhaps the
" land alone can fupply."

It muft be allowed, that the air, which is a
compound of almoft all the different bodies
we know, has many latent properties, by
which animals are varioufly affected ; and
thefe we neither can at prefent, nor perhaps
ever will be able to inveftigate. We do not
even know certainly what this *pabulum vitæ* is
in that fluid, which preferves and fupports animal life. The only means then we have to
judge of the exiftence of fuch an occult quality
as may be fuppofed peculiar to the air of the
ocean, muft be from its effects. Thefe, upon
this fuppofition, ought to be moft noxious,
and moft fenfibly perceived, in the middle of
the great oceans, and at the wideft diftance
from the continents and iflands, where there
is the greateft want of land-air, and of its vital
influences, which may be prefumed fo neceffary
to the fupport of the life of terreftrial animals.
But it is experienced, that fhips cruifing upon
certain coafts, at a very fmall diftance from the
fhore, where the air confequently differs widely from that of the main ocean, as being impregnated with many particles from the land,
and

and is almoft the fame with that of the fea-
port towns, are equally, if not more, afflicted
with this difeafe, than others are in croffing the
ocean.   And it will be found univerfally to
appear in a much fhorter time, and rage with
greater violence, (all circumftances being otherwife alike), in a fquadron cruifing in the narrow
feas of the *Baltic* and *Channel*, or upon the
coafts of *Norway* and *Hudfon's* bay, than in
another continuing the fame length of time in
the middle of the *Atlantic* ocean.   We often
obferved our *Channel* cruifers quickly over-run
with the fcurvy ; while their conforts, fitted out
at the fame port, and confequently with the
fame ftate of provifions and water, who foon
left them, ftretching into the main ocean upon a voyage to the *Indies*, or upon a much
longer cruife off the *Canaries* or *Cadiz*, kept
pretty free from it.   For my own part, I never could remark any alteration upon our fcorbutic patients, while we continued for many
days clofe in upon the *French* fhore, with the
wind or air coming from thence, or when, at a
greater diftance from any land, we kept the
middle of the *Channel :* and yet, in either of
thofe ftations, difference of weather had a remarkable influence upon fcorbutic ailments.

Nay,

Nay, fhips and fleets, without going to fea, are often attacked by this malady while in harbour. Thus, when Admiral *Matthews* lay long in *Hieres* bay with his fleet, many of the feamen became highly fcorbutic; on which account fome hundreds were fent to *Mahon* hofpital. And the fame has happened to our fleets when at *Spithèad,* and even when lying in *Portfmouth* harbour. This difeafe is not indeed peculiar to the ocean, there being many inftances of its raging with equal violence at land *(a)*.

FROM what has been faid, it appears, that the ftrong *predifpofing caufes* to this calamity at fea, are not conftant, but cafual, upon that element. For though it fhould be granted, that the fea-air gives always a tendency to the fcorbutic *diathefis,* yet the evil proves often, highly epidemic and fatal in very fhort voyages, or upon a very fhort continuance at fea, to crews of fhips who, at other times, have continued out much longer, cruifing in the fame place, and in parallel circumftances of water and provifions, and yet have kept entirely free

(a) Vid. the cafe of the *German* troops in *Hungary,* and of the *Ruffian* armies, part 3.

from

from it.   Thus, the great Lord *Anfon* cruifed
for four months, waiting for the *Acapulco* fhip,
in the *Pacific* ocean;   during which time, we
are told, his crews continued in perfect health:
when, at another time, after leaving the coaft
of *Mexico*, in lefs than feven weeks at fea, the
fcurvy became highly epidemic, notwithftanding plenty of frefh provifions and fweet water
on board.   And when it raged with fuch uncommon malignity in paffing *Cape Horn*, it deftroyed above one half of his crew, in lefs time
than he kept the feas in perfect health, in the
before mentioned cruife.

I had an opportunity in two *Channel* cruifes,
the one of ten weeks, the other of eleven, *ann.*
1746 and 1747, in his Majefty's fhip the *Salifbury*, a fourth rate, to fee this difeafe rage
with great violence.   And here it was remarkable, that though I was on board in feveral o-
ther long *Channel* cruifes; one of twelve weeks
particularly, from the 10th of *Auguft* to the
28th of *October*; yet we had but one fcorbutic
patient; nor in any other that I remember, had we the leaft fcorbutic appearance.
But in thofe two I have mentioned, the fcurvy
began to rage after being a month or fix weeks
at fea; when the water on board, as I took
particular

particular notice, was uncommonly fweet and good; and the ftate of provifions fuch as could afford no fufpicion of occafioning fo general a ficknefs, being the fame in quality as in former cruifes. And though the fcorbutic people were, by the generous liberality of that great and humane commander, the Hon. Captain *George Edgcumbe*, daily fupplied with frefh provifions, fuch as mutton-broth and fowls, and even meat from his own table; yet, at the expiration of ten weeks, we brought into *Plymouth* 80 men, out of a complement of 350, more or lefs afflicted with this difeafe.

Now, it was obfervable, that both thefe cruifes were in the months of *April*, *May*, and *June;* when we had, efpecially in the beginning of them, a continuance of cold, rainy, and thick *Channel* weather, as it is called whereas in our other cruifes, we had generally very fine weather; except in winter, when, during the time I was furgeon, the cruifes were but fhort. Nor could I affign any other reafon for the frequency of this difeafe in thefe two cruifes, and our exemption from it at other times, but the influence of the weather; the circumftances of the men, fhip, and provifions, being in all other refpects alike. I

O   have

have more than once remarked, that after great
rains, or a continuance of clofe foggy weather,
efpecially after ftorms with rain, the fcorbutic
people generally grew worfe ; but found a mi-
tigation of their fymptoms and complaints, upon the weather becoming drier and warmer
for a few days.   And I am certain it will be
allowed, by all who have had an opportunity
of making obfervations on this difeafe at fea
(b), or will attentively confider the fituation
of

(b) Extract of a letter from Mr Murray.

Of the feveral antecedent or efficient caufes of this difeafe,
it is not to be doubted, but a moift air, or hazy, cloudy weather, is among the principal.   A particular inftance of which
happened in a cruife we went upon in the *Canterbury,* along with
another fhip ; after having laid fix months in *Louifburg* harbour,
where the feamen had great plenty and variety of fifh, and where
we were properly victualled with found provifions, and very
good bread and water.   We cruifed not far from the *Bahama
Iflands*; the weather for moft part was ftormy, foggy, and very
wet.   Before we had been at fea a month, the fcurvy was very
epidemical on board both fhips ; and in fix weeks we had 50,
the other (the *Norwich*) 70 patients in this difeafe : whereas
at another time, in different weather, we were at fea nigh as
many months, before the like fymptoms and difeafes appeared ;
and even then were nothing near fo epidemical.   The particulars of that cruife were as follow.

We failed 29th *November* from *Cape Breton,* and in two days
were in lat. 43° 18′ ; and by the 11th *December* were in 29° 56′,
near which latitude we kept cruifing to the 7th of *January*. During which time the winds were fo variable, that it was hard to
tell

of feamen there, that *the principal and main predifpofing caufe* to it, is a manifeft and obvious quality of the air, *viz.* its *moifture.* The effects of this are perceived to be more immediately hurtful and pernicious in certain conftitutions; in thofe who are much weakened by preceeding ficknefs; in thofe who, from a lazy inactive difpofition, neglect to ufe proper

tell which point of the compafs they inclined moft to, or continued longeft in. The weather was extremely cold, foggy, and moift, the beginning of the month; but grew gradually warmer as we funk our latitude. But that its moifture continued, will appear from the following account of rainy days, which you have here, with the other ftate of the weather. *December.* Rain from the 1ft to the 5th; 7th, 11th, 16th, 18th, 21ft to 23d; 27th, 29th. Frefh gales 1ft, 2d, 3d, 4th, 6th, 7th, 10th, 11th, 14th to 25th; 27th to 31ft. Thunder and lightning 3d and 29th.——A fog the 1ft.——Moft part of the month cloudy and hazy. 174⁷₉, *January.* The weather this month was in general more moderate; but, confidering our latitude, not very warm. Rain the 2d, 6th, 10th, 13th, 15th, 16th, 18th, 19th, 24th, 25th, 26th, 31ft. Weather cloudy for feven days, but no fogs. Calm the 2d. Frefh breezes 6th, 7th, 9th, 10th, 12th, 16th to 20th; 24th, 25th, 26th, 31ft.

The difeafes depending upon this weather, were at firft, *plethoræ,* from the fudden change from cold to warmth; fome acute fevers; and particularly two ardent ones, which carried off the patients. About the end of *December,* people began to complain of the fcurvy; and before the middle of *January* we had 16 patients in that difeafe; and by the 25th, when we arrived at *St Thomas,* we had no lefs than 50 patients in it; and our confort the *Norwich* 70.

exercife;

exercise; and in those who indulge a discontented melancholy humour: all which may be reckoned the *secondary disposing causes* to this foul and fatal mischief.

As the atmosphere at sea may always be supposed moister than that of the land; hence there is always a greater disposition to the scorbutic *diathesis* at sea, than in a pure dry land-air. But, supposing the like constitution of air in both places, the inconveniencies which persons suffer in a ship during a damp wet season, are infinitely greater than people who live at land are exposed to; these latter having many ways of guarding against its pernicious effects, by warm dry cloaths, fires, good lodging, &c.: whereas the sailors are obliged not only to breathe in this air all day, but sleep in it all night, and frequently in wet bed-cloaths, the ship's hatches being necessarily kept open. And indeed one reason of the frequency of the scurvy in the above cruises, was no doubt the often carrying up the bedding of the ship's company to quarters; where it was sometimes wet quite through, and continued so for many days together, when, for want of fair weather, there was no opportunity of drying it.

No

No perfon fenfible of the bad effects of fleeping in wet apartments, or in damp bed-cloaths,
and almoft in the open air, without any thing
fufficiently dry or warm to put on, will be furprifed at the havock the fcurvy made in Lord
Anfon's crew in paffing *Cape Horn*, if their
fituation in fuch uncommon and tempeftuous
weather be properly confidered.

During fuch furious ftorms, the fpray of the
fea raifed by the violence of the wind, is di-
fperfed over the whole fhip; fo that the people
breathe, as it were, in water for many weeks
together. The tumultous waves inceffantly
breaking in upon the decks, and wetting thofe
who are upon duty as if they had been ducked
in the fea, are alfo continually fending down
great quantities of water below; which makes
it the moft uncomfortable wet lodging imagi-
nable: and, from the labouring of the fhip, it
generally leaks down, in many places, directly
upon their beds. There being here no fire or
fun to dry or exhale the moifture, and the
hatches neceffarily kept fhut, this moift, ftagnating, confined air below, becomes moft offenfive
and intolerable. When fuch weather continues
long, attended with fleet and rain, as it generally is, we may eafily figure to ourfelves the
condition

condition of the poor men; who are obliged to
fleep in wet cloaths and damp beds, the decks
fwimming with water below them; and there
to remain only four hours at a time; till they
are again called up to frefh fatigue, and hard
labour, and again expofed to the wafhing of
the fea, and rains. The long continuance of
this weather feldom fails to produce the fcurvy
at fea.

As to its breaking out fo immediately in thofe
fhips, upon their leaving the coaft of *Mexico*
(c), it was not only owing to their finding fo
few refrefhments, efpecially fruits and vegetables fit to be carried to fea, at the harbour of
Chequetan; but alfo to the inceffant rains they
had in their paffage to *Afia*, and the great inconveniencies that neceffarily muft attend fo
long a continuance of fuch weather at fea. To
which it may be added, that, by obfervations
made on this difeafe, it appears, that thofe who
are once infected with it, efpecially in fo deep a
degree as that fquadron was, are more fubject to
it afterwards than others. I remember, that many of them who returned to *England* with Lord
Anfon, and afterwards went to fea in other

(c) Part 3. chap. 2.

fhips,

fhips, were much more liable to the fcurvy than others.

It was however remarkable here, that though the calamity began fo very foon after their leaving land; yet, in fo tedious a paffage as four months, it did not rage with that mortality as in paffing *Cape Horn:* nor did it acquire fo great virulence, as appears by its being fo quickly removed upon their landing. And this was owing to the abfence of another caufe, which is found greatly to inforce and increafe the diftrefs, *viz.* cold; the combination of which with moifture is, upon all occafions, experienced to be the moft powerful predifpofing caufe to this malady; though indeed the latter of itfelf is found fufficient to produce it. And here frequent wafhing and cleaning of the fhip, as was obferved, did not ftop the progrefs of the difeafe; becaufe it did not remove the caufe, no more than *Sutton*'s machine is found to do; which only renews the air, without correcting its moifture.

Now, any perfon who has fufficiently confidered the fituation of a fhip's crew, expofed for many weeks to ftormy, rainy, or perpetual foggy clofe weather at fea, will not by this time be furprifed at our affigning dampnefs or

moifture,

moifture, as a principal caufe of the frequency and virulency of this difeafe upon the watry e-lement.   And this is not only agreeable to my own experience, but is confirmed by all juft obfervations that were ever made on this dif-temper.   In the very firft juft account we ever had of it in *Europe*, from *Olaus Magnus (d)*, it is remarked, That cold damp lodgings contri-buted greatly towards its production ; that its virulence was always increafed by cold and raw exhalations from the wet and damp walls of houfes; whereas people living in drier apart-ments, were not equally fubject to it.   And ac-cordingly we find, that petty officers, who fleep in clofe births, as they are called, with canvas hung round, by which they are fheltered from the inclemency of the weather ; as alfo feamen who go well clothed, dry, and clean, though ufing the fame diet with the reft of the crew, are not fo foon infected.   This is the principal reafon why officers obliged to live on the fhip's provifions, as the warrant-officers often do, (with this difference, that they drink a greater quantity of brandy and fpirits, which, as fhall be mentioned afterwards, fhould in a particular manner difpofe them to this difeafe), by lying

(d) Quoted at large, Part 3. chap. 1

in

in warm dry cabbins, and going better clothed, are feldom attacked by the fcurvy; unlefs upon its moſt virulent rage, and when the common failors have been previouſly almoſt deſtroyed by it.

It is obfervable, that fuch a fituation as has been defcribed, together with the ufe of fuch improper diet as ſhall hereafter be mentioned, produces the fcurvy in any climate: but its virulence will always be greatly augmented by the addition of cold. Thus we find it a much more frequent difeafe in winter than in fummer, and in colder than in warmer climates. Ships that go to the north, as to *Greenland*, and up the *Baltic*, are peculiarly fubjeft to it; whereas it is generally owing, in fouthern latitudes, to the continual rains which fall there at certain feafons, and more particularly to the great length of thefe voyages. But a combination of moifture with cold, is the moft frequent and genuine fource of this difeafe: and a very intenfe degree of cold, as in *Greenland*, &c. is experienced to have a moft pernicious influence in heightening its malignity.

What effefts are produced by thefe powerful caufes on the human body, it is not my pre-

P   fent

sent purpose to explain *(e)*. It may be sufficient here only to observe, that moisture is
the parent of corruption or putrefaction in nature; and, by the observation of all physicians
from the days of *Hippocrates*, a moist warm
air begets the most malignant putrid diseases,
even the plague itself. But moisture concurring with other peculiar circumstances, as a
gross diet, cold, &c. disposes in a particular
manner to the scorbutic corruption.

The qualities of the moist sea-air will certainly be rendered still more noxious, by being
confined in a ship without due circulation; as
air at all times in this state loses its elasticity,
and is found highly prejudicial to the health
and life of animals; but becomes much more
so where stagnating water is pent up along with
it, as it is from thence more speedily disposed
to putrefaction. It is likewise heated in ships
by passing through the lungs of many people,
and impregnated with various putrid effluvia.
Hence the eagerness and longings of scorbutic
people in such circumstances for the land-air,
and the high refreshment to their senses upon
being put on shore, are very natural; but no
more than what the vapour of fresh earth

(e) Vid. chap. 6.

would

would afford to a perfon after being long confined in a clofe, damp, unwholfome air; as
that of a prifon, dungeon, or damp apartment
at land; and what we all feel, upon taking in
the frefh country-air, perfumed with the various odours of nature, after having been obliged to breathe in a crouded, dirty, populous
city.

I come, in the next place, to an additional,
and extremely powerful caufe, obferved at fea to
occafion this difeafe, and which concurring
with the former, in progrefs of time, feldom
fails to breed it. And this is, the want of frefh
vegetables and greens; either, as may be fuppofed, to counteract the bad effects of their before mentioned fituation; or rather, and more
truly, to correct the quality of fuch hard and
dry food as they are obliged to make ufe of
Experience indeed fufficiently fhews, that as
greens or frefh vegetables, with ripe fruits, are
the beft remedies for it, fo they prove the moft
effectual prefervatives againft it. And the difficulty of obtaining them at fea, together with
a long continuance in the moift fea-air, are the
true caufes of its fo general and fatal malignity
upon that element.

The

The diet which people are neceffarily obliged
to live upon while at fea, was before affigned
as the *occafional caufe of the difeafe (f)* ; as in a
particular manner it determines the effects of
the before mentioned predifpofing caufes to
the production of it. And there will be no difficulty to conceive the propriety of this diftinction, or underftand how the moft innocent
and wholfome food, at times, and in peculiar
fituations, will with great certainty form a difeafe. Thus, if a man lives on a very flender
diet, and drinks water, in the fens of *Lincoln-
fhire*, he will almoft infallibly fall into an
ague.

All rules and precepts of diet, as well as the
diftinction of aliment into wholfome and unwholfome, are to be underftood only as relative
to the conftitution or ftate of the body. We
find a child and a grown perfon, a valetudina-
rian and a man in health, require aliment of
different kinds; as does even the fame perfon
in the heat of fummer and in the depth of
winter, during a dry or rainy feafon. Betwixt the tropics, the natives live chiefly on
fruits, feeds, and vegetables; whereas northern
nations find a flefh and folid diet more fuit-

(f) P. 93.

able

able to their climate. In like manner it appears, I think, very plainly, that fuch hard
dry food as a fhip's provifions, or the fea-diet,
is extremely wholfome; and that no better
nourifhment could be well contrived for labouring people, or any perfon in perfect health,
ufing proper exercife in a dry pure air; and
that, in fuch circumftances, feamen will live
upon it for feveral years, without any inconvenience. But where the conftitution is predifpofed to the fcorbutic taint, by the caufes
before affigned, (the effects of which, as fhall
be fhewn in a proper place *(g)*, are a weakening of the animal powers of digeftion), the influence of fuch diet in bringing on this difeafe,
fooner or later, according to the ftate and conftitution of the body, becomes extremely vifible.

The firft, generally, who feel its effects,
are thofe who are recovering from other difeafes, or fome preceeding fit of ficknefs, by
which the whole body, and the digeftive faculties, have been greatly weakened ; and are
in this condition obliged to ufe the fhip's fare.
Thus, in *May* 1747, when there prevailed feveral inflammatory diforders, particularly peri-

(g) Chap. 6.

pneumonic

pneumonic fevers, all who were recovering
from them became highly fcorbutic. The next
who complained, were the indolent and lazy;
fuch as are commonly called *fculkers*, and ufe
little or no exercife; a principal help to digeftion. As the difeafe gathered ftrength, it
attacked thofe who had formerly laboured under it, and had been our patients in *May* 1746;
where the conftitution had acquired a tendency
to it from being formerly deeply infected. It
afterwards became more univerfal; but was
confined to the common feamen, particularly
to the raweft and neweft failors. Impreft men
are extremely liable to its attack, by reafon of
their difcontented ftate of mind; and the marines, by not being accuftomed to the fea.

I obferved it increafed in frequency and virulence, upon the fhip's fmall beer being exhaufted, and having brandy ferved in its place;
and this laft obfervation I made in both cruifes.

But it will be now proper to inquire into the
diet which mariners are neceffarily obliged to
live upon at fea. And as it appears to be the
principal occafional caufe of their malady, it
may be worth while to confider fea-provifions
in their beft ftate; it being found by experience, that, notwithftanding the foundnefs and
goodnefs

goodnefs of both water and provifions, the calamity often rages with great fury, and can be
removed only by change of diet. Now, if in
this cafe they appear to have fo great an influence
in forming the diftemper, what ill confequences
may not reafonably be expected from a much
worfe ftate of them; as from putrid beef, rancid pork, mouldy bifcuit and flour, or bad
water, which are misfortunes common at fea?
all which muft infallibly have bad effects in fo
putrid a difeafe.

It muft be remarked in general, that the fea-
diet is extremely grofs, vifcid, and hard of digeftion. It confifts of two articles, *viz.* the
fweet farinaceous fubftances unfermented; and
falted, or dried flefh and fifh.

But more particularly, in our Royal navy,
whofe provifions, for goodnefs and plenty, exceed thofe of any other fhips or fleets in the
world, every man has an allowance of a pound
of bifcuit a-day; which, in the manner it is baked, will be found more folid and fubftantial
food, than two pounds of ordinary well-baked
bread at land. And this is a principal article of
their diet. But the fea-bifcuit undergoes little
or no fermentation in baking, and is confequently of much harder and more difficult digeftion,

geftion, than well-leavened and properly-fer-
mented bread. For it muft be here underftood, that the meally parts of vegetable feeds,
diffolved only in water, are by experience
found to make too vifcid an aliment, to be
conftantly ufed by the generality of mankind:
whereas, by fermentation, and the acid in the
leaven, the glutinous vifcidity and tenacious
oils of thefe meally fubftances are broken and
fubdued; and they become eafily diffolvable afterwards in water, with which before they
would only make a pafte or glue; and are now
mifcible with all the humours of the body.
Well-baked bread, which has undergone a
fufficient degree of fermentation, is of light
and eafy digeftion; and indeed the moft proper
nourifhment for man, as it is adapted by its
accefcency to correct a flefh-diet: whereas, on
the contrary, fea-bifcuit, not being thus duly
fermented, will in many cafes afford too
tenacious and vifcid chyle, improper for the
nourifhment of the body, where the vital digeftive faculties are weakened and impaired.

The next article in their allowance of
what is called *frefh provifions,* is one pound
and a half of wheat-flour in the week, which
is made into pudding with water, and a certain

tain proportion of pickled fewet. This laft does not keep long at fea, fo that they have often raifins or currants in its place. But flour and water boiled thus together, form a tenacious glutinous pafte; requiring the utmoft ftrength and integrity of the powers of digeftion, to fubdue and affimulate it into nourifhment. We find, that weak, inactive, valetudinary people, cannot long bear fuch food.

There remain two other articles of frefh provifions, of which the allowance to each man is more than they generally can ufe. The firft is, ground oats, boiled to a confiftence with water, commonly called *burgow*. Of this the *Englifh* failors eat but little; though in their circumftances it would feem to be wholfome enough, as being the moft acefcent part of their diet. The other is boiled peas; which are of a mild and foftening quality; but having hardly any aromatic parts, they are apt in weak ftomachs to breed flatulencies, and occafion indigeftion; and, like all other farinaceous fubftances, give a *lentor* or vifcidity to water in which they are boiled. It is evident, that in fome cafes they muft afford grofs and improper nourifhment.

This is the allowance of frefh provifions;

Q   and

and they have, befides, a proper quantity given them of falt butter and cheefe. The latter of which is experienced to differ extremely in its qualities, or in the eafe or difficulty with which it is digefted, according to its ftrength, age, &c. But the *Suffolk* cheefe will in many in-ftances, inftead of affifting digeftion, which o-ther cheefe is faid to do, prove a load to the ftomach itfelf; as well as the falt butter, or fweet oil, given fometimes in its place: neither of which indeed correct the qualities of their other food.

Laftly, Of flefh each man has for allowance, two pounds of falt beef, and two pounds of falt pork, *per* week. But thefe are found by every one's experience to be much harder, and more difficult to digeft, than frefh meats; and, after all, to afford a much more im-proper chyle and nourifhment. No perfon can long bear a diet of fuch falt flefh-meats, unlefs it is corrected by bread, vinegar, or ve-getables.

To the above articles, which are the provi-fions with which our navy is ufually fupplied, may be added, ftock fifh, falt fifh, dried or jerk-ed beef, often eat at fea; with whatever is of the like grofs, vifcid, and indigeftible nature: all
which

which will have ftill more noxious qualities when unfound, or in a corrupted ftate.

For drink, the government allows, where it can be procured, good found fmall beer; at other times wine, brandy, rum, or arrack, according to the produce of the country where fhips are ftationed. Beer and fermented liquors of any fort will be found the beft antifcorbutics, and moft proper to correct the ill effects of their fea-diet and fituation; whereas diftilled fpirits have a moft pernicious influence on this difeafe.

As I fhall have occafion elfewhere *(h)* to fhew the natural confequences of fuch diet, it will be fufficient here to obferve, that though the long continuance and conftant ufe of any one particular fort of food, without variety, has its inconveniencies, and is juftly condemned by phyficians *(i)*, nature having fupplied us with an ample variety, defigned no doubt for our ufe; yet the fact here truly is, that fuch food as has been mentioned, is at particular times, and in certain circumftances, not properly adapted to the ftate of the body, and the condition of the digeftive powers *(k)*.

Our

(h) Chap. 6. on the theory of the difeafe.

(i) *Vid. Celfum de medicina.*

(k) A learned Profeffor was pleafed to fend me the following queries.

" May

Our appetites, if they are not depraved, are, upon this and many other occasions, the moft faithful monitors, and point out the quality of fuch food as is fuited to our digeftive organs, and

" May not the fcurvy be owing to fuch a caufe as other epi-
" demical difeafes ; that is, fomething in the air which we do
" not know, nor will probably ever know, though we fee its
" various effects in fevers, fmall pox, meafles, plague, &c. ?
" And may not this be a modern *miafma*, as well as what pro-
" duces fome of thefe difeafes ? By obfervations the *caufæ pro-*
" *egumenæ* may be difcovered, and by diffections the effects
" may be obferved ; but the *caufa proxima* may yet be unknown.
" In the plains of *Stirlingfhire* the people live moftly on crude
" peafe-meal, have very bad water, and have great fogs from
" their own grounds, and from the Frith ; yet, among the nume-
" rous poor patients I have from that place when in the coun-
" try, I have not feen one with a genuine fcurvy."

Anfwer. As to its being a *modern miafma*, I think this can-not, with any colour of reafon, be inferred from the filence of ancient hiftorians, who have mentioned few or no camp-difea-fes; nor on account of its being imperfectly, if at all, defcribed by ancient phyficians, for reafons affigned part 3. chap. 1. The firft defcription of it I have met with, and a very accurate one, is in the year 1260 (vid. part 3. chap. 1.). There is no account of it again until after *ann.* 1490. Yet we cannot well fuppofe, that during that period there was no fuch difeafe in the world, or that people in fuch fituations as are now to be mentioned, would not contract the fcurvy.

It is demonftrable from the appearance of the calamity in e-very part of the world, that no ftate of air whatever is capable of producing it, without the concurrence of grofs vifcid diet, and abftinence from green vegetables. I have known the *Chan-nel* fleet bury a hundred men in a cruife, and land a thoufand

more

and to the ftate and condition of the body.
For where there is a difpofition to the fcorbutic
corruption from a long continuance in the moift
fea-air, concurring with the vifcous, glutinous,
and

more quite rotten in the fcurvy; yet, among the number, there
was not an officer, not even a petty officer.

In *Hungary*, where there muft have been the ftrongeft fcorbutic difpofition in the air (Vid. *Kramer*), not only the officers,
and natives of the country, but even the dragoons, by having
more pay, and confequently better diet, cloathing, and lodging, though equally fubject to the other difeafes of the country, yet kept free from the fcurvy. Who were attacked by it?
Only the *Bohemians*, who eat the coarfeft and moft grofs food.
The *Bohemians* ufed no other than what was the ordinary diet of
their own country, as we are informed by *Kramer*. The feamen in the *Channel* cruifers had the very fame provifions as other
fhips who went upon different ftations: yet it is evident one
caufe in both places was the diet; as a different diet prevented
the difeafe, and change of diet quickly cured it.

Now, there muft have been a quality in the air of *Hungary*
different from that of *Bohemia*; fomething which rendered a diet
harmlefs in the one country, hurtful in the other. The indifpofition of the air in *Hungary* was very obvious. The difeafe prevailed only in the fpring, and during a wet feafon; was much
more virulent in fome parts of the country than in others.
Kramer enumerates the different places where it raged moft,
viz. where-ever the foil was damp and marfhy. This obfervation has been made not only in *Hungary*, but in every other
part of the world; and I will venture to affirm, that, without
any one exception,

     Scorbutus locis aridis ignotus eft.   Steggius.

Moifture was difcovered to be one of the caufes of this malady
by *Ronffeus*, the very firft author who ever wrote exprefsly upon it.

                          The

and too folid diet ufed there, nature points out
the remedy.   In fuch a fituation, the ignorant failor, and the learned phyfician, will
equally long, with the moft craving anxiety, for
green

The facts he produces, feem demonftratively to prove it; befides
having the corroborating evidence of every accurate obfervation
made fince his time.   All which, *viz.* the experience of two
hundred years, we muft contradict, by excluding this caufe, and
referring the fcurvy to occult *miafmata*, or fuch latent caufes in
the air as produce fevers, and fome other epidemical difeafes.
There are indeed perhaps but few difeafes whofe caufes are
more evident to the fenfes, and admit of more exprefs proofs.
Stugart, in *Germany*, was formerly noted for being a place
where the fcurvy raged much; but, upon drying up a large
lake in the neighbourhood of the town, the difeafe has fince
quite difappeared.   Along the banks of the *Rhine*, from *Dour-
lach* to *Mentz*, particularly at *Philipfburg*, it often fucceeds large
inundations of that river.   *Sinopæus* obferved at *Cronftadt*, that
the appearance of the fcurvy, and its malignity, always depend-
ed upon the wetnefs of the feafon; a dry feafon inftantly ftopt it.

Where we have fuch undeniable proofs of the effects of moifture and drinefs, I cannot fee any reafon for having recourfe
to occult *miafmata* in the air, or the like imaginary and uncertain agents, for breeding a difeafe which a perfon contracts
from moift air, by lying in a damp lodging, and ufing at this
feafon too folid grofs food.   Such circumftances produce the
diftemper in every part of the world: and it may effectually be
prevented at any time, by living in dry apartments, going well
clothed, and having proper diet.

Though I have called the one *the predifpofing*, the other *the
cccafunal caufe* of the malady; yet, to fpeak more properly,
they are both of them *(viz. diet* and *moifture) caufæ proegume-
næ*, predifpofing caufes to the difeafe.   They are each but
half-

green vegetables, and the frefh fruits of the
earth; from whofe healing, attenuating, and
faponaceous virtues, relief only can be had.
And fuch people, in the height of the malady,

not

half-caufes, neither of them fingly being able to produce it: but
both of them concurring, conftitute the *caufa proxima*; *i. e.* all
that is requifite and fufficient to form the fcurvy.

As to the cafe of the people in *Stirlingfhire*; have they no
onions, coleworts, *&c.*? A mefs of broth twice a-week, fuch
as is made by the pooreft people in *Scotland*, of green coleworts, barley, and oats, would have preferved Lord *Anfon's*
fquadron from the fcurvy in paffing *Cape Horn*. It is to be remembered, that thefe caufes muft not only conjunctly fubfift,
and exert their influences together in a high degree; but muft
act likewife a confiderable time without intermiffion, efpecially
the diet. Change of food has not only a moft furprifing effect to recover from a very deplorable ftate in the fcurvy, but
even the fmalleft alteration of diet has a wonderful influence in
preventing the approach of it. This is evident from what is
faid (chap. 5.) of the prefent healthfulnefs of our factories at
Hudfon's bay; where fcorbutic *miafmata* (if any fuch there be)
are not wanting in the air, even at this day; as is plain by the
late afflicted condition of *Ellis's* people (fee part 3.), whilft the
perfons in thofe factories were quite healthy. It is farther confirmed by a fact which has more than once occurred. In our
fleet, when in conjunction with *Dutch* fhips, many of our men
have become fcorbutic; mean while the *Dutch* were quite free
from it; which was owing to a mefs of pickled cabbage given
them now and then.

And, for the fame reafon, *viz.* a very fmall difference in
the way of living or diet, even the frequent baths of the ancients, might have preferved their troops from the fcurvy when
quartered in *Pannonia*, the woody, marfhy parts of *Gaul, Germany*, and the *Low Countries*; as is evident from the late cafe of
the Imperial dragoons.

What

not only employ their thoughts all day long on
fatisfying this importunate demand of nature,
but are apt to have their deluded fancies tanta-
lifed in fleep with the agreeable ideas of feaft-
ing upon them at land.   What nature,
from an inward feeling, makes them thus
ftrongly defire, conftant experience confirms to
be the moft certain prevention and beft cure
of their difeafe.

MOREOVER, the fame caufes when fubfift-
ing at land, have been experienced at times to
give rife to as virulent and epidemic fcurvies as
at fea.   Thus, during the fiege of *Thorn* in
the year 1703, feveral thoufand *Saxons* fhut up
in that city were cut off by it.   But at the latter end of the fiege, they being blockaded for
five months, the feafon appears to have been
uncommonly tempeftuous and rainy, over moft
parts of *Europe:* fo that, in this fituation, the
inconveniencies and hardfhips they fuffered,
muft have been equal to thofe of feamen.
They were continually expofed to unwholfome
damp weather; their diet was grofs and vifcid,

What I have here faid, is not with defign to exclude the bad
effects of fome other caufes upon this diftemper.   But to breed
a difeafe, and to give vigour to it when bred, are very different
things.

viz.

viz. ammunition-bread, falt and dried meats, and other folid and coarfe food ; which they were at that time obliged to live upon, being deprived of vegetables. We are told *(l)*, that when fome few of the moft common and coar-feft greens were permitted to be brought into the town, by agreement entered into with the enemy, they were voracioufly devoured by the officers at the gates, as the greateft delicacies. The inhabitants, indeed, afcribed the calamity to the unwholfome beer in the city. But it was obfervable, it attacked and cut off firft the *Saxon* garrifon ; who were moft expofed to the inclemency of fuch weather, by doing hard duty night and day upon the walls. The in-habitants, who remained in warmer lodgings, were much later infeɛted with it; and probably only thofe, who, upon the garrifon's being al-moft deftroyed, were obliged to do duty. This was a real fcurvy ; as no fooner the gates were opened, and plenty of vegetables admitted up-on the furrender of the town, but the difeafe quickly difappeared, after having occafioned a very dreadful mortality.

2. THE next thing to be confidered, is the

(l) *Obfervationes circa fcorbutum,* &c. *auɛtore Fred. Bachftrom:*

peculiar

peculiar fituation and circumftances of fuch
places and countries where it is found to be a
conftant or endemic difeafe; which will ferve
further to illuftrate and confirm what has been
advanced.

It is obferved, that an intenfe degree of cold,
fuch as the inhabitants fuffer during the hard
winters in *Iceland, Groenland,* the northern
parts of *Ruffia, &c.* together with the diet
they are neceffarily obliged to ufe during that
rigorous feafon, infallibly gives rife to this diforder. And here we cannot but remark the
pernicious effects of cold in augmenting its malignity, and rendering it a much more frequent
and virulent diftemper in thefe northern countries, than in warmer climates. It may however be doubted, whether the moft intenfe degree of cold, provided the air is dry and pure
at the fame time, would breed this malady.
For all thefe northern countries are fubject to
great fogs, not only in fummer, but in winter;
and when the cold is exceffive, are peftered
with what is called *froft-fmoak;* a vapour which
rifes out of the fea like fmoak from a chimney,
and is as thick as the thickeft mift *(m)*.

(m) Vid. *John Edge*'s account of *Greenland,* a *Danifh* miffi-
onary, who refided there fifteen years.

Moreover,

Moreover, it is very certain, that the frequency of this evil in other places, as in the *Low Countries*, where it was formerly greatly endemic, and whofe authors have furnifhed us with the moft accurate obfervations, was not owing to their cold and northern fituation only; for in that cafe, all people living in the fame degree of cold, would, *cæteris paribus*, have been equally affeded: whereas, in the very fame climate of *Holland*, there were many villages and cities, living on a like diet with their neighbours, who kept entirely free; while others, at no great diftance from them, were extremely fubjed to it.

Thus, *Ronffeus* (*n*) takes notice, that in his time it was a much more frequent malady at *Amfterdam* and *Alcmaer*, than at *Goude* and *Rotterdam*; and at *Dort*, though in the fame climate, and where the inhabitants eat the fame food, it was hardly ever to be feen: but that, univerfally, in all parts of the country where the foil was fenny, damp, and marfhy, it raged with the greateft violence. This very accurate author obferves likewife, the great influence which the weather had upon it; as, that

(*n*) *Ronffeus de magnis Hippocratis lienibus,* &c. *feu vulgo dido fcorbuto.*

a long continuance of foutherly and wefterly winds *(o)* always occafioned a great frequency of this diftrefs ; but that rainy feafons efpecially, rendered the mifchief quite epidemic and malignant. When this phyfician wrote, his country was little better than a large morafs, expofed to frequent inundations from floods and high tides; which, together with the grofs coarfe diet ufed by the *Dutch* at that time, made the fcurvy perhaps the moft frequent endemic of their country. But now they are become a rich flourifhing republic, and have dried and improved their foil by dikes and drains, and alfo quite altered their way of living, the difeafe appears but feldom ; and is to be feen chiefly among the poorer fort, who inhabit the low damp parts of the provinces, and continue in their old grofs way of living *(p)*, upon falt, fmoked, often rancid pork, coarfe bread ; and are neceffitated to drink unwholfome ftagnating waters. They have indeed at times been fubject to violent returns of their old diftemper; as in feveral of their wars, when obliged to overflow their country with water.

(o) Thefe are obferved by *Muffchenbroek,* to be the moifteft winds that blow in *Holland. Vid. Element. philofophiæ naturalis.*
(p) *Vid. Brunneri tractat. de fcorbuto.*

The

The cafe is the fame in many other countries at prefent, *viz.* the *Lower Saxony*, and
other parts of *Germany*, *Sweden*, *Denmark*,
and *Norway*; where, in general, the difeafe is
much lefs frequent than it was formerly; the face
of all thefe countries, and the manner of their
living, being much improved within thefe laft
200 years. They now drink wine more freely,
brew better ale, live in drier, and more airy
commodious houfes, and have greatly drained
and improved their lands.

But here it may be worth while to remark,
that in all thofe parts where the fcurvy was formerly fo peculiarly endemic, by reafon of their
marfhy and damp fituation, together with their
grofs unwholfome diet, the cold of the climate muft certainly have contributed a great
deal towards its produ&ion. For we obferve,
that at *Venice*, whofe fituation is as damp as
moft places, the difeafe is unknown. This
feems owing principally to the heat of their climate, which raifes the watry vapours to a great
height above the furface of the earth, and there
difperfes them; giving the inhabitants almoft
conftantly ferene fine weather: unlefs it fhould
be rather fuppofed, that their light and wholfome diet, and the great quantity of vegetables

eat

eat by the *Italians*, are fufficient, in the moifteft parts of their country, to preferve them from this evil.

I SHALL now, in the third and laft place, conclude with obferving the effects of the different caufes affigned, in countries where they prevail lefs frequently; and fhall reftrict my obfervations to *Great Britain*.

In cold fea-port towns, where the fituation of the place is bleak, low, and damp, we generally obferve the inhabitants afflicted with putrid gums, œdematous fwelled legs with ulcers, *&c.*; whilft the neighbouring villages, fituated in a fandy dry foil, and purer air, are entirely free from all fcorbutic appearances. In places where they have continual rains, and much moifture, the fcurvy is endemic; as at *Fort-William (q)*.

They who live in fwampy inland foils, near moraffes, or incompaffed with thick woods and forefts; or in countries fubject to inundations from lakes or rivers; or where there are corrupted ftagnating waters, where the fun has not fufficient influence to elevate their va-

(*q*) Vid. Dr *Grainger's* account of it while there in the year 175½, chap. 2.

pours

pours to a proper height above the earth, being continually furrounded with unwholfome fogs and mifts, are fubject both to fcurvies and a-gues. Thofe who live in the higher apart-ments of a houfe, are obferved to be lefs liable to thefe diforders, than others who live on the ground-floors of the fame houfe. The poorer fort of people, who live in damp vaults and cellars under ground, are moft afflicted with fymptoms truly fcorbutic; as are likewife they who are confined in dungeons, damp and un-wholfome prifons, and fpend much of their time fleeping in apartments not fufficiently plaiftered or wainfcotted, where there is a con-tinual moifture and dewy dampnefs on the ftone-walls: an inftance of which I faw lately, in a perfon confined in a jail, who became highly fcorbutic (*r*).

Different aliments are found by experience to produce the moft different effects upon this dif-eafe. We fee it moft common among the poor-er fort of people in the before mentioned fitu-ations, who feed much on dried or falt fifh and flefh, and the unfermented farines, with-out ufing green vegetables and fruits (*f*); or upon bread made of peas, or a compofition of thefe

(*r*) Vid. chap. 2, (*f*) Vid. two cafes in *Fife*. chap. 2. & 5.

with

with oats; and, during the winter, eat what is called *broose*, which is oat-meal mixed with the fat of falt beef; and, for want of frefh and wholfome water, ufe what is either hard and brackifh, or putrid and ftagnating.

Different ways of life have likewife a different influence on this difeafe. The lazy and indolent, and thofe of a fedentary life, as fhoemakers, tailors, efpecially weavers, by reafon of their working in damp places, are moft fubject to it; while hard labourers, and thofe who ufe much exercife, though living on the fame, or even groffer food, keep entirely free. Fifhermen, from their way of life, grofs food, and habitual ufe of fpirituous liquors, are often fcorbutic.

The paffions of the mind are experienced here to have a great effect. Thofe that are of a chearful and contented difpofition, are lefs liable to it, than others of a difcontented and melancholy mind.

Laftly, It has always been remarked, that, in fuch circumftances as have been defcribed, the prefent ftate of the body has a powerful influence in difpofing to this affliction. They who are much exhaufted and weakened by preceeding fevers, and other tedious fits of ficknefs,

nefs, or they who have unfound and obftructed *vifcera* (as after agues of the autumnal
kind), are apt, by the ufe of improper diet, to
become fcorbutic. Others that labour under
a fuppreffion of any natural and neceffary evacuation, as women who have their *menfes*
fuppreffed, efpecially if the obftruction is occafioned by fear or grief, are more fubject than
others in fimilar circumftances to this difeafe;
as they are likewife at the time that thefe naturally leave them.

THE following abftract from the ingenious
Mr *Ives*'s journal, containing a hiftory of difeafes that occurred on board the *Dragon*, ferves
to confirm many things which have been advanced.

1743. *July*. We have been free from the fcurvy
ever fince the latter end of *April*.   Lay all this
month at *Mahon*, where the weather was exceffively
hot.   Our men wrought hard, and drank much wine
and fpirits. The diforders of the foregoing month increafed, with greater inflammation. Thefe were fevers with inflamed tonfils, pleurifies, and peripneumonies. Sent 17 men to hofpital.

Auguft. Continued at *Mahon*. The people received fome prize-money, which did not better their
health. The fame difeafes prevailed as in *July*, but

proved

proved fatal to none. Towards the end of the month fluxes took place of fevers. Sent 18 to hofpital.

September. Part of this month at *Mahon*, part at fea. The weather in the beginning was variable, with rains; towards the latter end moderate and hot. The difeafe peculiar to it was the dyfentery: it continued with the patient for moft part 5 or 6 weeks, but proved fatal to none. We had alfo fome flight fevers, rheumatifms, and agues.

October. Moftly at fea. The weather pretty moderate, though changeable. Rain and wind the 17th and 18th of the month My fick-lift was made up chiefly of men recovering from the fluxes of laft month. The diforder peculiar to this was the rheumatifm; which however did not prove obftinate. We had alfo 2 or 3 quartan agues, which continued for feveral months.

November Partly at fea, partly at *Gibraltar.* From the 1ft to the 10th frefh eafterly winds blew often, with rain. The whole month was fqually, but dry towards the latter end. On the 8th day, 6 or 8 people were taken with pains in their head, fhiverings, and fometimes a vomiting. The next day they were feverifh. On the 3d or 4th they complained of an univerfal prickling under the fkin, and had a fhort uneafy cough. On the 5th or 6th they were covered with little red fpots like flea-bites, with fore and watery eyes. On the 8th they either fweated plentifully, or had a loofenefs; and then they were fure to do well foon; though fome fpit, and others were relieved

ved

ved by urine.   20 feized with this fpecies of meafles, all recovered.   Rheumatifms ftill continue.

December. Lay at *Gibraltar.*   It was in general a cold, wet, ftormy month.   The fick-lift contained various, but not material complaints.   Towards the latter end of it we had appearances of an approaching fcurvy, although at *Gibraltar (t)*.   Sent 22 to hofpital.

1744. *January.* It was an extreme cold and ftormy month, with almoft conftant rain.   On the 8th *p. m.* we had a violent gale, with thick weather.   The ftorm continued the 9th, with much rain *a. m.*   From the 13th to the 27th the feafon was uncommonly tempeftuous, with rain.

On the 8th day we left *Gibraltar*, growing daily worfe in the fcurvy.   On the 10th day 50 fcorbutic patients were on the fick-lift, and by the 20th they were increafed to 80.   Many of them were now extremely bad, with hard contracted limbs, ulcerated legs, rotten gums, ftinking breath, offenfive ftools, fhortnefs of breath, &c.

On the 30th of *January* my lift ftood thus.   Very bad in the fcurvy 55.   Scorbutic fluxes 6.   Scurvy with cough 10.   Scurvy with ulcers 10.   Scorbutic afthma 1.   Scorbutic hæmoptoe 1.   Scorbutic hæmorrhoids 1.   Other diforders not fcorbutic, chiefly colds, 6. Sick in all 90.   The fhip at fea till towards the latter end of the month fhe arrived in *Hieres* bay.

(t) Not for want of the vital influences of land-air, as fhips here lie clofely embayed.

February

February was a cold, ftormy, and rainy month. The weather, efpecially in the beginning and latter end of it, was extremely rough and uncomfortable.

From the 3d of this month to the 10th, the fick were on the ordinary days on which they are allowed falt beef and pork, ferved with frefh meat, and broth with greens in it; in all about 5 times.

Upon coming into the bay of *Hieres*, our men underftood the enemy's fleets and ours were very foon to engage. There appeared not only in the healthy, but alfo in the fick, the higheft marks of fatisfaction and pleafure: and thefe laft mended furprifingly daily; infomuch that on the 11th of *February*, the day we engaged the combined fleets of *France* and *Spain*, we had not above 4 or 5 but what were at their fighting-quarters. From the 11th to the 15th few or none took notice of their illnefs. On the 15th my lift ftood thus. Recovering from the fcurvy 30. Scorbutic complaints in the firft ftage 5. Bad in the fcurvy 4. Ulcers 4. Pleurify 1. Flux 1. *Lumbagines* 3. Agues 2. Coughs and cold 11. Sick in all 61 *(u)*.

N. B. No perfon has been fent on fhore for cure

(u) A furprifing inftance of the influence of the paffions of the mind on this difeafe! For I think no perfon can afcribe the alteration of the fick-lift from 30th *January* to 15th *February* to five fervings or meffes of broth. May not the relapfes afterwards have been much occafioned by the unfortunate engagement on the 11th *February?* The *Dragon* however that day did her duty.

fince *December*; and I do not find that above 1 has
died. When we got to *Mahon* the latter end of
the month, my fick-lift was greatly increafed; thofe
who were fo much mended before, having relapfed.
I here put all the fick to hofpital.

March. It was in general a cold, windy, and rainy month. When it did not rain, it was commonly
cloudy and hazy. In the latter part of it the wind was
more moderate: but on the laft day of the month we
had a ftrong gale, though without rain. We fpent all
this month at *Mahon*; where we now and then had a
frefh patient in the fcurvy, whom I always put on
fhore. 5 or 6 fcorbutic men who had coughs, are
now in deep confumptions. Towards the latter end
of the month coughs and flight fevers prevailed.

April. On the 1ft and 2d day the weather was
ftormy. From the 3d to the 7th fqually, with rain.
From the 8th to the 12th moderate and fair. From
the 12th to the 20th frefh gales, with rain. From
20th to 26th calm and fair. From thence to the end
of the month clofe rainy weather, but warm. We
were this month at fea on the coafts of *France, Savoy,*
and *Genoa.* In the beginning of the month the coughs
and colds increafed; and towards the middle and latter end of it, they were attended with inflammation
and danger. 4 or 5 had peripneumonic fymptoms,
1 of whom died. 3 or 4 had high fevers with delirium,
&c. 1 of whom died alfo. In the latter end of the
month we had 2 troublefome ophthalmias.

May. The weather was very warm; fometimes fair,

at

at other times hazy and rainy. We fpent this month at fea as in the laft, and on our paffage to *Mahon*.

The diforders differed little from thofe in *April*, though not fatal to any. I fhould have mentioned, that in the latter end of laft month 2 or 3, who in other refpects were perfectly healthy, complained of an univerfal cutaneous itchy eruption. More were feized with it this month, and it proved very trouble-fome. One of them catched cold, fell into a fever, and had near died; but at laft was faved by nature throwing out a fecond time the peccant matter on the fkin.

June. Although we were at *Mahon*, where the weather was very hot, and our men worked hard; yet our inflammatory complaints did not increafe, but rather leffened. Towards the middle, and in the end of the month, a gentle diarrhæa prevailed throughout the fhip's company.

Left *Mahon* the 14th *June*, and arrived at *Gibral-tar* the 30th.

July. The weather was exceffive warm, and for moft part clear and dry. On the 3d we left *Gibral-tar*, and on the 19th or 20th arrived at *Lifbon*.

A few have ftill gentle diarrhæas; but, in general, a very healthy month.

Auguft. The weather was for moft part hot and dry, except the 21ft day, which was fqually, with heavy rains. We lay all this month at *Lifbon*, where the men were ferved with frefh provifions and greens twice a-week from the city. They had here the
finest

fineſt opportunity of being provided with all manner of vegetables. We continued ſtill healthy, with now and then a ſlight diarrhæa.

September. From the 1ſt to the 4th we had high winds; but from the 5th to the 14th the wind was very moderate. All this firſt part of the month the weather was cloudy, hazy, and rainy, with a good deal of lightning. From the 15th to the end of the month the winds were moderate, and weather very changeable, being for moſt part cloudy and rainy, with ſome intermediate days fair, and generally warm. Left *Liſbon* the 3d; got to *Gibraltar* the 15th.

Though a healthy month, yet, towards the middle and latter end of it, we had now and then a ſcorbutic complaint. Sent 9 to hoſpital, for different ailments.

October. Except a few days of good weather and eaſy gales, it was a very windy, rainy, and foggy month; ſometimes hot, at other times cold.

We were much alarmed at the ſudden appearance of the ſcurvy (*x*). On the 13th I put on ſhore 24 people. We left *Gibraltar* the 14th; and when we came the length of *Minorca,* having received orders to proceed further, I ſent 20 men in the ſcurvy alſo, by the *Portſmouth* ſtoreſhip, to *Mahon* hoſpital.

November. From the 1ſt to the 11th, we had cold fair weather, with variable winds. The remaining

(*x*) Not owing to abſtinence for ſo very ſhort a time from vegetables. Their late ſupply at *Liſbon* was a thing uncommon to them.

part of the month was remarkably bad, with high, piercing, cold winds, much rain, and some snow.

We arrived at *Vado* the 20th, and sailed from thence the 29th. Upon our arrival there we had 50 men in the scurvy *(y)*.

December was also a very cold, windy, and wet month; with but few intermissions of little wind, and fair weather.

1745. *January* was much the same as the former month. We had but 8 days in it that were moderate and fair.

When we arrived at *Vado*, as before mentioned, on the 20th of *November*, I gave to every scorbutic patient one *China* orange, and three apples; and continued to do so daily till the 5th of *December*, when the apples being all gone, they had only the continuance of an orange, which lasted to the 7th of *December*. On the 22d *November* they had fresh flesh-broth. On the 27th they had the same with turnips boiled in it; and again on the 29th *November*, 1st and 2d *December*; which was the whole supply of fresh meat and vegetables we got at *Vado*. On the 8th of *December*, being then off *Sardinia*, Captain *Watson*, now Rear-Admiral of the Blue, agreeable to his wonted humanity, gave mutton-broth to 21 of our men; the 13th he did the same to 45. Now follow the remarks in my diary.

[*November* 29. The scorbutic people in general,

(y) Putrid air could have but little influence during so cold a season.

mend

mend much. Thofe whofe limbs were contracted, grow pliable; their rotten gums become founder; fhortnefs of breath, &c better *(z)*.

December 2. They continue to mend much.

December 5. The weather not fo cold fince we left *Vado*.

December 6. All are recovering from the fcurvy.

December 25. My fick-lift contained but 30 ; and thefe almoft well, and recovered from the fcurvy.

January 6. We are ftill at fea; the weather cold and wet; and for 9 days paft have been in want of wine for the people. The fcorbutic patients are re-lapfed, and more are added to the fick-lift, being unfit for duty.

January 8. Anchored at *Mahon*; put to hofpital 59 in the fcurvy.]

February A cold uncomfortable month, which we fpent at *Mahon*; where we had now and then a cafe in the fcurvy; but more towards the end of it, with feverifh fymptoms. Sent 5 to hofpital.

March. The weather this month was warmer, but inconftant. The winds moderate. Left *Mahon* the 17th; arrived at *Gibraltar* the 22d. The lift was pretty numerous, compofed of valetudinarians taken from *Mahon* hofpital, and one or two fevers. Put to hofpital at *Gibraltar* 14.

April. The one half of this month was fair, the o-ther half rainy, cloudy, and foggy; but generally warm.

(z) This Mr *Ives* juftly afcribes to the oranges and apples.

T   We

We had fome, though not many, ill of coughs and colds. One old man died of a fever. Left *Gibraltar* the 6th, carrying along with us all our people from the hofpital, where they were badly fupplied with vegetables and frefh meat. We were in hopes of doing better for them at *Lifbon*, or on the coaft of *Portugal*; where we continued cruifing all this month.

May. The weather was moderate and warm, without much rain, though fometimes hazy. Spent this month at fea.

In the middle and latter end of it, feveral were ill of fcurvies, others of fluxes. We got no refrefhments from the land for the poor people brought from hofpital. And the fick muft have fuffered much, had not Captain *Watfon* fupplied them. He caufed four of his fheep to be killed for their ufe; and gave up entirely (as indeed was his wonted cuftom under fuch diftrefs) every drop of milk his cow afforded, for their benefit.

June. Boifterous winds blew continually from the north, which occafioned very uncomfortable weather at fea; and kept the air pretty cool, until the 13th we arrived at *Lifbon*, very ill in the fcurvy *(a)*. Here 3 or 4 died of it.

July. We continued at *Lifbon*. All have not yet got free of their fcorbutic ailments; feveral have fcorbutic fluxes; others have diarrhœas and dyfenteries,

---

(a) This weather muft have proved very hard upon the weakly men taken from *Gibraltar* hofpital.

without

without any symptom of the scurvy. Towards the latter end of the month, several were in fevers.

August. Slight fevers, but especially diarrhæas and dysenteries, still prevail. Mr *Mauberty* our carpenter died of the dysentery. I called to his assistance Dr *Kennedy* physician at *Lisbon,* and Dr *Lind,* then surgeon of the *Kennington.* 22d of this month we left *Lisbon,* and sailed for *England.* Had then 20 sick on my list.

C H A P. II.

The diagnostics, or signs.

IN order to observe greater accuracy in the description of a disease attended with so many and various symptoms, these might have been properly enough ranged under three classes.

The *first,* Containing the most common and constant symptoms; such as may be said to be essential to the nature of the malady.

The *second,* Such as are more casual and accidental; proceeding not so much from the genius of the distemper, as from the epidemical constitution of the air, the state or habit of the body at the time, or from the determination of other causes.

And

And the *third*, Some extraordinary and uncommon fymptoms, that fometimes, though but feldom, have happened in it; and which occur only in the higheft and moft virulent ftate of this difeafe, from the peculiar *idiofyncrafy* of the patient, its combination with other malignant difeafes, or from other incidental circumftances.

But, for the fake of greater perfpicuity, I chufe rather to defcribe the fymptoms in the order in which they generally appear, and as peculiar to the feveral ftages of the difeafe; and fhall diftinguifh, as I go along, thofe which are more conftant or eflential, from the lefs frequent or adventitious.

The firft indication of the approach of this difeafe, is generally a change of colour in the face, from the natural and ufual look, to a pale and bloated complexion; with a liftleffnefs to action, or an averfion to any fort of exercife. When we examine narrowly the lips, or the caruncles of the eye, where the blood-veflels lie moft expofed, they appear of a greenifh caft. Mean while, the perfon eats and drinks heartily, and feems in perfect health; except that his countenance and lazy inactive difpofition, portend a future fcurvy.

This

This change of colour in the face, although it does not always preceed the other symptoms, yet conftantly attends them when advanced. Scorbutic people for the moft part appear at firft of a pale or yellowifh hue, which becomes afterwards more darkifh or livid *(a)*.

Their former averfion to motion degenerates foon into an univerfal laffitude, with a ftiffnefs and feeblenefs of their knees upon ufing exercife; with which they are apt to be much fatigued, and upon that occafion fubject to a breathleffnefs or panting. And this laffitude, with a breathleffnefs upon motion, are obferved to be among the moft conftant concomitants of the diftemper.

Their gums foon after become itchy, fwell, and are apt to bleed upon the gentleft friction. Their breath is then offenfive; and upon looking into their mouth, the gums appear of an unufual livid rednefs, are foft and fpungy, and become afterwards extremely putrid and fungous; the pathognomonic fign of the difeafe.

(a) Mr Murray's remark.——They commonly appear of a melancholy and fullen countenance; fuch alfo is their difpofition of mind. So that dejection of fpirits may juftly be reckoned a caufe as well as fymptom of the future malady.

They

They are subject not only to a bleeding from the gums, but prone to fall into hæmorrhages from other parts of the body.

Their skin at this time feels dry, as it does through the whole course of the malady *(b)*. In many, especially if feverish, it is extremely rough; in some it has an anserine appearance; but most frequently it is smooth and shining. And, when examined, it is found covered with several reddish, bluish, or rather black and livid spots, equal with the surface of the skin, resembling an extravasation under it, as it were from a bruise *(c)*. These spots are of different sizes, from the bigness of a lentil to that of a handbreadth, and larger. But the last are more uncommon in the beginning of the distemper; they being usually then but small, and of an irregular roundish figure. They are to be seen chiefly on the legs and thighs; often on the arms, breast, and trunk of the body; but more rarely on the head and face.

(b) Mr Murray.——Except in the last stage, when a cold clammy moisture may be often observed on the skin, especially if the patient is subject to faintings.

(c) Mr Murray.——The skin begins to look in spots with a yellow rim. From thence the deepness of the dye gradually increases, till it becomes of a deep purple, and sometimes quite black.

Many

Many have a fwelling of their legs; which
is firft obferved on their ancles towards the e-
vening, and hardly to be feen next morning:
but, after continuing a fhort time in this manner, it gradually advances up the leg, and the
whole member becomes œdematous; with this
difference only in fome, that it does not fo eafily yield to the finger, and preferves the impreffion of it longer afterwards than a true œ-
dema.

Thefe are the moft conftant and effential
fymptoms of this malady in the progrefs of its
firft ftage. But a diverfity is fometimes obferved in the order of their appearance. Thus,
when a perfon has had a preceeding fever, or
a tedious fit of ficknefs, by which he has been
much exhaufted, the gums for the moft part
are firft affected, and a laffitude conftantly attends; whereas, when one has been confined
from exercife by having a fractured bone, or
from a bruife or hurt, thefe weak and debilitated
parts become almoft always firft fcorbutic *(d)*.

As

(d) Mr *Ives.*——As was the cafe of *John Thomas* marine, belonging to the *Dragon*, who, on the 18th of *Auguft* 1742, got,
by a mufket-ball from the *Spaniards*, a very bad fracture of the
os humeri, with great comminution. Eight or ten large pieces
of the bone were cut in upon, and taken away, and the bones
fhivered

As for example, if a patient labours under a strain of the ancle, the leg, by becoming swelled, painful, and œdematous, and soon after covered with livid spots, gives the first indication of the disease. And as old ulcers on the shin are very frequent among seamen, in this case likewise the legs are always first affected, and these ulcers put on the scorbutic appearance, although the patient seems otherwise perfectly healthy, and preserves a fresh good colour in his face.

The distinguishing characteristics of scorbutic ulcers are as follow. They afford no good digestion, but a thin, fœtid, sanious stuff, mixed with blood; which at length has the true appearance of coagulated gore lying caked on the surface of the ulcer, and is with great

shivered quite to its head. By the end of *November* following, a union was brought about by means of an interveening *callus*, and a sound skin brought over almost all the incisions. He had nearly recovered his flesh and strength lost under the discharge and confinement, being daily supplied with fresh provisions by the bounty of the officers. Upon the scurvy breaking out in *December*, his supply of fresh provisions was stopt, and given to more necessitous objects, as was thought, he being then pretty healthy. Upon which he fell into a bad scurvy: the first symptom of which that appeared, was the breaking out of the late wounds in his arm. He sunk under the discharge, and died at *Mahon* hospital.

difficulty

difficulty wiped off, or feparated from the parts below. The flefh underneath thefe floughs feels to the probe foft or fpungy, and is very putrid. No detergents or efcharotics are here of any fervice: for though fuch floughs be with great pains taken away, they are found again at next dreffing, where the fame fanguineous putrid appearance always prefents itfelf. Their edges are generally of a livid colour, and puffed up with excrefcencies of proud flefh arifing from below under the fkin. When too tight a compreffion is made, in order to keep the *fungus* from rifing, they are apt to have a gangrenous difpofition; and the member never fails to become œdematous, painful, and for moft part fpotted. As the difeafe increafes, they at length come to fhoot out a foft bloody *fungus*, which the failors exprefs by the name of *bullocks liver :* and indeed it has a near refemblance, in confiftence and colour, to that fubftance when boiled. It often rifes in a night's time to a monftrous fize; and although deftroyed by cauteries, actual or potential, or cut fmooth with a biftory, (in which cafe a plentiful hæmorrhage generally enfues), is found at next dreffing as large as ever. They continue how-

U

ever

ever in this condition a considerable time, without affecting the bone.

The slightest bruises and wounds of scorbutic persons degenerate into such ulcers. Their appearance, on whatever part of the body, is so singular and uniform, and they are so easily distinguished from all others, by being so remarkably putrid, bloody, and fungous, that we cannot here but take notice of the impropriety of referring most of the inveterate and obstinate ulcers on the legs, with very different appearances, to the scurvy; which are generally best cured by giving mercurial medicine: whereas that medicine, in a truly scorbutic ulcer, is the most dangerous and pernicious that can be administered.

But to proceed: The first remark to be made upon this disease, is, that whatever former ailment the patient has had, (especially rheumatic pains, aches from bruises, hurts, wounds, &c.), or whatever present disorder he labours under; upon being afflicted with this distemper, his former and old complaints are renewed, and his present malady, whatever it may be, rendered worse. Scorbutic people, as the disease advances, are seldom indeed free from complaints, especially of pains; though
they

they have not the same seat in all, and even in the same person often shift their place. Some complain of universal pain in all their bones, as they express it; most violent in their limbs, and small of the back, and especially on their joints and legs when swelled. But the most frequent seat of their pain is in some part of the breast; a tightness and oppression there, with stitches felt upon coughing, being usual symptoms in this disease. And as scorbutic pains in general are very liable to move from one place to another, so they are always exasperated by motion of any sort, especially the pain of the back; which, upon this occasion, proves very troublesome.

The next thing observable here, is, that whatever diseases are epidemical at the same time with the scurvy, or even whatever inter-current diseases prevail, these scorbutical habits are very liable to be seized with. And this some-times happens when such distempers would appear to be of a pretty opposite genius to the scurvy; in which case it is lucky for the pa-tient. But, on the contrary, if the prevailing distempers are of a putrid nature, such as the small pox, measles, dysenteric fever, &c. it is then, that, co-operating with the scorbutic acri-

mony,

mony, they produce the most fatal and malignant symptoms.

I observed a considerable difference in the genius of the disease in the two cruises *ann.* 1746 and 1747. In the latter, when fevers from cold of the pleuritic and peripneumonic sort prevailed, it tended chiefly to affect the breast with a tightness, oppression, and a hard bound cough, by which a very viscid phlegm was with great difficulty brought up. The fits of coughing were not constant, but extremely fatiguing; and this was a universal complaint. Several at this season were feverish; we had none in a salivation, and the fluxes were mild and manageable. Whereas in the year 1746, when a different species of diseases prevailed, occasioned by the unwholsome newness of the ship's timbers, and diarrhæas were frequent, the scurvy proved more virulent and fatal. Its worst, most common, and troublesome symptoms, were salivations and dysenteries, especially the latter; in which one *Nichols* died, and eight or ten more were landed at *Plymouth* in a very low and exhausted condition by it. I did not at that time remark any of them to be feverish, and their breasts were but slightly affected. *John Hearn* was our patient
in

in both cruifes. His cafe begins in my diary, under the 24th of *June* 1746, thus. He
has been afflicted with the fcurvy for fome time
paft. It firft appeared with fore fpungy gums,
pain and œdematous fwellings of his legs,
weaknefs, *&c.* Has taken *elixir vitriol* twice
a-day for a confiderable time, but grows daily
worfe. Has a continual falivation, at the rate of
two quarts in twenty four hours, attended with
fevere gripes and *tenefmus.* The falivation
foon ftopt; but was followed with a violent
dyfentery, which continued until he was landed. I find him again mentioned under the
15th of *May* 1747. *J. Hearn* complains of
a laffitude and ftiffnefs of his limbs, with pain
in his back. Upon examination, we find his
legs covered with red, black, and livid fpots;
his gums are fwelled; his chief complaint is a
troublefome fatiguing cough. And this laft was
what afflicted him moft during the whole
cruife.

I believe indeed it will univerfally be
found, that, in the progrefs of this diftrefs,
the breaft is always more or lefs affected, unlefs the belly is very open. The pain fhifts
from one part of it to another, often to oppofite fides, and is at firft perceived upon coughing

ing only: but when the malady is farther advanced, it commonly fixes in a particular part,
most frequently in the side; where it becomes
extremely severe and pungent, so as to affect
the breathing; a dangerous symptom in this
disease *(e)*.

The head is seldom or never affected with
pain, unless the patient is feverish. As to fevers, it may indeed be doubted whether there
be any such as are purely and truly scorbutical;
the disease being altogether of a chronic nature, and fevers may be justly reckoned a-
mongst its adventitious symptoms. I have been
told by a very intelligent surgeon, who has had
opportunity of seeing some hundred scorbutical cases, and those of the worst kind, that he
remarked very few of them to be attended with
fevers; which, to the best of his remem-
brance, always proved mortal. And I am convinced, that fevers of any sort do prove fatal,

---

(e) Mr Murray's remark.——This pain in some measure an
swers to the description of the *pleuritis notha* ; and, like it, is
sometimes, but not always, to be relieved by blisters: the application of which however is not here safe, as there is some
danger of a gangrene from them. I have likewise often observed a pain of the breast, I think mostly in the left side, in scorbutic fluxes, and always found it mortal.

though

though they very seldom occur, in the last stage of the malady *(f.)*

I observed before, that, in the year 1746, none of our scorbutical patients were feverish: but, in the cruise in the year 1747, several had the fever in the beginning of the distemper. The symptoms were not so violent nor inflammatory in scorbutical people, as in others. In two or three it assumed an intermitting form; and in this state I observed it to be altogether mild, and without danger.

One *Daniel Harlyhee* having an obstinate ulcer on his shin, his legs, about the beginning of *May* 1747, became painful and œdematous, and his ulcer truly scorbutic. On the 12th of that month he was seized with a pretty smart fever; which abated the next day,

---

(f) Ives.——I cannot say I have ever seen an instance of it: for I do not remember, nor can I find in my journals, one case of a person advanced in the scurvy being seized with a fever. I entirely agree with you, that this disease is purely chronic. Ulcerated lungs is a common consequence of the scurvy; and where there has been a violent cough and stitches preceeding, 'tis certain I may have perceived the pulse to have quickened, and possibly too an increase of heat in the skin: yet these circumstances seemed to me altogether symptomatic, and not properly to be denominated a fever with the scurvy; for, after a rupture in the pulmonic texture, the commotion of the blood, and heat of the body, generally cease.

but

but returned regularly every third day for five weeks, till he arrived at *Plymouth*. His gums were putrid; he had a pain in his breast, together with a cough, and the other scorbutic symptoms usual at that season.

But of all species of fevers that may be superadded to this disease, the most terrible, more so perhaps than even the plague itself, is that of the petechial fever, or jail-distemper, as it is called; which has sometimes been contracted in large, crouded, and sickly ships; either from infection, or by keeping scorbutical patients long confined in a foul putrid air *(g)*.

Lastly,

(g) Of this indeed I have never seen an instance; but have been favoured with the following account of it from Mr *Murray*, when surgeon of the *Canterbury*.

He observed in that ship, during an epidemical rage of the scurvy, when at the same time they had on board some petechial fevers, that several were seized with a slight fever, which was abated the third or fourth day, upon the appearance of a miliary, erysipelatous, or herpetical eruption, for the most part on the inferior extremities. These eruptions gradually grew livid, from thence black and gangrenous; attended with, or producing sordid and sanious ulcers, *spinæ ventosæ*, and *caries* of the most obstinate and dangerous kind; spreading always upwards, seldom or never downwards. The gums were in this case lax, not much swelled, but often bleeding; and soon attended with *caries* of the jaw, from the sockets of which the already loosened teeth easily dropped out. The patient was continually thirsty; the skin dry and hot; the pulse small and quick; the eyes sometimes staring, oftener moving quick, and
looking

Lastly, According to the habit and constitution of the patient, there will occur likewise some little diversity in the state of the body in this disease: some through the whole course of it being regular enough in their belly, while others are apt to be very costive; but generally scorbutic persons are inclinable to loose stools at times, which in all are remarkably fœtid. The urine I found to be extremely various at different times, even in the same patient; except that it is generally high coloured, and soon becomes rank and fœtid *(h)*. The pulse likewise varies according to the habit of the patient, and state of the malady; being most commonly slower and feebler than when in health *(i)*.

The

looking wild, with a despairing moving aspect; the tongue moist and tremulous; the patient restless, and sometimes delirious. This dreadful evil soon carried off the unhappy sufferer, if remedies were not immediately administered; or rather Nature had not strength enough to disburthen herself upon some of the extremities, especially the inferior, as before remarked, generally a little below the knee; where carious or cancerous ulcers made quick ravage, were attended with the most exquisite pain, and often quickly dispatched the patient, blessing him with death.

(h) Mr Murray's remarks.——The urine of almost all scorbutic persons, when let stand, gathers an oily saline scum a-top.

(i) Mr Murray.——Where there is fever, the pulse is generally small, but hard and quick. You say, that *Eugalenus,* and

X   the

The true scorbutic spots, as was said before, are always flat, and equal with the surface of the skin. I have, however, observed the legs, at the same time when greatly swelled, sometimes covered with a dry scurf or scales. At other times, though very rarely, there appear on the skin small eruptions of the dry miliary kind.

In the second stage of this disease, they most commonly lose the use of their limbs; having a contraction of the flexor tendons in the ham, with a swelling and pain in the joint of the knee. Indeed a stiffness in these tendons, and a weakness of the knees, appear pretty early in this disease, generally terminating in a contracted and swelled joint. They are subject to frequent languors; and when long confined from exercise, to a proneness to faint upon the least motion of the body; which are the most pecu-

the authors who have followed him, tell us, that in scorbutic faintings, the pulse rises and becomes stronger. This singularity, I think, I must have observed, had it been so. In such cases the pulse is for most part obscure and small; sometimes rising all of a sudden for a few strokes, soon sinking, and always intermitting. In the fever mentioned, unless a flux accompanied it, faintings were less frequent: the pulse was quick and serrated, and sometimes run like quick-silver in a flexible tube, pushed along by starts.

liar,

liar, conftant, and effential fymptoms of this ftage.

Some have their legs monftroufly fwelled, and covered with one or more large livid fpots, or *ecchymofes* ; others have hard fwellings there in different places, extremely painful; and others I have feen, without any fwelling, have the calf of the leg *(k)* quite indurated.

They are apt, upon being moved, or expofed to the frefh air, fuddenly to expire. This happened to one of our people, when in the boat, going to be landed at *Plymouth* hofpital. It was remarkable he had made fhift to get there without any affiftance, while many others were obliged to be carried out upon their beds. He had a deep fcorbutical colour in his face *(l)*, with complaints in his breaft. He panted for about half a minute, then expired *(m)*.

Scorbutic people are at all times, but more efpecially in this ftage, fubject to profufe hæmorrhages from different parts of the body; as from the nofe, gums, inteftines, lungs, &c.

(k) Mr Ives.——And thighs too.

(l) Mr Murray's remark.——In this ftage I have feen livid *maculæ*, or fpots, on the face.

(m) Mr Ives.——Of this I have feen many inftances, when they are imprudently brought up from the orlope to the frefh air. The utmoft caution and circumfpection are here requifite.

and

and from their ulcers, which generally bleed very plentifully. Many at this time are afflicted with violent dyfenteries, accompanied with exquifite pain; by which they are reduced to the loweft and moft weakly condition: while others I have feen, without a diarrhæa or gripes, difcharge great quantities of pure blood by the *anus*.

The gums are for the moft part exceffively fungous, with an intolerable degree of ftench, putrefaction, and pain; fometimes deeply ulcerated, with a gangrenous afpect. But I never remarked, except in cafes of falivations, the back part of the throat, or upper part of the mouth, much affected; and I believe the lips feldom or never are. The teeth moft commonly become quite loofe, and often fall out; but a *caries* of the jaw does but rarely follow.

Upon this occafion it muft be noted, that a fcorbutic *caries* happens only in two cafes. *Firft*, If the outer *lamella* of a bone has been broken off, fo as that the fcorbutic corrofive humour, ftagnating in any of the cavities of the body, has accefs to the internal cellular fubftance, it fpeedily corrupts and gangrenes it. But otherwife ulcers continue long on the fpine of the *tibia* and other parts, without affecting the

the bone; except in another and rare cafe; which is, when, by the deepeft and moft virulent infeftion, this cellular fubftance becomes tainted; which is commonly attended with excruciating pain, and always with an enlargement of the bone, or rather an *exoftofis*, often the *fpina ventofa*, followed with painful fpreading ulcers, and an internal *caries* of the moft malignant kind *(n)*.

Moft, although not all, even in this ftage, have a good appetite, and their fenfes entire, though much dejefted, and often low fpirited. When lying at reft in their beds, many make no complaint, either of pain or ficknefs, unlefs afflifted with the dyfentery, or a troublefome falivation. This laft indeed I am inclined to think would happen but feldom, were it not occafioned by the exhibition of fome mercurial medicine *(o)* in the cure of ulcers, or other

fcorbutical

(n) Mr Murray.——I never obferved a carious bone to follow, but where there was a fever and moft virulent fcurvy.

(o) Mr Ives.——Did you in 1746 exhibit mercurials? If not, how do you account for the falivations that happened then? They would appear to me to have been purely fcorbutic. I do not remember an inftance of any confiderable falivation in the fcurvy. *Anfwer.* It appears from my diary, that we had then three patients in a falivation, *viz. Rice Meredith, Robert Robifon.* and *John Hearn.* The two firft had taken gentle dofes of

mercurius

scorbutical complaints, where it is often injudiciously administered; which, in such cases,
in extreme small quantity, induces a copious
and dangerous salivation, almost always attended with the dysentery. These succeed
each other alternately; so that the spitting
generally ceases for a day or two, while
the patient is racked with gripes, and bloody
stools; which being stopt for a little, the salivation again returns.

IT is not easy to conceive a more dismal and
diversified scene of misery, than what is beheld
in the third and last stage of this calamity; it
being then that the anomalous and more extraordinary symptoms most commonly occur. It
is not unusual at this time, for such persons as
have had ulcers formerly healed up, to have
them break out afresh: while in others the skin
of their swelled legs often bursts, particularly
where soft, painful, livid swellings, have been
first observed; and these degenerate into such
crude, bloody, fungous ulcers, as formerly
described. Some few at this period (though
very rarely) fall into colliquative putrid fevers,

mercurius alcalisatus, and about half a dram of mercurial pill: but
there is no mention of their having been given to *Hearn.* I
am pretty clear he took no mercury.

attended

attended almost always with *petechiæ*, fœtid sweats, *&c.* or rather sink under profuse evacuations of rotten blood, by stool and urine, from the lungs, nose, stomach, hæmorrhoidal veins, *&c. (p)* : while the disease more frequently in others, by occasioning obstructions and putrefaction in the abdominal *viscera*, gives rise to a jaundice, dropsy, and the *affectio hypochondriaca*, or the most confirmed melancholy and despondency of mind, attended with severe nervous rigors; as also to violent colics, obstinate costiveness, *&c.*

Towards the close of this malady, the breast is most commonly affected with a violent and uneasy straitness and oppression, and an extreme *dyspnæa*; accompanied sometimes with a pain under the *sternum*, but more frequently in either of the sides: while others, without any complaint of pain, have their respiration become quickly contracted and laborious, ending in sudden, and often unexpected death.

Many more symptoms might be here added that at times have been observed, especially towards the close of this most virulent disease. And we shall have no occasion to be surprised, even at the most extraordinary which have been

(p) *Ives.*——All which I have often seen, except the fever.

related

related by authors, when we come, in its proper place *(q)*, to view the true state of the body at this period, with the high degree of putrefaction in the blood, the other humours, and *viscera.*

I have been told by some practitioners, that this is a disease not met with in people living at land in *Great Britain.* To such gentlemen I would recommend the serious perusal of an excellent chapter *(r)* in Dr *Huxham*'s late essay on fevers, where they will be made better acquainted (as is very necessary) with what is truly the scorbutic *diathesis.* Whatever number or diversity of symptoms may occur in this evil, from difference of constitution, and especially at sea, from the influence of such powerful causes as subsist there; yet putrid gums, bluish and black spots on the body, constitute its characteristic and pathognomonic signs every where.

As the before mentioned learned author, my honoured friend, has published several very curious and truly scorbutical cases which occurred in *England*; I shall conclude this chapter, after giving a case somewhat more out of

(q) Chap. 7. dissections.
(r) Chap. 5. on the putrid and dissolved state of the blood.

the

the common road, with an account of fome
fcurvies in *Scotland.*

(f) Lieutenant *John A*——of marines, aged
40, was formerly extremely healthy, though
much at fea ; where he had feldom or never eat
of falt provifions, officers tables being generally well provided with better fare. He had
lately returned from fome *Channel* cruifes to
the weftward; where, as ufual, he had not eat
of any thing falt, having a natural averfion to
fuch food. One day, to his great furprife, he
obferved on about the middle of one of his legs
a confiderable bunching up from over the *tibia* ; and, taking down his ftocking, found a
bluifh infenfible fwelling. Next morning it
was increafed to the fize of a large walnut;
and in two or three days the fkin broke, and
it became a genuine fcorbutic ulcer, with the
liver-like *fungus.* After which began alfo o-
ther fymptoms ; change of colour, tightnefs in
the breaft, rotten gums, and, what was very
threatening to his life, an obftinate conftipa-
tion of the bowels, attended with intolerable
gripings.

He took country-lodgings; and, being pro-

(f) Communicated by Mr *Ives.*

Y   perly

perly treated, in about fix weeks, or two
months, recovered.

Letter from Dr James Grainger *(t)*, *furgeon to*
Lt-Gen. Pultney's *regiment.*

I Have extracted from my notes the following
brief defcription of the fcurvy, which prevailed *ann.* 175$\frac{1}{2}$, among the fix companies of
our regiment quartered at *Fort-William.*

I had then an opportunity of feeing it in no
lefs than near 100 patients; and muft ingenuoufly own, it was there I learned my firft
leffon upon the difeafe.

My predeceffor had not informed me, that
this was a diforder of that garrifon; it was a
fubject of which I had read much, but knew
little; fo that the firft I treated, had well nigh
fallen a martyr to improper prefcription. The
pains this foldier complained of, appeared to me
rheumatic. This I the more eafily gave into, as
at that time this difeafe was actually frequent.
He was bled, and treated accordingly; upon
which his pains grew worfe than ever, and no
wonder. I began to talk ferioufly to him, and

(*t*) The ingenious author of *Hiftoria febris anomal. Batav.*
ann. 1746, *&c.*

upbraided

upbraided him with having pretended complaints more than real.   But he foon gave me evident marks of real diftrefs.   Livid fpots on the thighs, rotten, bleeding gums, and his ftinking breath, quickly convinced me, that I had miftaken his cafe, and confequently his method of cure.

At aliquis malo fuit ufus in illo.

The fcurvy now began to fpread, and I profited by my former inattention.

Its firft appearances were, *laffitudo,* breathleffnefs upon the leaft quicknefs of motion, and a tafte in the mouth peculiarly difagreeable. which were foon followed by rotten, fpungy, painful gums, bleeding from the flighteft touch; fœtid breath; pains always of their thighs, frequently of their legs, fometimes of their loins, feldom of their arms.   All thefe parts were fometimes difcoloured with purple *maculæ,* which, as the malady increafed, grew black and broad.   The anterior parts of the legs and thighs chiefly fuffered.   The former I have feen all livid, the latter very clofely fpotted.   Neither were much fwelled, yet both were harder than ufual; and fo extremely painful, that the gentleft touch gave agony.   Unlefs thefe were

Y 2   fpeedily

speedily checked, the contagion spread, their faces grew strangely sallow, their teeth loosened, palate and *fauces* ulcerated, asthma increased; they fell away, slept little, old ulcers broke out again, cried out when turned a-bed, and sometimes fainted upon motion of their body.

What surprised me most, was, that their appetite, even in these deplorable circumstances, was not greatly impaired; and that none of them could properly be said, though thirsty, to be in a fever. All of them were rather costive; and their urine, though not copious, was always vastly fœtid and thick, in those especially who complained of their loins. Most of them were continually spitting; and a small quantity of mercury occasioned a dreadful salivation.

A soldier who laboured under the venereal disease, used but a dram of crude mercury, by way of unction, one evening. Next morning I found him in a true mercurial salivation. The spitting went on, increasing until the tenth day; when the inside of his mouth, lips, and cheeks, became monstrously swelled. The stench of his mouth was intolerable to all about him. He every day spit out a quantity of fœtid blood, part of his gums, and teeth. He lost almost all the latter; and what was very remarkable, they

were

were found preternaturally enlarged. His urine was extremely fœtid, thick, and almoft black-ifh. He often fainted away. In fhort, the poor fellow was reduced to the moft deplorable condition, and with great difficulty efcaped. It was three months afterwards before he was fit for duty.

The fcurvy began in *March*, raged in *April*, declined in *May*, and left us before the middle of *June*. Ninety during that period had fcur-vies at *Fort-William*; while there were only two foldiers out of four companies feized with it at *Fort-Auguftus*, and but one in a Captain's command at the barracks of *Bernera*. Thefe three indeed were very bad. No officer had it in any one of thefe garrifons.

I imputed the malady to the following cau-fes. 1*mo*, Conftant moift, rainy weather. 2*do*, Salt provifions from *December* till near the end of *May*, falt butter, cheefe, oat-meal. 3*tio*, Few or no vegetables; little, bad, or no milk. 4*to*, Indifferent water. 5*to*, Hard duty. The 1ft, 3d, 4th, 5th caufes prevailed lefs at *Fort-Auguftus* and *Bernera*; and therefore thefe places had not their proportion of fcor-butical patients.——— *(u)*

(u) See the remainder of this letter, chap. 5.

This

This difeafe is in feveral parts of *Scotland* called by the name of the *black leg*. It has often been very epidemic and fatal to the miners at *Strontian* in *Argylefhire*. Not long ago many of them died of it, with this remarkable fymptom, that the hypochondria and lower belly were at length covered with large fcorbutic *maculæ*. This *Dodonæus (x)*, a good author on the fcurvy, long ago obferved to be a mortal fymptom.

I am informed of a certain Noble family, whofe feat in the country is bleak, and expofed to the fea, where they have been univerfally afflicted with fpungy, rotten gums, fwelled legs, ulcers, *&c.*

Lately a gentleman confined in jail at *Edinburgh*, complained of a fwelling of his legs. Upon examination, they were found covered with black and bluifh fpots; foon after his gums became extremely putrid and fungous. His cafe being neglected, a *caries* of the lower jaw enfued; for which he was put under my care.

A navy-furgeon refiding in *Fife*, in paffing by *Backhaven*, was defired to vifit two poor fellows who were extremely bad. He found them in a

(*x*) Vid. Part 3.

miferable

miserable condition indeed! Their gums were monstrously putrid, their bodies spotted, and they were altogether deprived of the use of their limbs, by a swelling in the joint of the knee; in one of them the tendons in the ham were contracted, and quite indurated. The gentleman acquainted them with the nature of their malady, and by a proper prescription re-stored them soon to health *(y)*.

C H A P.   III.

The prognostics.

FOR the better understanding of this, and some of the following chapters, it be-comes necessary to make a distinction, which is to be attended to. It is, That this disease may be either adventitious, or constitutional; arti-ficial, (if I may be allowed the term), or natu-ral to the patient. The first is the case of most seamen, and of all sound constitutions, either at sea or land, who have contracted the taint from such obvious external causes as were be-fore mentioned *(a)*; in whom it is an artificial

(y) See the prescription, chap. 5   *(a)* Part 2. chap. 1.

or adventitious difease. But there are likewife many to be met with, living at land, who, from very flight caufes, are liable to become fcorbutic; and that from a certain indifpofition of their own body: and in fuch the malady is to be deemed conftitutional, or natural to the patient. Though in whatever manner it is induced, the diftemper is ftill the fame, and the like method of cure is proper for its removal; fo I fhall have no occafion to mention this diftinction again ; but am here to advertife the reader, that feveral of thefe prognoftics are chiefly applicable to the artificial fcurvy.

Perfons who have been weakened by other preceeding diftempers, fuch as fevers or fluxes; or by tedious confinement and cures, as thofe who have undergone a falivation, are of all others moft fubject to this difeafe. Intermitting fevers in a particular manner difpofe the conftitution to it.

Thofe who have formerly been afflicted with it, are much more liable to it, in parallel circumftances, than others.

Different feafons varioufly affect fcorbutic ailments. At land they become troublefome, when the winter's rain and cold begin to fet in towards the autumnal equinox; cold,

moift,

moist, open winters greatly inforce the disease; but by the return of warm dry weather, these scorbutic complaints are much mitigated.

Where the indisposition is but beginning, and even when the gums have been pretty much affected, there are numerous instances of a perfect recovery, without having the benefit of fresh vegetables; provided the patient is able to use due exercise. But when confined to bed, or prevented from using exercise, by swelling of the legs, weakness, or from other causes, the evil, where no green vegetables or fruits can be procured, infallibly increases; and when it is advanced to what I have called the *second stage*, is not to be cured without them. Of which many instances might be produced, particularly from the hospital at *Gibraltar*; where several died most piteous objects in this distress, notwithstanding they had the benefit of the land-air, and plenty of excellent fresh flesh-broths; when a small quantity of greens every day, would in all probability have saved their lives.

This disease, when adventitious, may in its first, or even its second stage, be cured by fresh greens and proper treatment, (especially

Z   by

by the use of oranges and lemons), on board
a ship, either in harbour or at sea.

The symptoms related to occur in the last
stage, are of all others the most dangerous;
viz. oppression on the breast, obstinate costiveness, stitches in the side, and frequent faintings; but especially great difficulty of breathing.

At sea, where no greens, fresh meats, or
fruits are to be had, the prognostics in this difease are sometimes deceitful; for people that
appear to be but slightly scorbutic, are apt to
be suddenly and unexpectedly seized with some
of its worse symptoms.

Their dropping down dead upon an exertion
of their strength, or change of air, is not easily foretold; though it generally happens after
a tedious confinement in a foul air.

The first promising appearance in bad cases,
when fruits or greens are first allowed, is the
belly becoming lax; these having the effect of
very gentle physic: and if in a few days the skin
becomes moist and soft, it is an infallible sign
of their recovery; especially if they bear gentle
exercise, and change of air, without being
liable to faint. If the vegetable aliment restores them in a few days to the use of their
limbs

limbs *(b)*, they are then paſt all danger of dying at that time of this diſeaſe; unleſs afflicted with the ſcorbutic dyſentery, or the pectoral diſorder. Theſe two often prove fatal, and are the moſt obſtinate to remove of all the ſcorbutic ſymptoms.

The blackneſs of the ſkin, or ſpots, upon recovery, go off nearly in like manner as other *ecchymoſes*, growing gradually yellow, from the circumference to the center; the natural colour of the ſkin returning in the ſame manner.

A deep ſcorbutical taint, where the breaſt has been much affected, often ends in a conſumption. Others have contracted a dropſical diſpoſition from this diſeaſe; or, what is more frequent, ſwelled, œdematous, and ulcerated legs. Such perſons are likewiſe ſubject, in different periods of their life afterwards, to chronic rheumatiſms, pains and ſtiffneſs in their joints; and ſometimes to cutaneous eruptions, or a foulneſs of the ſkin *(c)*.

C H A P.

(b) Mr Ives.——The contraction of their knees ſometimes can never be cured; as happened to one of our marines, *Samuel Norton*, who, although he recovered from the other ſymptoms of a deep ſcurvy, yet never did of this contraction; and upon that account was diſcharged as an invalid from the ſervice, with his heel almoſt touching his buttock.

(c) Mr Murray's remark.——The gums eſpecially are left

confiderably

C H A P.   IV.

The prophylaxis, *or means of preventing this difeafe, efpecially at fea.*

FOR the prevention of this difeafe at land, a warm, dry, pure air, with a diet of eafy digeftion, confifting chiefly of a due mixture of animal and vegetable fubftances, (which is found to be the moft wholfome food, and agreeable to the generality of conftitutions), will for the moft part prove fufficient.

Thofe who are liable to it by living in marfhy wet foils, and in places fubject to great rains and fogs; and others who inhabit unwholfome damp apartments, as the lower floors and cellars of a houfe in winter, fhould remedy thefe inconveniencies by keeping conftant fires, to correct this hurtful moifture; which will ftill prove more effectual for the purpofe, if made of aromatic woods. But it is rather advifable for perfons threatened with this malady, to remove into dry, chearful, and better-aired

considerably affected, either by being eat away, and leaving the teeth too bare; or remaining lax, and covering too much of them; and being fubject to bleed on the flighteft touch.

habitations.

habitations. Their principal food in fuch a cafe fhould be broths made of frefh flefh-meats, together with plenty of recent vegetables, if they can be procured; otherwife of preferved roots and fruits. Their bread ought to be made of wheat-flour, fufficiently leavened, and well baked; and at their meals they are to drink a glafs of good found beer, cyder, wine, or the like fermented liquor. The obfervance of thefe directions, together with moderate exercife, cleanlinefs of body, eafe and contentment of mind, procured by agreeable and entertaining amufements, will prove fufficient to prevent this difeafe from rifing to any great height, where it is not altogether conftitutional.

In towns or garrifons when befieged, officers fhould take care that the beds, barracks, and quarters for the foldiers, be kept dry, clean, and warm, for their refrefhment when off duty; and that their men be fufficiently provided with thick cloaks and warm cloaths, for fhelter againft the inclemency of cold, and rains, when neceffarily expofed to them. The ammunition-bread fhould be light, and well baked, and their other provifions as found and wholfome as poffible. To correct the too grofs and

folid

folid quality of thefe, they would do well to join vegetables, even the moft common, and fuch as are to be met with on the ramparts, with their other food. This precept becomes ftill more neceffary when the garrifon's provifions in ftore are fpoiled or unfound; in which cafe the ufe of vinegar is recommended by feveral authors. *Bachſtrom's* advice, of fowing the feeds of the antifcorbutic plants *(a)*, fo that thefe may grow up with the grafs on the ramparts, will, upon this occafion, be found very beneficial. They can indeed be under no difficulty in procuring fome of the moft falutary of them at all times, if they are provided with their feeds, fuch as the garden-creffes; which, in a few days, even in their apartments, will fupply them with a frefh antifcorbutic falad. When the army is in the field, they generally meet with fuch plenty of wholfome vegetables as are fufficient to prevent this difeafe becoming fatal to many of them, except in defert and depopulated countries.

But the prevention of this calamity at fea, and the prefervation of a truly valuable part of mankind, *viz.* the feamen of all nations, from its fatal and deftructive malignity in long voyages

(a) Vid. Obfervationes circa fcorbutum, &c. p. 36.

and

and cruifes, is what in a particular manner demands our attention, and has exercifed the genius of fome of the moft eminent phyficians in all parts of *Europe* for above a century paft.

A *German* who had acquired a confiderable fortune in the *Eaft Indies*, by being *Dutch* Governor of *Sumatra*, was fo affected with pity and humanity for the many afflicted failors he had obferved in this malady, that, imagining the art of chemiftry, which at that time made a great noife in the world, might probably furnifh fome remedy for their relief, he erected and endowed a perpetual profefforfhip of that fcience at *Leipfic*. He nominated his countryman Dr *Michael*, a very great chemift, who was the firft univerfity-profeffor of chemiftry in *Europe;* and remitted him a confiderable fum of money, in order to bear the expence of his experiments, with the promife of a much greater, in cafe he fucceeded in the difcovery of a remedy for prevention of the fcurvy at fea. The Doctor fpent an incredible deal of time and labour in preparing the moft elaborated chemical medicines. Volatile and fixed falts, fpirits of all forts, effences, elixirs, electuaries, *&c.* were yearly fent over to the *Eaft Indies;* nay even the *quinta effentia* (which
became

became afterwards a celebrated *noftrum* for the scurvy in *Germany*) of the chemical oil of the feeds of fcurvy-grafs. But all proved ineffectual.

Bontekoe recommended to the *Dutch* failors an acrid alcaline fpirit; *Glauber (b)* and *Boerhaave*, a ftrong mineral acid, *viz. fp. falis.* The Royal navy of *Great Britain* has been fupplied, at a confiderable expence to the government, by the advice of an eminent phyfician, with a large quantity of *elixir* of *vitriol*; which is the ftrong mineral acid of vitriol combined with aromatics. Wine-vinegar was likewife prefcribed upon this occafion by the college of phyficians at *London*, when confulted by the Lords of the Admiralty; which differs from all the former, being a mild vegetable acid procured by fermentation. Vinegar has been indeed much ufed in the fleet at all times. Many fhips, efpecially thofe fitted out at *Plymouth*, carried with them cyder for this purpofe, upon the recommendation of the learned Dr *Huxham*. The lateft propofal to the Lords of the Admiralty was a magazine of dried fpinage prepared in the manner of hay. This was to be moiftened and boiled in their food. To which it was objected by a very

(b) In his book, intitled, *Confolatio navigantium, &c.*

ingenious

ingenious physician *(c)*, That no moisture whatever could restore the natural juices of the plant lost by evaporation, and, as he imagined, altered by a fermentation which they underwent in drying.

Moreover, all the remedies which could be used in the circumstances of sailors, that at any time have been proposed for the many various diseases going under the name of a *scurvy at land*, have likewise been tried to prevent and cure this disease at sea: the effects of several of which, besides the before mentioned, I have myself experienced, *viz.* salt water, tar-water, decoctions of guajac and saffafras, bitters with *cort. winterani;* and such warm antiscorbutics as can be preserved at sea, *viz.* garlic, mustard-feed, *pulv. ari comp. et spirit. cochlear.;* which last was formerly always put up in sea-medicine chests. I have also in various stages, and for different symptoms of this distemper, made trial of most of the mineral and fossil remedies

(c) Dr Cockburn.——The Doctor's judgment is fully confirmed by experience. We find the college of physicians at *Vienna* sent to *Hungary* great quantities of the most approved antiscorbutic herbs dried in this manner; which were found to be of no benefit. Many of these would have their virtues as little impaired by drying as spinage, *e. g.* marsh trefoil. *Kramer* tried almost every species of dried herbs to no purpose, Vid. part. 3, chap. 2.

which have been recommended for the scurvy
at land; such as mercurial, chalybeate, anti-
monial, vitriolic, and sulphureous medicines.
But, before I mention the result of these experiments, and the observations made upon the
effects of several remedies that have been most
approved of in this disease, it may not be amiss
to take notice, that the want of success hitherto in preventing this fatal malady at sea, seems
chiefly owing to these two causes.

1*st*, The methods of preservation have been
put in practice too late; that is, when the difease was already bred; it being generally then
that *elixir vitriol*, vinegar, cyder, and other
antiscorbutics, were administered: whereas certain precautions seem necessary to prevent the
first attacks; it being found, that almost all
diseases are easier prevented than afterwards
removed.

2*dly*, Too high an opinion has been enter-
tained of certain medicines recommended by
physicians at land, rather from a presumption
founded on their theory of the disease, than
from any experience of their effects at sea. Indeed the causes which they were supposed to
obviate, were often none of the true and real
occasions of the distemper. Thus lime-water
has

has been long since prescribed to correct the too great quantity of sea-salt necessarily used by sailors. And the college of physicians at *London* gave it as their opinion, that *Lowndes*'s salt made from brine was preferable for salting sea-provisions, to that made of sea-water, even to the bay-salt; from a suspicion of some noxious qualities in this salt which might occasion the scurvy. *Sp. sal, el. vitriol,* and vinegar, were deemed proper antidotes to the rank and putrid state of sea-provisions, and water; or perhaps to the putrescent state of the humours in this disease.

But whatever good effect for the last purposes these may be supposed to have had in a smaller degree; yet experience has abundantly shewn, that they have not been sufficient to prevent this disease, much less to cure it. And the same may be said of many others. The consequence of which is, the world has now almost despaired of finding out a method of preventing this dreadful evil at sea; and it is become the received opinion, that it is altogether impossible there, either to prevent or cure it. But it is surprising, that this ill-grounded belief, so fatal in its consequences, should have gained credit, when we see people recovering from this disease every day, (even in the most deplo-

rable

rable condition, and in its laſt ſtages), in a
ſhort time, when proper helps are adminiſter-
ed.   I have already given an inſtance of ſeventy
people cured in the bad air of a ſhip, without
being landed *(d)*.   I ſhall hereafter produce
other inſtances of this diſeaſe being cured at
ſea, though theſe muſt have occurred to every
perſon who has had occaſion there to be converſant with ſcorbutical caſes *(e)*.

It may be proper, in order fully to remove this prejudice, to obſerve, that an epidemical ſcurvy,   either at ſea or land, is an adventitious, not a natural diſeaſe: that is to ſay, it
is not owing to any ſpontaneous degeneracy of
the human body,   from a healthful condition
into this morbid ſtate; but to the influence of
very powerful and active,   but ſuch plain and
obvious cauſes as have been before aſſigned *(f)*.
And it is conſtantly experienced, that when
theſe cauſes do not ſubſiſt, or are corrected and
guarded againſt,   the diſeaſe may be effectually
prevented.   This will admit of a demonſtration from many facts.   Officers are ſeldom or

(d) P. 99.
(e) Many inſtances have already been given in Mr *Ives*'s
journal, part 2. chap. 1.
(f) Part 2. chap 1.

never

never affected with the scurvy; even the sub-
altern and petty officers generally keep free
from it, while it commits great ravage among
the common seamen. There have occurred
frequent instances of *English* and *Dutch* ships
being in company together, where the former were in great distress from this disease;
while the latter, by a very small difference in
their diet, were quite healthy. But what is
sufficient to convince the greatest sceptic, that
this calamity may be effectually prevented,
is the present healthfulness of *Newfoundland*,
the northern parts of *Canada*, and of our factories at *Hudson*'s bay. In those parts of the
world, the scurvy was formerly more fatal to
the first adventurers and planters, than it was
ever known at sea; which facts I shall have
occasion presently to mention, and account for.
And as it is a satisfaction to know that this disease may effectually be prevented, so it is likewise an encouragement to the utmost diligence
in discovering, and putting in practice, the means
proper for that purpose.

It being of the utmost consequence to guard
against the first approaches of so dreadful an e-
nemy, I shall here endeavour to lay down the
measures proper to be taken for this end, with
that

that minutenefs and accuracy which the importance of the fubject, and the prefervation of fo many valuable and ufeful lives, juftly demand; and at the fame time fhall, as much as poffible, avoid offering any thing that may be judged impracticable, or liable to exception, on account of the difficulty or difagreeablenefs of complying with it. And, *laftly*, I fhall propofe nothing dictated merely from theory; but fhall confirm all by experience and facts, the fureft and moft unerring guides.

What I propofe is, firft, to relate the effects of feveral medicines tried at fea in this difeafe, on purpofe to difcover what might promife the moft certain protection againft it upon that element.

The medicine which fucceeded upon trial, I fhall afterwards confirm to be the fureft prefervative, and moft efficacious remedy, by the experience of others.

I fhall then endeavour to give it the moft convenient portable form, and fhew the method of preferving its virtues entire for years, fo that it may be carried to the moft diftant parts of the world in fmall bulk, and at any time be prepared by the failors themfelves: adding fome farther directions, given chiefly

with

with a view to inform the captains and commanders of ships and fleets, of methods proper both to preserve their own health, and that of their crews.

It will not be amiss further to observe, in what method convalescents ought to be treated, or those who are weak, and recovering from other diseases, in order to prevent their falling into the scurvy; which will include some necessary rules for resisting the beginnings of this evil, when, through want of care, or neglect, the disease is bred in a ship.

As the salutary effects of the prescribed measures will be rendered still more certain, and universally beneficial, where proper regard is had to such a state of air, diet, and regimen, as may contribute to the general intentions of preservation or cure; I shall conclude the precepts relating to the preservation of seamen, with shewing the best means of obviating many inconveniencies which attend long voyages, and of removing the several causes productive of this mischief.

The following are the experiments.

On the 20th of *May* 1747, I took twelve patients in the scurvy, on board the *Salisbury* at sea. Their cases were as similar as I could

have

have them. They all in general had putrid
gums, the fpots and laffitude, with weaknefs
of their knees. They lay together in one
place, being a proper apartment for the fick in
the fore-hold; and had one diet common to
all, *viz.* water-gruel fweetened with fugar in
the morning; frefh mutton-broth often times
for dinner; at other times puddings, boiled
bifcuit with fugar, *&c.*; and for fupper, barley
and raifins, rice and currants, fago and wine,
or the like. Two of thefe were ordered each
a quart of cyder a-day. Two others took
twenty-five gutts of *elixir vitriol* three times
a-day, upon an empty ftomach; ufing a
gargle ftrongly acidulated with it for their
mouths. Two others took two fpoonfuls of
vinegar three times a-day, upon an empty ftomach; having their gruels and their other food
well acidulated with it, as alfo the gargle
for their mouth. Two of the worft patients,
with the tendons in the ham rigid, (a fymptom none of the reft had), were put under a
courfe of fea-water. Of this they drank half a
pint every day, and fometimes more or lefs as
it operated, by way of gentle phyfic. Two o-
thers had each two oranges and one lemon given them every day. Thefe they eat with gree-
dinefs,

dinefs, at different times, upon an empty fto-mach. They continued but fix days under this courfe, having confumed the quantity that could be fpared. The two remaining patients, took the bignefs of a nutmeg three times a-day, of an electuary recommended by an hofpital-furgeon, made of garlic, muftard-feed, *rad. raphan.* balfam of *Peru*, and gum myrrh; ufing for common drink, barley-water well acidulated with tamarinds; by a decoction of which, with the addition of *cremor tartar*, they were gently purged three or four times during the courfe.

The confequence was, that the moft fudden and vifible good effects were perceived from the ufe of the oranges and lemons; one of thofe who had taken them, being at the end of fix days fit for duty. The fpots were not indeed at that time quite off his body, nor his gums found; but without any other medicine, than a gar-garifm of *elixir vitriol*, he became quite heal-thy before we came into *Plymouth*, which was on the 16th of *June*. The other was the beft recovered of any in his condition; and being now deemed pretty well, was appointed nurfe to the reft of the fick.

Next

Next to the oranges, I thought the cyder *(g)* had the best effects. It was indeed not very sound, being inclinable to be aigre or pricked. However, those who had taken it, were in a fairer

(g) Extract of a letter from Mr Ives.

I judge it proper to communicate to you, what good effects I have observed in the scurvy, from the use of cyder and sea-water, during the last cruise I made in the western squadron, with my honoured benefactor Admiral *Martin.* But as I do not pretend to have taken notice of any thing, more than merely a palliative benefit from them, I think, without mentioning particular cases, it will be sufficient for me to inform you, that, in our preceeding cruise with the western squadron, his Majesty's ship *Yarmouth*, of 70 guns and 500 men, was not only troubled with the scurvy in common with other ships, but, in spite of all my endeavours, lost in it a proportioned number of men. Upon our return from that cruise, I took an opportunity to represent to the Admiral, that as vegetable juices of all sorts were from experience found to be the only true antiscorbutics, and I had myself formerly experienced the good effects of apples, it was reasonable to presume that cyder must certainly be of service. This suggestion agreed with some accounts the Admiral had received from others; and he with great readiness bought, and put under my care, several hogsheads of the best *South-Ham* cyder. During the next cruise, each scorbutic patient had daily a quart or three pints of cyder; and as many of them as I could prevail on, took twice a-week three quarters of a pint of sea-water in a morning. In all other respects I treated them as I used to do people in the scurvy; which you well know, from the conversation which has often passed betwixt us on this subject, was with squill vomits, pills composed of soap, squills, garlic, *&c. elixir vitriol,* and other medicines suited to the different stages and symptoms of the malady. In one word, we had this cruise as many scorbutic patients as any other ship.

fairer way of recovery than the others at the end of the fortnight, which was the length of time all these different courses were continued, except the oranges. The putrefaction of their gums, but especially their lassitude and weakness, were somewhat abated, and their appetite increased by it.

As to the *elixir* of *vitriol*, I observed that the mouths of those who had used it by way of gargarism, were in a much cleaner and better condition than many of the rest, especially those who used the vinegar; but perceived otherwise no good effects from its internal use upon the other symptoms. I indeed never had a great opinion of the efficacy of this medicine in the scurvy, since our longest cruise in the *Salisbury*, from the 10th of *August* to the 28th *October* 1746; when we had but one scurvy in the ship. The patient was a marine, (one *Walsh*); who, after recovering from a quotidian ague in the latter end of *September*, had ta-

in proportion to our complement of men. But although all the rest buried a great many, some to the number of 20, others 30, 40, 50, and upwards; yet the *Yarmouth* did not bury more than two or three; and these at the latter end of the cruise, all our cyder having been expended for a week or ten days before. Upon our arrival at port, we sent to the hospital a great many in very dreadful circumstances.

ken

ken the *elixir vitriol* by way of restorative for three weeks; and yet at length contracted the disease, while under a course of a medicine recommended for its prevention.

There was no remarkable alteration upon those who took the electuary and tamarind decoction, the sea-water, or vinegar, upon comparing their condition, at the end of the fortnight, with others who had taken nothing but a little lenitive electuary and *cremor tartar*, at times, in order to keep their belly open; or a gentle pectoral in the evening, for relief of their breast. Only one of them, while taking the vinegar, fell into a gentle flux at the end of ten days. This I attributed to the genius and course of the disease, rather than to the use of the medicine. As I shall have occasion elsewhere to take notice of the effects of other medicines in this disease, I shall here only observe, that the result of all my experiments was, that oranges and lemons were the most effectual remedies for this distemper at sea. I am apt to think oranges preferable to lemons, though perhaps both given together will be found most serviceable.

It may be now proper to confirm the efficacy of these fruits by the experience of others.
The

The first proof that I shall produce, is borrowed from the learned Dr *Mead (h)*.

" One year when that brave Admiral Sir
" *Charles Wager* commanded our fleet in the
" *Baltic,* his sailors were terribly afflicted
" with the scurvy: but he observed, that the
" *Dutch* ships then in company were much
" more free from this disease. He could im-
" pute this to nothing but their different food,
" which was stock-fish and gort; whereas
" ours was salt fish and oat-meal *(i)*. He
" was then come last from the *Mediterranean,*
" and had at *Leghorn* taken in a great quantity
" of lemons and oranges. Recollecting, from
" what he had often heard, how effectual these
" fruits were in the cure of this distemper, he
" ordered a chest of each to be brought up-
" on deck, and opened, every day. The men,
" besides eating what they would, mixed the
" juice in their beer. It was also their con-
" stant diversion to pelt one another with the
" rinds, so that the deck was always strewed
" and wet with the fragrant liquor. The

(h) Discourse on the scurvy, p. 111.
(i) The first is seldom now put on board ships of war, and of the last *English* sailors eat but little.

" happy

" happy effect was, that he brought his sail-
" ors home in good health."

I have been favoured upon this occasion, by
different gentlemen, with many instances of
the like good effects of these fruits in this difease at sea; particularly by Mr *Francis Ruffel*,
in a cruise performed by the *Princess Caroline*
off the islands of *Sardinia* and *Corsica*; where,
according to his relation, some of these fruits
got at *Vado*, preserved great part of the crew,
which otherwise must undoubtedly have perished.

An ingenious surgeon of great merit and experience in the *Guernsey* when extremely distressed by the scurvy *(k)*, has the following
observation in his letter upon it. " I have
" great reason to believe, that several lives
" were absolutely preserved, when we were at
" sea, by a lemon squeezed into six or eight
" ounces of *Malaga* wine mixed with water,
" and given twice a-day."

I am informed, it was principally oranges
which so speedily and surprisingly recovered
Lord *Anson's* people at the island of *Tinian*.
Of which that noble, brave, and experienced commander was so sensible, that, before

(k) See the case of that ship, chap. 1. p. 98.

he

he left the ifland, one man was ordered on
fhore from each mefs to lay in a ftock of them
for their future fecurity.

My ingenious friend Mr *Murray,* who has
favoured me with fo many ufeful obfervations
upon this difeafe; and has had the greateft opportunities of being acquainted with it, as he
for a confiderable time attended the naval hofpital at *Jamaica* whilft our great fleets were
in the *Weft Indies,* and was likewife furgeon
of the *Canterbury,* expreffes himfelf thus in his
letter. " As to oranges and lemons, I have
" always found them, when properly and fuf-
" ficiently ufed, an infallible cure in every
" ftage and fpecies of the difeafe, if there was
" any degree of natural ftrength but left;
" and where a diarrhæa, lientery, or dyfen-
" tery, were not joined to the other fcorbutic
" fymptoms. Of which we had a moft convin-
" cing proof, when we arrived at the *Danifh*
" ifland of *St Thomas (l)*; where fifty patients
" belonging to the *Canterbury,* and feventy to
" the *Norwich,* in all the different ftages of
" this diftemper, were cured, in little more
" than twelve days, by limes alone; where

(*l*) See the former part of this letter, chap. 1. p. 107.

" little

" little or no other refreshments could be ob-
" tained."

It was reasonable to ascribe this to the eminent virtues of these fruits; as it is well known,
and daily experienced, that without such remedies scorbutic people will infallibly die in the
purest land-air. But what cures such deplorable cases, must still more powerfully prevent
them. Perhaps one history more may suffice
to put this out of doubt.

" In the first voyage made to the *East In-*
" *dies (m)*, on account of the *English East-*
" *India* company, there were employed four
" ships, commanded by Captain *James Lanca-*
" *ster* their General, *viz.* the *Dragon* having the
" General and 202 men, the *Hector* 108
" men, the *Susan* 82, and the *Ascension* 32.
" They left *England* about the 18th of *April;*
" in *July* the people were taken ill on their
" passage with the scurvy; by the 1st of *Au-*
" *gust*, all the ships, except the General's, were
" so thin of men, that they had scarce enough
" to hand the sails; and, upon having a con-
" trary wind for fifteen or sixteen days, the
" few who were well before, began also to fall

(m) Vid. *Harris*'s collection of voyages, and *Purchas*'s
collection, vol. 1. p. 147.

" sick.

" sick. Whence the want of hands was so
" great in these ships, that the merchants who
" were sent to dispose of their cargoes in the
" *East Indies*, were obliged to take their turn
" at the helm, and do the sailors duty, till
" they arrived at *Saldania* (*n*) ; where the Ge-
" neral sent his boats, and went on board him-
" self, to assist the other three ships ; who were
" in so weakly a condition, that they were
" hardly able to let fall an anchor, nor could
" they hoist out their boat without his assist-
" ance. All this time the General's ship con-
" tinued pretty healthy. The reason why his
" crew was in better health than the rest of
" the ships, was owing to the juice of lemons ;
" of which the General having brought some
" bottles to sea, he gave to each, as long as it
" lasted, three spoonfuls every morning fast-
' ing. By this he cured many of his men,
" and preserved the rest: so that although his
" ship contained double the number of any of
" the others ; yet (through the mercy of God,
" and to the preservation of the other three
" ships) he neither had so many men sick, nor
" lost so many as they did."

(*n*) A bay near the Cape of *Good Hope.*

Here

Here indeed is a remarkable and authentic proof of the great efficacy of juice of lemons against this disease; as large and crouded ships are more afflicted with it, and always in a higher degree, than those that are small and airy. This little squadron lost 105 men by the scurvy. Upon its afterwards breaking out among them when in the *East Indies*, in a council held at sea it was determined, to put directly into some port where they could be supplied with oranges and lemons, as the most effectual and experienced remedies to remove and prevent this dreadful calamity.

I cannot omit upon this occasion observing, what caution is at all times necessary in our reasoning on the effects of medicines, even in the way of analogy, which would seem the least liable to error. For some might naturally conclude, that these fruits are but so many acids, for which tamarinds, vinegar, *sp. sal. el. vitriol*, and others of the same tribe, would prove excellent *succedaneums*. But, upon bringing this to the test of experience, we find the contrary. Few ships have ever been in want of vinegar, and, for many years before the end of the late war, all were supplied sufficiently with *el. vitriol*. Notwithstanding which, the *Channel*

fleet

fleet often put on shore a thousand men miserably over-run with this disease, besides some hundreds who died in their cruises. Upon those occasions tar-water, salt water, vinegar, and *el. vitriol* especially, with many other things, have been abundantly tried to no purpose: whereas there is not an instance of a ship's crew being ever afflicted with this disease, where the before mentioned fruits were properly, duly, and in sufficient quantity, administered.

I elsewhere observed the uncertainty of such theories as are founded upon the chemical principles of acid and alcali *(o)*: for although acids agree in certain properties; yet they differ widely in others, and especially in their effects upon the human body. Of theory in physic the same may perhaps be said, as has been observed by some of zeal in religion, That it is indeed absolutely necessary; yet, by carrying it too far, it may be doubted whether it has done more good or hurt in the world.

Some will perhaps say, that these fruits have been often used in the scurvy without success; as appears from the experience of physicians, who prescribe them every day in that disease at land. And here we may again ob-

(o) Part 1. chap. 2.

serve

serve the fatal confequence of confounding this malady with others. Legions of diftempers (according to *Willis* and others) very different from the real and genuine fcurvy, have been claffed under its name: and becaufe the moft approved antifcorbutics fail to remove fuch difeafes, hence we are told by authors *(p)*, that it is the mafterpiece of art to cure it. But this is contradicted by the daily experience of fea-men, by the journals of our fea-hofpitals, and by the yearly experience of our *Englifh Eaft-India* fhips at *St Helena*, and the Cape of *Good Hope*. So that nothing can be more abfurd, than to object againft the efficacy of thefe fruits in preventing and curing the real fcurvy, becaufe they do not cure very different dif-eafes.

Some new prefervative might here have been recommended; feveral indeed might have been propofed, and with great fhew of the probability of their fuccefs; and their novelty might have procured them a favourable reception in the world. But thefe fruits have this peculiar advantage above any thing that can be propo-fed for trial, that their experienced virtues

(*p*) *Boerhaave,* and many others.

have

have stood the test of near 200 years. They were providentially discovered, even before the disease was well known, or at least had been described by physicians. *Ronsseus*, the first writer on this subject, mentions them *(q)*; and observes, that in all probability the *Dutch* sailors had by accident fallen upon this remedy, when afflicted with the scurvy, in their return from *Spain* loaded with these fruits, especially oranges. Experience soon taught them, that by thus eating part of their cargo, they might be restored to health. And if people had been less assiduous in finding out new remedies, and trusted more to the efficacy of these fruits, for preventing this fatal pestilence to seamen, the lives of many thousand sailors, and others *(r)*, (especially during the last war), might

(q) Epist. 2.

(r) Vid. *Kramer*'s observations, part 3. chap. 2. the best ever made on this disease; which abundantly confirm all that is here advanced. In a book published afterwards he makes the following remarks. The scurvy is the most loathsome disease in nature; for which no cure is to be found in your medicine-chest, no not in the best-furnished apothecary's shop. Pharmacy gives no relief, surgery as little. Beware of bleeding; shun mercury as a poison: you may rub the gums, you may grease the rigid tendons in the ham, to little purpose. But if you can get green vegetables; if you can prepare a sufficient quantity of the fresh noble
antiscorbutic

might in all probability have been preserved. But some have been misled to recommend many other things, as of equal, if not superior antiscorbutic qualities to these; and have reduced them to a level with other acids, and many falsely supposed antiscorbutic medicines: from whence the many unhappy disappointments hitherto met with in preventing this disease at sea, seem to have arisen.

We are told, that at the siege of *Thorn*, when this calamity raged with great violence in the town, it was the last and most earnest petition of the diseased, that some of these fruits might be permitted to enter their gates, as the only hopes of life, and last comfort of the dying patient (*f*). In this disease, when drugs of all sorts are nauseated and abhorred, the very sight of these fruits raises the drooping spirits of the almost expiring patient. I have often observed, (upon seeing scorbutic people landed at our naval hospitals), that the eating of them was attended with a pleasure easier

antiscorbutic juices; if you have oranges, lemons, or citrons; or their pulp and juice preserved with sugar in casks, so that you can make a lemonade, or rather give to the quantity of three or four ounces of their juice in whey, you will, without other assistance, cure this dreadful evil. *Krameri medicina castrensis.*

(*f*) *Bachstrom observ. circa scorbutum, p.* 15.

to be imagined than to be defcribed. Hence Lord *Delawar*, a very great fufferer in this malady, (in the relation of his cafe to the Lords and others of the council of *Virginia*), very pathetically expreffes himfelf thus. " Heaven " has kindly provided thefe fruits as a fpecific " for the moft terrible of evils *(t)*."

As oranges and lemons are liable to fpoil, and cannot be procured at every port, nor at all feafons in equal plenty; and it may be inconvenient to take on board fuch large quantities as are neceffary in fhips for their prefervation from this and other difeafes; the next thing to be propofed, is the method of preferving their virtues entire for years in a convenient and fmall bulk. It is done in the following eafy manner.

Let the fqueezed juice of thefe fruits be well cleared from the pulp, and depurated by ftanding for fome time; then poured off from the grofs fediment: or, to have it ftill purer, it may be filtrated. Let it then be put into any clean open earthen veffel, well glazed; which fhould be wider at the top than bottom, fo that there may be the largeft furface above to favour the evaporation. For this purpofe a china bafon

(t) Purchas, vol. 4. p. 16.

or punch-bowl is proper; or a common earthen bafon ufed for wafhing, if well glazed, will be fufficient, as it is generally made in the form required. Into this pour the purified juice; and put it into a pan of water, upon a clear fire. Let the water come almoft to boil, and continue nearly in a ftate of boiling (with the bafon containing the juice in the middle of it) for fevera hours, until the juice is found to be of the confiftence of oil when warm, or of a fyrup when cold. It is then to be corked up in a bottle for ufe. Two dozen of good oranges, weighing five pounds four ounces, will yeild one pound nine ounces and a half of depurated juice; and when evaporated, there will remain about five ounces of the extract; which in bulk will be equal to lefs than three ounces of water. So that thus the acid, and virtues of twelve dozen of lemons or oranges, may be put into a quart-bottle, and preferved for feveral years.

I have fome of the extract of lemons now by me, which was made four years ago. And when this is mixed with water, or made into punch, few are able to diftinguifh it from the frefh fqueezed juice mixed up in like manner; except when both are prefent, and their
different

different taftes compared at the fame time; when the frefh fruits difcover a greater degree of fmartnefs and fragrancy.

The learned Dr *Mead* afcribes fome falutary effects to the fragrancy of the frefh fruits, when he obferves, that by the failors pelting each other with the rinds in Admiral *Wager's* fhip, the decks were ftrewed and wet with this wholfome liquor. Was any thing to be expected from perfuming the air with the fragrancy of thefe fruits, it is eafily done at any time by a few drops of their effence, or the aromatic oil contained in the rinds. An addition of a fmall quantity of this to the extract, will give it the fmell and fragrancy of the frefh fruit in great perfection. And if it is alfo required to be taken inwardly, a few drops of it upon fugar may be given along with the extract. But perhaps fo hot an oil may rather prove prejudicial. It is the faponaceous juice alone, of thefe fruits, that is here requifite; and their entire falutary virtues may be obtained by taking that inwardly; as appears plainly by the relation of Captain *Lancaster's* voyage, where the juice of lemons kept in bottles, not only prevented the difeafe, but cured it, at fea. This juice muft either have been mixed up with fpi-

rits,

rits, or something else, to preserve it *(u)*; and consequently differed much more in quality from the fresh fruit than what is proposed.

However, if it be judged of any consequence to preserve the perfect fragrancy of the fruit, I have found, upon experiment, that there are several other ways of doing it. They who intend this extract for acidulating punch, may infuse some of the fresh peel of the oranges or lemons in the spirit before it is used. I have known some who distil brandy themselves from their spoiled wines, throw these peels into the still. Either of the methods makes a most agreeable and fragrant punch with the extract. The essential oil of the rind is thus so subtilised, and incorporated with the spirit, as to be itself converted as it were into a purer spirit. And it will not then have the heating quality, nor affect the head afterwards so much as the simple oil may do. The water of these peels drawn in a cold still, keeps a considerable time in a separate bottle from the extract; and when mixed with it at using, restores the perfect fragrancy of these fruits as when fresh.

(u) The lime-juice brought home from the *West Indies*, is commonly either mixed with rum, or covered a top with oil; notwithstanding which, it generally turns musty.

But,

But, for this purpose, I find it is sufficient to add a very small quantity of the outer peel to the extract a little before it is taken off the fire, and there will be all that is requisite to make it entirely equal to the fresheft fruit; in so much that the niceft tafte will not be able to diftinguifh any difference. Its virtues (as muft appear to any one so far converfant in chemical principles, as to know there is nothing more loft here than water, with a fcarce perceptible acid) will be found nothing inferior to the frefh fruit *(x)*.

In this manner prepared, it muft be kept in bottles, where it will remain good for several years. When made in a proper place and feafon, it will come very cheap; and our navy may be fupplied with it at a much eafier rate than any thing as yet propofed. It will be found extremely wholfome on all occafions, but efpecially to correct bad brandy, and other noxious fpirits, often drank by failors in immoderate quantity. Rum in the *Weft Indies*, ar-

(x) This I think cannot be doubted by any perfon who has ufed it, or who will take the pains to make proper comparifons and trials with it, and the frefheft orange or lemon juice. Indeed the benefit prefumed to be derived from the flavour is fo fmall, that the plain extract is quite fufficient. Officers, by putting in a little of the candied peel in their punch, will give it the agreeable flavour wanted.

rack

rack or brandy, when ferved them by way of allowance, fhould always be firft mixed up with the extract. This will not only make them more palatable, but, what is a matter of much greater moment, will convert thefe poifonous pernicious draughts into a fovereign remedy, and a prefervative againft a fcorbutic habit, the bane of feafaring people.

I fhall add one obfervation in its favour. The ifland of *Jamaica* is much lefs liable to ficknefs at prefent than formerly. Our fleets in the *Weft Indies* in the beginning of the war, were much more fickly than in the latter end of it, when indeed they were furprifingly healthy. This, with great reafon, has been univerfally afcribed to the drinking a great quantity of this acid, by making their punch four and weak.

I proceed to fome farther directions given for the information of commanders of fhips, and thofe who have proper conveniencies, who may relieve the fick, upon occafion, with their ftores. And it may be proper to acquaint them, that moft berries, and feveral fruits, when gathered two thirds ripe on a dry day, while the fun fhines, if put into earthen pots, or rather in dry bottles, well corked, and fealed up, fo that

that no air or moisture can enter, will keep a long time, and, at the end of a year, be as fresh as when new pulled. These the captains may supply themselves with at every port in *England*, from the pastry-cooks shops, with proper directions for their preservation. Green gooseberries will keep for years, if, after being put into dry bottles, their moisture is exhaled, by putting the bottles slightly corked into a pot of water, which is allowed to come nearly to boil, and continue so for a little; when a very small quantity of juice yielded by them is to be thrown away, and they are afterwards kept close stopt. These would prove a sovereign remedy for the sick: and, by such methods, ships in long voyages, when touching at any place for water and provisions, may likewise lay up a sea-store of berries and fruits.

Various wholsome herbs and roots may likewise be preserved at sea, according to the different directions given for that purpose in books of confectionery; such as small onions in a pickle of vinegar, &c. Most green vegetables, as cabbage, *French* beans, and others, are preserved, if put when very dry in clean dry stone-jars, with a layer of salt at bottom; then a thin layer of the vegetable covered with salt,

and

and so alternately, till the jar is full; when the
whole is to be covered with salt, and well press-
ed down with a weight, and its mouth close
stopt, that no air or moisture may enter. At
using, the salt is to be washed off by warm
water; when the vegetable, after keeping a
year, will be found fresh and green. I have
been told, that in this manner that sovereign,
never-failing remedy, the *Greenland* scurvy-
grass-(*y*), may be preserved, and that pots of
it have been brought over quite fresh and green.

Every common sailor ought to lay in a stock
of onions. I never observed any that used
them fall into the scurvy at sea. When this
stock is exhausted, the captains may have recourse to their pickled small onions; and with
fowls, mutton, or portable soop, and the pickled cabbage before mentioned, of which the
Dutch (*z*) sell great quantities, they will be
able

(*y*) Vid. Mr *Maude*'s letter concerning it, chap. 5.; also, the
extraordinary case of a sailor related by *Bachstrom.*
(*z*) The *Dutch* sailors are much less liable to the scurvy than
the *English*, owing to this pickled vegetable carried to sea.
Vid. Krameri epistolam de scorbuto. A mess of this given twice a-
week boiled in their peas, seems all the addition requisite to be
made to the present victualling of the navy for the effectual prevention of the scurvy. It may be objected, That its saltness would
rather prove hurtful in this disease. But this objection is founded

able to make a broth at fea, almost the same
with what is used in our naval hospitals for recovery of scorbutic people.   I have known several

ed upon a very false opinion, that sea-salt breeds the scurvy :
the contrary of which has been fully demonstrated chap. 1. and
is confirmed by numberless instances of giving salt water in very
bad scurvies, both at sea and land, with great benefit to the patient. See Mr *Ives*'s letter, p. 194.   Dr *Grainger*'s, chap. 5.

The fact here truly is, that vegetables preserved in this manner, so far from being salt after duly washing them in warm
water, require to be eat with salt : they are thus preserved quite
succulent and green.   Their virtue is the same as if taken fresh
out of the garden, and the method infinitely superior to the drying of them, as was proposed, like hay; which would entirely
destroy their antiscorbutic quality ; as will be made appear when
we come to inquire (chap. 6.) into the properties and virtues peculiar to green succulent vegetables, so essentially requisite for
the prevention, and in the cure of this malady.   To the surgeon's necessaries in long and sickly voyages, it would not be a-
miss to add some boxes of portable soop ; and at all times some
pots of preserved small onions.   It is demonstrable from the most
incontestable experience, that a soop of boiled cabbage and o-
nions will cure an adventitious scurvy in its first stage, either at
sea or land, in any part of the world.   By a like soop, with addition of fresh flesh-meat, seventy people were perfectly cured
in the *Guernsey* (see p. 98.), without one of them setting foot on
shore.   This was not owing to the flesh in their soop, but to the
vegetables : for I have known some favourites of the Captain's
who had fresh mutton-soop given them almost every day, without the least benefit, until they arrived at port ; where they were
cured in a few days by the same soop, with addition of vegetables.   And that vegetables have the same effect at sea as at
land, is plain from Mr *Ives*'s journal (see p. 144. & 145.),
where the people continued to recover at sea from the 29th

veral captains, who, by carrying out boxes filled with earth, which stood in their quarter-
galleries, were supplied with wholsome salads,

November that they left *Vado*, until the 25th *December*, by means
of fruits given them.

A gentleman on board the Commodore at that time told me,
that the whole squadron was greatly distressed with the scurvy,
and in particular the Commodore's ship; in so much, that, after
having used all means, to no purpose, that could be thought of
to put a stop to the malady, he was at last obliged, for the preservation of his people, to stretch over to the coast of *Italy*,
and leave his station for a while. At this time many were extremely bad. Upon his arrival at *Vado*, he found the whole
country covered with snow; and such was the severity of the
winter, that there was hardly any kind of greens to be got for
the relief of his distressed crew. Upon which this excellent
commander (now Adm. *Osborn*) very wisely directed his people to buy up all the oranges and lemons in the town. His
boats brought on board a considerable quantity of them. He
likewise supplied his squadron with some fresh beef. Being obliged to make but a very short continuance at *Vado*, he directly returned to his station with a store of these fruits, but with
his men still in a bad condition. He continued cruising at sea
for three weeks, in very rough weather. Notwithstanding
which, by means of these fruits, many who were very bad,
and all who were in the first stage of the disease, were perfectly
recovered while at sea, and the lives of the whole crew preserved.

N. B. This relation given me by Mr *Russel* (see p. 198.),
does not entirely agree with Mr *Ives*'s as to the fruits got at *Vado*. It seems different ships got different fruits. However,
there must be many people who are well acquainted with those
facts, as it was a considerable squadron, consisting of very large
and capital ships.

after

after being some months out of harbour. A cask of rich garden-mould put occasionally in boxes on the poop, and sown with the seed of garden-cresses, would furnish these at any time. Such seeds will likewise grow in wet cotton.

Besides fresh and preserved fruits and vegetables, fermented liquors of all sorts are found beneficial in this disease. Some of them however are more antiscorbutic than others. By my own experience, I found cyder the best of any I have had occasion to try. And it would seem an excellent method of preserving other vegetable juices, (gooseberries, blackberries, currants, elderberries, or even *Seville* oranges), to ferment them into made wines or beer. These I am persuaded will be found preferable to many medicated antiscorbutic ales and wines by infusion, that might here be recommended.

It is pretty remarkable, that the first northern colonies in *America* were extremely subject to this disease. The *French* especially, upon their first planting *Canada* and *New-France*, suffered so much by the mortality it occasioned in the winter-season, that they had often thoughts of abandoning their settlements; even the natives were not exempted from the

ravage

ravage of this cruel evil *(a)* : whereas not only these colonies, but others in a colder and more northern situation, are at present quite healthy. One would be apt to ascribe this, to the many hardships and inconveniencies infant-colonies are necessarily exposed to; were it not, that we see many poor people wintering yearly in *Newfoundland*, where this disease was formerly so fatal, who from poverty suffer equal, if not greater hardships, than the first planters during the severity of winter. They are, for almost eight months in the year, destitute of fresh vegetables, and live entirely on salt and dried fish, coarse bread, and much worse fare than a ship's provisions. Their air is likewise grosser, colder, and moister, than is commonly the case at sea. Notwithstanding which, they keep pretty free from the scurvy. And this is ascribed to their common drink, which is spruce beer.

It is indeed matter of surprise, and was taken notice of before as the most convincing proof that this calamity may be prevented any where, that the people who reside at our factories in *Hudson*'s bay, are so very healthy; where, according to *Ellis*'s account, they sometimes do not bury one man in seven years out

(a) See part 3. chap. 1.

of

of a hundred that are in their four factories *(b)*: whereas the first adventurers to that part of the world, who wintered in the same places, were almost all destroyed by the scurvy, *viz.* Capt. *Monck's* people in 1619 *(c)*, Capt. *Thomas James's* at *Charleton* island in 1631 *(d)*, and most others who attempted it. A set of sailors, consisting of seven men, was left two winters successively, in the years 1633 and 1634, at *Greenland* and *Spitzbergen*, by way of experiment: but every man of them next spring was found to have died of the scurvy *(e)*. The unhappy fate of those people, who all perished in this great misery, and left behind them a journal of their piteous misfortunes, seems to have been owing to the world's ignorance of the distemper at that time, and the pernicious methods recommended to them for preservation; which we find were chiefly purging antiscorbutic potions, distilled spirits, *viz.* brandy, and the like; all which infallibly increased the malady, and hastened their unhappy end.

From these unsuccessful trials it was judged

(b) See voyage to *Hudson's* bay.
(c) *Churchill's* collection of voyages, vol. 1. p. 541.
(a) *Harris's* collection of voyages, vol. 2. p. 406.
(e) *Churchill's* collection, vol. 2. p. 347.

impracticable

impracticable to pass the winter in those parts. But the following accident afforded the most convincing evidence of this mistake. A boat's crew, consisting of eight men, was by chance left behind, and obliged to winter in almost the same place *(f).* The season proved equally rigorous and severe. The poor fellows had nothing to trust to for sustenance but what their guns procured. Thus luckily were every one of them preserved alive, by being unprovided with what might have been deemed necessary (though in effect pernicious) means of subsistence and preservation. They had no brandy, no coarse hard biscuit, nor salt flesh-meats, *&c.*

But what deserves particular consideration, is, that those who live on the coarsest food, with a salt diet, and use spruce beer at the same time, are seldom or never afflicted in the coldest and most northern countries. It was observed in *Holland,* that when the custom of drinking wine more freely was practised, this distemper became less frequent *(g).* And among the first cures recommended to the world was wine, with wormwood infused in it *(h);*

(f) Churchill, vol. 4. p. 745.
(g) Bruneri tract. de scorbuto.
(h) See part 3. chap. 1. Olaus Magnus.

which

which was afterwards long used by way of prevention in *Saxony*, where this evil was peculiarly endemic *(i)*. Fermented vinous liquors of any kind are indeed very beneficial. But it appears by the experience of the northern *American* colonies, as also of several countries up the *Baltic* in *Europe*, &c. that genuine spruce beer is, above all others, not only an effectual preservative against it, but an excellent remedy.

The antiscorbutic virtue of the fir was, like many other of our best medicines, accidentally discovered in *Europe (k)*. When the *Swedes* carried on a war against the *Muscovites*, almost all the soldiers of their army were destroyed by the true marsh or marine scurvy, having rotten gums, rigid tendons, &c. But a stop was put to the progress of this disease, by advice of *Erbenius* the King's physician, with a simple decoction of fir-tops; by which the most deplorable cases were perfectly recovered, and the rest of the soldiers prevented from falling into it. It also proved

(i) See part 3. chap. 2.

(k) Vid. Moellenbroek de arthritide vaga scorbutica, p. 116. *Etmulleri opera*, p. 2. said by some to have occurred in the army of *Uladislaus* King of *Poland*.

an excellent gargle for the putrid gums. From thence this medicine came into great reputation, and the common fir, *picea major*, or *abies rubra*, was afterwards called *pinus antiscorbutica*. *Pinus sylvestris*, the mountain-pine, has likewise been found highly antiscorbutic.

I am inclined to believe, from the description given by *Cartier* of the *ameda* tree, with a decoction of the bark and leaves of which his crew was so speedily recovered, that it was the large swampy *American* spruce tree *(l)*. For although the pines and firs, of which there is great variety, differ from each other in their size and outward form, the length and disposition of their leaves, hardness of wood, *&c.* ; yet they seem all to have analogous medicinal virtues, and great efficacy in this disease. The shrub spruce, of that sort vulgarly called the *black*, which makes this most wholsome drink, affords a balsam superior to most turpentines, though known only to a few physicians.

A simple decoction of the tops, cones, leaves, or even bark and wood of these trees, is anti-

(l) See part 3. chap 1. *Hackluit*'s collection of voyages, vol. 3. p. 225. Some have believed it to be the sassafras, others the white thorn; but, in his third voyage, he mentions the white thorn, and makes the *ameda* to be three fathom in circumference.

scorbutic:

scorbutic: but it becomes much more so when
fermented, as in making spruce beer; where
the *moloses* contributes, by its diaphoretic
quality, to make it a more suitable medicine.
By carrying a few bags of spruce to sea, this
wholsome drink may be prepared at any time.
But where it cannot be had, the common fir-
tops used for fuel in the ship, should be first
boiled in water, and the decoction afterwards
fermented with *moloses*, in the common method
of making spruce beer; which will be found
the most efficacious antiscorbutic perhaps of
any fermented liquor, as being of a diuretic
and diaphoretic quality. In extremity tar-water may be tried, fermented in like manner; by
which it will certainly become much more antiscorbutic.

We come now to observe what treatment is
proper for convalescents, or those who are recovering from tedious fits of sickness, by which
they have been greatly exhausted and weakened. Here the prevention of the scurvy will
depend much upon two articles, *viz.* a proper
diet, and exercise. The former must be adapted to the weakness of their digestive powers,
and the sharp and acrimonious condition of the
blood and juices. The latter must be suited to
the

the debilitated ſtate of their body. We find, that when people in this condition at land, and much more ſo in the moiſt ſea-air, are put di-rectly upon a groſs viſcid diet, they are very apt to become ſcorbutic. For theſe, in the firſt place, we would recommend an allowance of flour inſtead of ſalt beef and pork; and (ſea-biſcuit being too groſs food for them) this muſt be well leavened, and baked into freſh bread, inſtead of being cooked into puddings and dumpling, as is common; which will be found an excellent antiſcorbutic; and is, toge-ther with vegetables, eagerly longed for by ſcorbutic perſons. It may appear a direction not eaſily to be complied with, to people unac-quainted with ſea-conveniencies. But many ſhips, eſpecially all ſhips of war, have an oven; and it is a practice with moſt captains, to have their own bread baked twice or thrice a-week, while at ſea. When the patient is extremely weak, a little of this freſh bread ſhould be boil-ed in water, and made into panada; adding a few drops of the juice or extract of lemons, and a ſpoonful of wine.

The other parts of diet ſhould be oat-meal and rice gruels, flumery, roaſted or ſtewed apples, if they can be got, ſtewed barley, with

raiſins

raisins or currants, sago and wine, &c. but particularly the pickled green cabbage, and small onions, boiled with the portable soop made weak. Most food and drink ought to be acidulated with the orange or lemon juice; which at such times proves highly grateful, both to the palate and stomach of the patient; who by degrees, as his appetite, but especially as his strength increases, is to be indulged with more solid food: though he would do well to abstain for some time from grosser animal substances, and take no other restorative but wine, with the proper vegetable and lightest farinaceous substances. A caution is here requisite, that to the convalescents nourishment should be given often, but in a small quantity at a time, so as not to oppress the organs of digestion.

It is likewise a matter of great importance, that the body weakened by preceeding sickness, be by degrees habituated to exercise. Nothing can be more inhumane, than to oblige a poor weak man to undergo more fatigue than his strength can bear; nor any thing more prejudicial to his recovery, than, under the notion of preserving him from the scurvy, to force him too soon to do the ship's duty. On the other

hand,

hand, a total neglect of exercise is peculiarly productive of this disease. The rule then is, to proportion the continuance and degree of it, to the strength and condition of the patients; to begin with the most gentle and easy at first, and proceed gradually to the more violent, as they acquire strength. Thus, after being accustomed to sit up some hours through the day in bed, they are then to be allowed to get out of it, and continue so, as long as their strength, without great weariness or fatigue, will permit. They may next be put into a sling hung below the forecastle, or betwixt decks; which will affect them not only by causing a change of air, but at the same time give spirits and refreshment. They will afterwards be able to bear riding on a crofs deal laid betwixt two chests, where the succeffive concuffions of the body will be more sensibly perceived. And it is to be remarked, that as weak persons at land generally find the greatest benefit from exercise in a coach, chaise, or on horseback; so the convalescents in a ship, especially scorbutical people, will receive much more advantage from this exercise, than from walking, running, or any kind of muscular motion in
which

which a great exertion of ftrength is required. The reafon feems to be, becaufe thefe latter are attended with a wafte and diffipation of fpirits; and are generally followed with wearinefs and fatigue: whereas, by the frequent fucceeding agitations of a jolting machine, the circulation is promoted, the fibres of the body ftrength-ened, and the weakened animal functions invi-gorated, without any confiderable lofs of fpirits, which fuch people cannot well bear.

Thefe and the like exercifes are abfolutely neceffary to prevent the fcurvy in thofe who have hurts, fprained joints, ulcers on their legs, and other ailments, which confine them below, and difable them from walking; in which cafe they foon become fcorbutic, when living on the grofs fea-diet.

Others upon recovery may, at the fame time they practife thefe exercifes, be made to walk a little upon deck, fo as not to over-fatigue them-felves: and afterwards be put upon fuch duty as their condition will permit them to perform: having recourfe, if needful, to *elixir vitriol,* bitters, the bark, or fteel, according as they may be requifite to perfect their ftrength and recovery. To which, however, nothing will contribute fo much, and at the fame time more

effectually

effectually prevent the scurvy, than bodily exercise; which will be found to agree best with them when the stomach is not full, or rather just before meals. It is observed, that when scorbutic people use no exercise, the disease advances very fast upon them at sea: therefore, if they can bear only the most gentle motions, these are often to be practised; and the body is not to be permitted continually to rest, without some sort of action. When confined to bed, frictions may be used upon their limbs and body. Let it however be remembered, that too violent exercise is as dangerous and pernicious in this disease as too little.

I proceed now to point out the means of correcting or removing many inconveniencies which occur at sea, especially those which are observed to be productive of this malady. A most powerful and principal cause of which (*m*), and indeed of many others at sea, is the moisture of the air, and consequently the dampness of their lodging; especially during a long continuance of thick close weather, or a stormy and rainy season. As this is found to be the most frequent cause of this fatal disease, whose effects are rendered still more pernicious when

(*m*) See Part 2. chap. 1.

combined

combined with cold ; thefe require in a particular manner to be guarded againſt. And they
are either immediately to be corrected, or their
effects and confequences prevented.

As to the firſt: Although we cannot at once
remove a perfon into another climate, or into
the land-air; yet we can eafily give to the air
he breathes, a more falutary quality, by rendering it at any time warmer or colder, moiſter
or drier, as the exigency of the cafe and circumſtances may require. I obſerved elfewhere *(n)*, that the noxious qualities of the
moiſt air at fea were greatly heightened by
being confined in fo clofe a place as a fhip, without a fucceſſion, or frefh fupply of it. But
as that inconvenience is fufficiently guarded a-
gainſt by the excellent invention of *Sutton*'s
machine, which extracts all fuch foul and putrid air, and thus will prevent many infectious
malignant fevers caufed from thence; fo there
feems nothing wanting to make it likewife an
excellent prefervative againſt the fcurvy, but
that it fhould correct the moiſture of the fea-
air, and dry or warm it betwixt decks when
needful.

This I conjecture it might be made to do by

(n) Part 2. chap. 1. p. 114.

fome

some additional contrivances, which may invert its operation; that is, instead of drawing up the air from below, the air warmed by the fire in the galley or fire-place, may be forced betwixt decks through its pipes when requisite. I mention it only (for experiments alone must make this improvement, and with such caution as to prevent detriment by it) to induce something of this kind to be thought of by proper judges. If the additional machinery were but small, and not incommodious in the ship, the advantages derived from it would be very great. These are evident from what has been said in discoursing on the causes of the scurvy *(o)*. It must prove highly serviceable in cold climates, and in northern voyages in the winter, (where the sailors not only become terribly scorbutic, but are often chilled to death with the cold, and at other times have their limbs mortified), if, by a simple contrivance of this sort, the fire used for dressing their victuals, could be made to warm them even when in bed.

Fire made with any of the aromatic woods, or even with common fir or pine, juniper, and the like, effectually corrects this disposition of

(o) Chap. 1.

the

the air, and at the fame time renders it more
falutary in other refpects. It is obfervable,
that betwixt the tropics, the rainy feafons prove
the moft unhealthy and dangerous, not only
at land, but in fhips; giving rife to malignant
fevers, fcurvies, &c. In this cafe, without
any inconvenience or danger, a clear open fire,
properly fecured, might be lighted betwixt
decks, to ftand upon the hatchways in a ftove;
which would greatly purify the air, and deftroy
its hurtful moifture, without much increafing the
heat, if burnt in an open hatchway. There
is certainly lefs danger, nay lefs heat, attending
a fire burning for an hour or two in the day
there, guarded by a centinel, than having fifty
or fixty candles lighted in an evening; or burning them conftantly night and day in the orlope,
and other dark places: whence fuch parts of
the fhip are continually replete with the naufe-
ous effluvia of rank corrupted tallow. It
would feem indeed no difficult matter, to convert even thefe into medicinal prefervatives a-
gainft the fcurvy, and other putrid difeafes from
bad moift air, by the addition of fome proper
aromatic in their compofition. The burning
of fpirits will be of fervice in the fick-apart-
ment. The captains, or thofe who can afford

ford them, will find the myrtle wax candles the best for use in a moist sea-air.

Next to be considered, are the best means of preventing the effects and ill consequences of such air, when not corrected by the methods proposed.

Fire, as before observed, is the most certain consumer and drier of humidity. We moreover find, that the exhalations of aromatics, though, properly speaking, they do not dry up moisture, yet prevent the pernicious effects of it upon the human body, by diffusing through the air a subtile acid, of an antiseptic and astringent quality, opposite to the putrid and relaxing tendency of moisture. Thus we often observe many asthmatic persons greatly affected with a moist wind, and in a damp season hardly able to breathe; but upon throwing a little benzoin, or the like aromatic gum, on a red-hot iron, by which their chamber is well perfumed, and the air replete with these aromatic particles, they are sensible of relief, and breathe much more freely. So here I would recommend a most simple and easy operation, to be performed in such damp seasons in a ship; which is, putting a red-hot loggerhead in a bucket of tar, which should be moved about, so that all

the

the ship, once or twice a-day, may be filled with this wholsome antiseptic vapour.

Persons for proper security, during a scorbutic and moist constitution of air, should go well cloathed, and shift often with dry linen. Driness and cleanliness of body are excellent preservatives against this malady. They should use the flesh-brush, or frictions with a dry cloth on their skin; eat a bit of raw onion, or a head of garlic, in a morning before they are exposed to the rains and washings of the sea. Whatever promotes perspiration is useful; and perhaps nothing will do it more effectually at this time than a raw onion. Nor ought these farther precautions to be omitted, of using proper exercise in the day, and having their bedding kept always dry, not binding it up close together till sufficiently aired and dried.

When they are threatened with the approach of this disease, they ought, at going to bed, to promote a gentle *diaphoresis*, by draughts of water-gruel and vinegar, with the addition of lemon-juice, or the extract. They should use plenty of mustard and onions with their victuals; and may then indulge more freely in the use of fermented vinous liquors, *viz.* cyder, beer, and wine: but when of necessity

G g   obliged

obliged to drink fpirits, they ought always to acidulate them with the acid of oranges or lemons. Thefe directions will preferve feamen not only from the fcurvy, but from many other difeafes, as coughs, catarrhs, &c. arifing from an obftructed perfpiration in a moift air.

The water and provifions being often in fuch an unfound and corrupt condition, as may be fuppofed to increafe the virulence of this evil, it will not be improper to add fome confiderations for preventing and remedying thefe inconveniencies.

Water is with difficulty preferved fweet at fea *(p)*; and fometimes cannot even be procured wholfome at places where fhips may touch. There are two forts of bad water. The firft is, putrid and ftinking; the other, a hard heavy water that is not putrid, but which will not incorporate with foap, or break peas when boiled in it. Both are very unwholfome.

Water at fea will fooner or later putrify, according to its various contents, and the man-

(p) See the manner of preferving water good and wholfome at fea by quick-lime, part 3. chap 2.; alfo, Dr *Hales*'s curious philofophical experiments, and his directions to preferve water and provifions at fea.

ner

ner in which it is kept. It has been experienced, that, by fuming the casks with burning
brimstone, water will keep longer sweet.
Some add a little oil of vitriol to it; which
likewise preserves it a longer time from putrifying. It is a common practice, and a very
good one, to throw a little salt into water
while warming; and as it grows hot, there
will arise a thick feculent unwholsome scum,
which is carefully to be taken off as it casts up.
And this should always be done in boiling peas
and oat-meal.

When the water is become putrid and stinking, one manner of sweetening it is, by taking
out the bungs of the casks, exposing it to the
air, and shaking, and pouring it from one vessel into another. Another way is, by letting
it quickly come to boil; taking care not to boil
it too long, which would expel the most active
parts of the water. This will still be rendered
sweeter, and more wholsome, when a little of
the juice or extract of lemons is added to it;
which is much safer for common use, than the
mineral acids of *vitriol*, or salt, ordered by
some on this occasion. The acid will likewise contribute to precipitate the earthy particles of the water, and the various *animalcula*

with

with their sloughs, now destroyed by the boiling.

But as this may be found troublesome to do for a whole ship's company, there is another method of sweetening putrid water. Sometimes, as is observed by my learned friend Dr *Home* (*q*), by keeping such water close and warm in a large vessel, it will become fit for use when the process of putrefaction is once over; by which the noxious and putrescent particles having been made quite volatile, will fly off of themselves; as is often the case of the *Thames* water. A large cask of stinking water closely bunged up, should be put into the galley, and kept in a degree of warmth sufficient to promote this process of putrefaction: the effect of which will be, that the heterogeneous putrescent particles rendered thus volatile, will all quickly escape; and the putrefaction by this means being stopt, the water becomes wholsome, and fit for use.

Besides this putrid water, sailors are often obliged to use, for want of better, a hard water, as it is called, replete with foreign, saline, and terrestrial particles; which is found to be very unwholsome, though fresh and sweet.

(*q*.) In his ingenious essay on the *Dunse* Spaw, p. 119.

To

To make this wholfome and falutary, the ftone filtre ufed on board feveral fhips is very proper, where the water does not abound with vitriolic or marine falts. But its operation is tedious, and it can never pafs a fufficient quantity for the ufe of a fhip's company. Sand is the fitteft body for feparating thefe heterogeneous and unwholfome particles from water. Upon this occafion, I muft again refer to the ingenious effay on the *Dunfe* Spaw *(r)*.

(r) P. 120. The *Auftrian* army, when incamped in *Hungary,* find no good water, unlefs when on the banks of fome great river. So, when obliged to ufe lake-water, they purify it in this manner. A long fmall boat is divided into feveral different apartments by crofs partitions. They fill them all, except the laft, with fand. The boat is put into the lake. A hole level with the furface of the water is made in the end of the boat, which lets the water into the firft divifion; from this it gets into the fecond, by a hole made in the bottom of the firft partition; from the fecond it runs into the third, through a hole in the top of the fecond partition; and fo alternately above and below, that it may be obliged to pafs through all the fand. At the top of the laft divifion there is a pipe, through which the water comes, at pleafure, as pure as from a fine fpring. And thus feamen when abroad meeting with fuch water, may purify even the hardeft kind of it. And for the fame purpofe in a houfe he propofes fome cafks divided in the middle, and filled with fand; into the firft of thefe divifions the water may be thrown as into a ciftern; the cafks ought here to be joined by pipes; and by making it thus circulate through eight or ten divifions filled with fand to the top, a pure fpring may be had any where.

When

When the provisions of beef and pork are putrid and rancid, it will be most advisable not to eat of them; or at least to correct their bad qualities, by using at the same time plenty of vinegar, oranges, lemons, and vegetables. I am afraid any method that might be proposed to sweeten putrid flesh, will be found not easy to be put in execution at sea.

There are several ways generally known of recovering spoiled beer, wines, and other fermented liquors; and as these liquors are all of them antiscorbutic, they are well worth preserving. Yeast should be carried to sea for this and other purposes. When it has grown stale by keeping, a little flour, sugar, salt, and warm beer, are to be mixed with it; or even hot water and sugar only. By adding to it the grounds of strong beer, and letting the mixture stand a little before the fire, it will serve either to work beer, or bake bread. In case there is no yeast on board, honey, sugar, leaven, or molosses, may be used to renew the fermentation of liquors.

The dry provisions, oat-meal, peas, and flour, are apt to be corrupted and spoiled by weevils, maggots, and by growing damp and mouldy. These destructive vermine may be

killed

killed by the fumes of brimstone in a close place. But even then the weevils, when eaten, are found to be very unwholsome, and are said to have such a caustic quality, as, when applied to the skin in the form of a poultis, to raise blisters like the *cantharides.* When no better provisions can be procured, the flour, oat-meal, or peas, should be put in a heap, and then these vermine will come to the top of it; so that a great number of them may be taken away, and sifted out with the dust. The parcel is to be stirred and heaped again, until as many of them as possible are removed. The groats and peas may be turned over into a wire-sieve, which will let the dust and weevils pass through it.

Sound good bread is a most important article at sea. The biscuit, when mouldy and spoiled, should be put into a warm oven, or under the fire-place, till the putrid moisture is quite exhaled, and the *animalcula* destroyed. These are afterwards to be well beat out of it, and then it may be eat dipt in vinegar. Close casks preserve biscuit and other dry provisions best; and all possible care should be taken to keep them dry, and free from dampness.

CHAP.

C H A P. V.

The cure of the difeafe, and its fymptoms.

IF proper precautions were taken for the prevention of this difeafe, and the rules which
have been laid down for that purpofe were complied with, we fhould feldom have occafion to
meet with it in a high degree either at fea or
land. It is indeed difficult to perfuade fome
to practife, when in health, what is neceffary
to preferve fo valuable a bleffing. All mankind have not the benefit of a pure wholfome
air, warm dry lodgings, with proper conveniencies to guard againft the inclemency of different weather and feafons. Many are alfo
of neceffity obliged to live upon fuch grofs
food as is not properly adapted to their digeftive
powers, to their conftitution, and the exercife
they ufe, fo that from thence they may be apt
to contract this evil. It is proper therefore to pre-
fcribe the cure for it, as well as the prevention.

Indeed the general method of it, and the
beft remedies, have already been taken notice
of in the former chapter. Experience fhews,
that the cure of the adventitious fcurvy is very
fimple,

simple, *viz.* a pure dry air, with the use of green herbage or wholsome vegetables, almost of any sort; which for the most part prove effectual.

Hence the first step to be taken towards its removal, when contracted either at sea or land, is change of air. We are upon this occasion informed by several authors, of an odd custom practised in some parts of *Norway* for the recovery of scorbutic people. They expose them in a neighbouring desart island in the summer-season, where they live chiefly on cloud-berries; and it is remarked, that, by eating plentifully of these berries, together with the change of air, they are restored to perfect health in a very short time. In that country, the fruits gathered by the diseased themselves, are reputed of the greatest virtue. It no doubt is the case, as by this means the patient breathes the salutary country-air in the open fields. Thus a free and pure country-air, with such moderate exercise as at the same time conduces to the agreeable amusement of the mind, is requisite.

Their food should be of light and easy digestion. The most proper is, broths or soops made with fresh meat, and plenty of vegetables, *viz.* cabbage, coleworts, leeks, onions, &c. Fresh and well-baked wheat bread must be gi-

ven

ven them. Salads of any kind are beneficial; but especially the mild faponaceous herbs, dandelion, forrel, endive, lettuce, fumitory, and purflain. To which may be added, scurvy-grafs, creffes, or any of the warmer fpecies of plants, in order to correct the cooling qualities of fome of the former; as experience fhews the beft cures are performed by a due mixture of the hotter and colder vegetables. Summer-fruits of all forts are here in a manner fpecific, *viz.* oranges, lemons, citrons, apples, *&c.* For drink, good found beer, cyder, or Rhenifh wine, are to be prefcribed.

Thus, we have numberlefs inftances of people, after long voyages, by a vegetable diet and good air, miraculoufly as it were, recovered from deplorable fcurvies, without the affiftance of many medicines. For which indeed there is no great occafion; provided the green herbage and frefh broths keep the belly lax, and pafs freely by urine, fweat, or perfpiration. But when otherwife, it will be neceffary to open the belly, every other day or fo, by a decoction of tamarinds and prunes, adding fome diuretic falts; and upon the intermediate days, to fweat the patient in a morning with camphorated bolufes of theriac, and warm draughts of *decoct.* *lign.*;

lign.; and, as has been ufual in fome of our hofpitals, give twelve or fifteen grains of *pil. fcillit.
pharm. Edin.* twice or thrice through the day.

But it is here to be obferved, that though
the recovery of fuch perfons feems promifing
and fpeedy at firft, yet it requires a much longer continuance of the vegetable diet, and a proper regimen, to perfect it, than is commonly
imagined. There are many inftances of feamen who have been fent from the hofpitals,
after having been three weeks or a month on
fhore, to their refpective fhips, who in all appearance were in perfect health; yet, in a fhort
time after being on board, relapfed, and became
highly fcorbutic. It were to be wifhed, that
either a longer continuance was allowed fuch
men at the hofpital, or that their cure was rendered more perfect by a fweating courfe.

It is indeed frequently experienced, that people once deeply infected, are extremely apt to
relapfe into fymptoms of this difeafe, in different periods of their life afterwards. There
are likewife fome particular conftitutions, who,
from the peculiar tendency and difpofition of
their humours to the fcorbutic corruption, are,
from much flighter caufes, more liable than o-
thers to fall into the fcurvy. In fuch cafes,

thefe

thefe people, in order to purify their blood from this deep-feated fcorbutic taint or tendency, befides the diet and regimen before recom-mended, fhould alfo have recourfe to other me-dicinal helps; fome of the beft of which have been already mentioned in the foregoing chapter.

But in this place I fhall more particularly deliver,

1*ft*, The method proper to remove a fcor-butic habit of body, whether acquired by a deep infection, or conftitutional.

2*dly*, The different treatment of fcorbutic patients, adapted to the various fymptoms of their difeafe; when the urgency of fuch fymp-toms requires a particular attention; but efpe-cially when the general method of cure cannot be complied with.

3*dly*, I fhall obferve what remedies have been recommended upon good authority, and are ufed in different countries.

And, 4*thly*, Conclude with fome neceffary cautions and obfervations.

To begin with the *firft* of thefe: In order thoroughly to fubdue a fcorbutic taint, the phyfical intentions muft be, to keep the outlets and emunctories of the body open and clear, for the gentle evacuation of the fcorbutic acrimo-

ny,

ny, *(viz.* the belly, urinary paſſages, and ex-
cretory duſts of the ſkin): mean while, the remaining maſs of humours is rendered mild,
ſoft, and balſamic, by proper antiſcorbutic
food and medicine.   And it is to be remarked,
that all the above evacuations are moſt ſucceſſ-
fully promoted, when the medicines for theſe
intentions are joined with antiſcorbutics.

Here milk of all ſorts, where it agrees
with the conſtitution, is beneficial; as being
a truly vegetable chyle, an emulſion prepared
of the moſt ſucculent wholſome herbs: but
whey, by reaſon of its more diuretic and clean-
ſing quality, is rather preferable.   And upon
this occaſion the *ſal polychreſt.* will be found a
very uſeful addition, as it is a mild purgative,
an excellent diuretic; and when taken in a
ſmall quantity, well diluted, evacuates plentifully, either by perſpiration or urine, according as its operation is direſted to the ſkin or
kidneys, by exerciſe, lying in bed, or keeping
the body warmer or cooler.

Goats, of all animals, afford the richeſt whey,
poſſeſſed of the greateſt antiſcorbutic virtues.
It contains a moſt noble, reſtorative, vegetable balſam, which in a ſingular manner ſweet-
ens and correſts the ſcorbutic acrimony.

The

The *succi scorbutici* of the *Edinburgh* and *London pharmacopœia's*, where the volatile acrimony of the hotter species of plants is qualified by a due quantity of the juice of *Seville* oranges, are likewise proper in their season. They will be experienced yet more serviceable, when made farther diuretic and cleansing, by being clarified with whey. Besides taking them in this manner through the day, the patient ought to be sweated in a morning, twice or thrice a-week, by draughts of the said juices mixed with sack-whey.

This method cannot be sufficiently recommended. It is an evacuation, which, of all others, scorbutic persons bear the best, and from which they find the greatest benefit; what nature pointed out to the northern *Indians* for the cure of this their endemic evil *(a)*, and which experience confirms to be a most efficacious remedy. It is practised with remarkable success by the surgeons at the Cape of *Good Hope*, who have the greatest opportunity of treating scorbutic seamen *(b)*; is recommended by the first and best writers on this disease *(c)*;

(a) Vid. Part 3. chap. 1.
(b) Vid. *Kolben's* account of the Cape of *Good Hope*
(c) *Wierus, Albertus, &c.*

and

and seems to have been the most usual way of their giving these juices.

There are, besides, other herbs, whose juices are here of eminent virtue. Such especially, from their saponaceous and mild aperient quality, are *dens leonis* and *fumaria*. And an antiscorbutic inferior to none, is the juice of the tender sprouting tops of green wheat, in the months of *June* and *July*, mixed with the juice of *Seville* oranges.

But, during all these courses, scorbutic habits will find great benefit by warm baths, (provided there be no danger from a hæmorrhage), in which the aromatic and fragrant plants have been infused, *viz.* rosemary, marjoram, thyme, *&c.:* and these are preferable to the usual manner of sweating them in stoves or bagnios.

In the winter-time, for the cure of this disease, genuine spruce beer, with lemon and orange juice, is to be prescribed; or an antiscorbutic ale by infusion of wormwood, *rad. raphani*, mustard-seed, and the like, made gently laxative by addition of senna. It must be drank when pretty fresh or new. But the spring is the most favourable season for a perfect recovery from a scorbutic habit.

HAVING

HAVING said this much on the cure of the disease in general, I come, *secondly*, to observe what is proper to be done for the relief and removal of its most urgent symptoms.

When first the patient complains of an itching and spunginess of the gums, with loose teeth, aluminous medicines will be found most serviceable in putting a stop to the beginning laxity of these parts. But, upon the putrefaction increasing, a gargle is to be used of barley-water, and *mel rosat.* acidulated with some of the mineral acids. The *sp.* or *elix. vitriol* is generally prescribed; but some have imagined *sp. salis* less hurtful to the teeth. The quantity of the acid must be proportioned to the greater or lesser degree of putrefaction in the parts. The *fungus* must be often removed, or, if needful, cut away; and, by frequent gargarising, the mouth kept as clean as possible. Where the ulcers appear deep and spreading, they are to be checked with a touch of *ol. vitriol*, either by itself, or diluted, according as the patient bears it.

In a spontaneous salivation; or, as is much oftener the case, when a copious spitting has unfortunately been induced by some mercurial medicine, where immediate danger is apprehended,

hended, fpeedy revulfion muft be made from
the falivary glands, by epifpaftics applied to different parts of the body, finapifms to the foles
of the feet and hams; and by opening the
belly with glyfters, and fuch gentle purgatives
as operate only in the firft paffages. But the
impetus of the blood, and colliquated humours,
is here to be determined, particularly to the
pores of the fkin: a defect of perfpiration,
generally attended with a ftricture and fpafm
on the *cutis* in fcorbutic habits, being the true
caufe why the force of the mercury fo powerfully falls upon the falivary glands. For this
purpofe, bolufes of theriac, with camphire,
and *flor. fulph.* are to be given, and repeated
every four or fix hours, in order to force a
fweat; which proves the beft means of abating
the ftrength of the falivation, and refcuing the
patient from the danger of being choked by
it. Gargles at the fame time muft be ufed,
with *oxym. fcill.* to attenuate the thick and vifcous *faliva.* When by this management the
moft threatening danger is prevented, there
generally continues, for a confiderable time,
a troublefome falivation, with great putrefaction in the mouth; which it is very difficult
to put a ftop to. It may however be palliated

by

by keeping the belly and urinary paſſages o-
pen with glyſters, or by diuretic and gentle
phyſic; avoiding all ſtrong cathartics, or whatever may farther promote the diſſolution of the
blood.   Inviſcating and glutinous medicines
are ſometimes ſerviceable, *viz. gum Arabic,*
ichthyocolla, &c. · diſſolved in common drink.
Aſtringent gargariſms of alum, and a decoction of the *cortex quercûs,* are indiſpenſa-
bly neceſſary: as alſo the *cort. peruv.* and *e-*
lixir vitriol. taken inwardly.   Mean while, the
ſtrength of the patient muſt carefully be ſup-
ported by warm mulled wines, *&c.*   Such perſons, when much exhauſted, are to be confined altogether to a milk and vegetable diet.
    When the legs are ſwelled and œdematous,
gentle frictions are to be uſed at firſt, with
warm flannel, or woollen cloths charged with
the fumes of *benzoin.* and amber, or any o-
ther of the aromatic gums; provided the ſwelling be ſmall, ſoft, and not very painful; roll-
ing up afterwards with an eaſy bandage
from below upwards.   But if the legs are
much ſwelled, ſtiff, and painful, they muſt
be fomented with a warm diſcutient fomentation; which will afford ſome momentary relief,
without putting a ſtop to the progreſs of the
ſwelling:

fwelling: or what I have found preferable,
is the fteam of the fomentation received by the
member well covered round with a blanket or
cloths.   And this operation muft be repeated
night and morning.   It is generally followed
with remarkable fupplenefs and eafe in the ftiff,
painful, and contracted joints.   Upon this occafion, I have indeed often prefcribed the
fteam of warm water only, with the addition of a
little vinegar, or crude *fal ammoniac.* After receiving the fume on their joints clofely covered
up for half an hour, they are to be anointed
with *ol. palmæ.*   If fuch fwellings are not removed foon after being put upon a vegetable
diet, the limb fhould be fweated by burning
of fpirits, or with bags of warm falt.

Ulcers on the legs, or any other part of the
body, require pretty much the fame treatment,
viz. very gentle compreffion, in order to keep
under the *fungus,* and fuch antifeptic applications as have been recommended for the putrid
gums, *viz. mel rofat.* acidulated with *fp. vitriol.*
ung. Ægyptiac. &c.   But nothing will avail
where the patient cannot have vegetables or
fruits.

In dangerous hæmorrhages from thefe ulcers, or from the gums, nofe, *&c.* the mine-

ral acids, *viz. sp.* or *el. vitriol.* are to be given, and often repeated, in small quantities at a time, so that they may more certainly and easily enter the lacteals, and get into the blood; together with small doses of the *cort. peruv.* when it agrees with the stomach. These likewise, with red wine, are the principal medicines to be relied upon in their putrid and colliquative fevers.

For pain of the limbs, in the small of the back, and breast, and universally in most of their pains, whether fixed or wandering, the *oxym. scill.* is to be administered in a warm diaphoretic mixture; where wine must supply the place of a spirituous cordial: and the patient, upon going to bed, should, by warm draughts of water-gruel, with vinegar, or, in place of the latter, the *acetum theriacale*, endeavour to force a sweat. But most of these complaints yield readily to the general method of cure, and can only be palliated until that is undergone *(d)*.

There

(d) Extract of a letter from Mr Murray.

N. B. The letters *(a)*, *(b)*, *(c)*, *(d)*, refer to some remarks subjoined.

Untoward fortune has too often placed me among a number of scorbutic patients, where vegetables and proper diet, and even many necessary medicines, were wanting, and where the
very

There remain two symptoms of this disease, which are, of all others, the most obstinate to remove, even though the patient enjoys the benefit of the purest air, with the most proper antiscorbutic

very elements were our enemies; and I have spent many melancholy hours considering what was best to be done to overcome this enemy, and stop the progress of this often fatal, and always loathsome distemper. And although I have seldom cured my patient without vegetables; yet the relief I have given to many, amply rewarded my labour, and the reflection to this day gives me pleasure. I shall first give you my method in general, and then I can produce an instance of its success.

Many at the time had a miliary fever, which I then judged to be purely scorbutic. But, since the receipt of your last letter, I have altered my opinion; and submit to your decision, that there is no such thing as a fever that may be so termed. I was always averse to bleeding, for the reasons you give: yet if the scurvy was the primary disease, (as I then judged it), preceeded by high febrile symptoms, and the habit was originally found or plethoric, I never observed any hurt from the loss of a small quantity of blood; which made a succeeding vomit always more safe; and this was followed by a purge, either cooling or warm, as symptoms indicated. Of the first sort was the purging salts, with *sal tartar.* or *tartar. vitriolat.* dissolved in *decoct. lignorum;* or *infus. sennæ et tamarindor. &c.* Of the last kind was *infus. amar. cum senna,* with the addition of a proper quantity of *canella alba.* And these were repeated occasionally.

So soon as the symptoms of scurvy appeared, I discharged the use of salt meat; and confined my patients to the vegetable articles of diet on board, with what fresh victuals could be had from the officers tables. Their common drink was *decoct. lignor.* with their allowance of rum (*a*) put into it. The medical course I put them under, was for most part a neutral mixture of vinegar and *sal tartar;* of which I gave from two to

four

antiscorbutic food and medicines. These are,
the scorbutic dysentery in some; and in others,
a hard bound cough, accompanied with *dyspnœa*,
pain and disorder in the breast. This last
often

four ounces twice or thrice a-day. *Spirit. mindereri* was beneficial to some; but the small quantity of volatile salts or spirits
carried to sea, prevented that from being a general medicine. I
have also given a mixture of *cremor* and *sal tartar.* with success,
and sometimes *tartar. vitriolat. (b)*. In violent scorbutic
pains, diaphoretic anodynes of *acet. theriacal.* or *theriac.
andromach.* with *spirit. minderer.* and *oxym. scillit.* I have found
very serviceable : as likewise the last in particular for disorders
of the *thorax*. In visceral obstructions, I gave the ferulaceous
gums, with *gum. guajac.* soap, and *tartar of vitriol*; and
sometimes added only *gum. guajac.* and *tartar of vitriol* to the squill
pills. The liver or spleen, perhaps both, are sometimes affected,
especially that lobe of the first which stretches over the *pylo-
rus*. Hence I have known violent pain at the pit of the stomach ; and the hardness and pain I have sometimes observed at
the *fundus* of that *viscus*, leave no doubt of the *pancreas* being also obstructed. The mesenteric glands share the same fate.
Hence, as observed in your description of this disease, towards the
close of it, from these obstructions proceed violent colic-pains,
jaundice, &c.; all which I have seen ; as also great tension of
the *abdomen*, lienteries, &c. The appetite then begins to fail, the
lungs are affected, respiration becomes contracted, the motion
of the heart less vigorous, the circulation languid, and placid
death closes the scene.

But to return to my practice at sea : Where there was any topical pain, I fomented with a ley of wood-ashes, in which was
boiled camomile and elder flowers, wormwood, rue, &c. and
lemon-peel, when it could be got. For the fungous gums, I
made a powder of *bol. armen, alum. rup. tart. vitriol.* and *g.
myrrh.*

often ends in a confumption: while the former, or flux, is very troublefome to ftop, and fometimes alfo proves fatal.

Scorbutic

myrrh. wafhing them with *infuf. falviæ* ; to which I added *alum. rup.* and *el. vitriol.* or *fp. fal.* ; which ferved alfo in ulcers, when I added honey. Thefe laft I touched frequently with a rag dipt in *mel Ægyptiac. rofat. fp. fal. d. et tinɛt. myrrh.* I dreff- ed ulcers of the extremities chiefly with *ung. Ægyptiac. mercu- rial.* and *liniment. arcæi* mixed together. When the patient was altogether free from feverifh fymptoms, I gave three or four ounces twice a-day, along with *decoɛt. lignorum,* of the *tinɛt. ad fto- machicos (c) Phar. Ed.* ; to which I added muftard-feed and *canel- la alba.* When he began to recover, I ftrenuoufly infifted on his ufing exercife, and embrocated the contraɛted joints or tendons as you direɛt. Such was my general praɛtice; and the follow- ing is an inftance of its fuccefs.

Benjamin Lovelay, aged 25 years, had a continual fever in *September* 1746; for which he was fent to the hofpital at *Louif- burg*; and from thence returned, to all appearance well, the 13th *Oɛtober* following. On the 30th *November,* (being taken ill the day before), he was feverifh, and complained of violent pain in his bones and joints. Upon account of the fcurvy being then epidemic, he was very fparingly blooded, took a vomit, and was purged. Upon which the fever fubfided a little; and there appeared a miliary eruption, foon after followed with the feveral fcorbutic fymptoms in the greateft degree; to which was added a violent pain in the pit of his ftomach, inclining to the right fide, often fo violent as to make him fhriek out. The fymptoms continued upon the increafe for fome time; and at laft he grew fo bad, as to faint away upon the leaft motion. The antifcorbutic regimen above defcribed was fteadily purfued. His common drink was *decoɛt. lignor.* acidulated with *elixir vi- triol.* His diet was water-gruel, rice, fago with wine, and

fometimes

Scorbutic diarrhœas at sea are not suddenly to be stopt; as the acrimonious humour must

sometimes a little fresh broth or meat from the officers table. The several forms of medicines already mentioned were administered as symptoms required; and I think he had almost every symptom belonging to the disease, attended with feverishness, all along till the decline of the distemper; when I added aloes and *extract. gentian.* to his pills, and begun the use of the *tinct. ad stomachic.* The bile in most chronical diseases, especially in the scurvy, is defective either in quality or quantity, and something must be given to supply its defects. The disease took a turn for the better in the beginning of *January*, and he returned to his duty on the 22d of *February (d)*.

I shall use the freedom with my ingenious friend to make some remarks on his letter.

(a) Wine would probably have been better: for whatever effects rum diluted in this manner with an antiscorbutic medicine might have had; yet all distilled spirituous liquors may be suspected as hurtful.

(b) The medicines were no doubt properly adapted in the cases to which they seem to allude; which were fevers and scurvies: these saline neutral draughts being certainly preferable in such cases to the soap, squill, and garlic pills, commonly prescribed in scurvies without a fever.

(c) The medicine recommended, is truly an excellent restorative; proper for prevention of the scurvy in such as are recovering from other diseases, and to confirm the strength of scorbutic persons when in the convalescent state. But I must own a like medicine did not agree with those who were in neither of these situations to whom I gave it. Bitters of the terebinthinated kind, though dry and kept; also all fresh and succulent plants and fruits of this quality, are nevertheless most efficacious antiscorbutics.

(d) The case is curious and singular.

some

some way or other be discharged; and it may as well pass off by the guts as by any other outlet. They, however, are to be moderated. The tone of the intestines must be strengthened: mean while, the peccant humour is gently evacuated by small doses of rhubarb, occasionally repeated; to which a little *theriac.* or *diascord.* is always to be joined, with a view to keep up perspiration; an important point. For this purpose, *decoctum fracastor.* or boluses of *diascord.* with other warm diaphoretic and strengthening medicines, are principally to be given; and *opium* more freely, in extreme cases. Mean while, the patient is supported with strong rough red wine, diluted, and a glutinous subastringent diet. I have sometimes given four or five grains of crude alum in a *diascord.* bolus, where the blood was evacuated in great quantity; and when it passed the stomach without ruffling, it generally did service. In this last case, *tinct. rosar.* well acidulated, and other styptics, are necessary.

I know no peculiar treatment proper in the scorbutic dysentery, different from what has been recommended by authors on that disease, farther than that the use of greens, and especially of the austere and acid fruits, is to be per-

mitted

mitted. I am informed by Mr *Christie,* formerly surgeon to the naval hospital at *Port-Mahon,*
that, after trial of many medicines, he found an
infusion of *ipecacuan.* in brandy, given in small
quantities, often repeated, the most effectual
remedy to remove it. Rhubarb-purges, stomachic bark-bitters, *elixir vitriol.* or the use of
some light steel mineral water, will serve to perfect a recovery here; as in all other scorbutic
cases, where the patient has been much exhausted by colliquative evacuations and hæmorrhages, usual in this disease.

For scorbutic pectoral disorders, blistering
and issues are proper at land; as also riding on
horseback in the country-air; an entire milk
and vegetable diet; keeping the breast open by
expectorants. Such are *oxym. scillit. gum. ammoniac.* and *bals. copaiv.*

When the scorbutic taint has been entirely
subdued, it sometimes leaves behind it other
disorders; which require the same treatment as
is proper for them when proceeding from o-
ther causes; together with a mixture of antiscorbutic medicines for farther security.

Besides the consumptive disposition now mentioned, a dropsical habit is now and then contracted; or, what is more frequent, the legs remain

main swelled, œdematous, and ulcerated. In
this last case, if the ulcers have been of long
standing, sufficient provision being made for
healing them up, by purging, and issues near
the part, an electuary of the prepared crude antimony may be given, with the addition of æthiops
mineral; and at the same time an antiscorbutic
diet-drink used: or, provided they are obstinate, and the gums sufficiently hardened, the
patient may undergo a slow and gentle course
of mercury. In scorbutic habits, I generally
kill the mercury with a small quantity of *balf.*
sulph. tereb. and find it succeed well, where
the intention is not to raise a copious salivation.
A bottle of decoction of the woods must be
drank every day at the same time. This, by
promoting a diaphoresis, will assist the operation of the mercury, and determine the dissolved humours more particularly to the cutaneous secretion. After this course, a few grains
of *sulph. aur. antim.* will perhaps be necessary
evening and morning, or Dr *Plummer*'s medicine *(e)*, and the continuance of the decoction
of woods; which in all probability will complete the cure.

Those that are troubled, after having been

(e) Vid. Medical Essays, vol. 1.

afflicted

afflicted in the scurvy, with numbness and pain in their joints, or chronic rheumatic pains, must practise riding, swallow a spoonful of un-beat mustard-feed once or twice a-day, or undergo the mercurial course as above directed, and be well sweated.

It may be now proper to observe, in the *third* place, what other remedies have been recommended for this disease, and are reputed in different countries. I elsewhere *(f)* took notice of the *pinus antiscorbutica,* the spruce shrub, and their virtues. The learned *Boerhaave* is said to have prescribed, for the most part, new churned milk. *Cort. winteran.* first came into repute, from the good effects it was supposed to have had in Captain *Winter*'s crew, belonging to Sir *Francis Drake*'s squadron.

There is a remarkable observation given us by *Bernard Below (g)*, of the great virtue of *herba vermicularis*, wall-pepper, in this disease. He boiled eight handfuls of the herb in eight pints of old ale, to half the quantity, in a close vessel. Of this a warm draught, *viz.* three or four ounces, was taken every morning, or every o-

(f) Page 222.

(g) Miscell. curios. medico physic. academ. natur. curios. ann. 6. *et* 7. *obs.* 22.

ther

ther morning, on an empty stomach, as the patient bore it: which had the happy effect to cure almost all the soldiers of the army afflicted in this disease; excepting a few, who, by the severity of the preceeding winter, were reduced into a condition past recovery. He remarked, that those who were vomited easily and most plentifully by the medicine, soonest recovered. He made use of this decoction, with the addition of alum and *mel rosat.* by way of gargle for the gums, which were in all affected and putrid; and by this simple remedy cured above fifty, who had the tendons in the ham contracted, applying the boiled herb warm to the part. He bathed their ulcers with the same decoction, and applied the warm herb to them in like manner.

There is an instance given by *Etmuller (h)*, of the soldiers in a besieged garrison greatly over-run with this disease, who were all perfectly cured by *ruta muraria*, white maiden hair.

Chelidonium minus, pilewort, or little celandine, for its supposed great virtues, has by the *Germans* been called *schorbock rout*. But the

(h) *Schroderi dilucidati phytologia.*

Danes

Danes (i) efteem moft *trifolium paluſtre*, marfh trefoil; which they adminifter fometimes by it-felf, at other times with the addition of fcur-vy-grafs.

We are informed *(k)*, that the *Swedes*, e-ver fince the furprifing recovery of their troops, when afflicted with this malady, by the ufe of a decoction of fir-tops, efteem it altogether fpe-cific in the fcurvy.

In *Groenland*, where this difeafe is extremely frequent, we are told by a gentleman *(l)* who twice vifited the country, that the natives make ufe of fcurvy-grafs *(m)* and forrel toge-ther;

(*i*) *Vid. Act. Haff. vol.* 3. *obf.* 75.   *Etmul. Schrod. dilucid. phytol. p.* 104.   *Simon. Pauli digreff. de vera caufa febrium fcor-buti*, &c.

(*k*) *Vid. Moellenbroek, p.* 116.   *Etmul. Schroderi dilucidati phy-tolog: p.* 2.   See the account of it, chap. 4.

(*l*) *Hermannus Nicolai.   Vid. Act. Haffn. vol.* 1. *obf.* 9.

(*m*) Communicated by the ingenious Mr *Thomas Maude*, fur-geon in *Brookſtreet, Holborn.*

The fhips who are annually employed in the whale-fifhery, are of all others the beft fitted out, both as to the variety and quality of their food; the voyage is fhort, and the feamen kept much in action: fo that bad water and decayed provi-fions can fcarcely fall to their fhare.   Yet it is notoriously known, that there is no part in the world where fhips crews are fo liable to the fcurvy, as in the polar circle.   Thofe who are feized on their firft entrance into the cold, find an increafe of their fymptoms when got into the ice.   The attack of the ma-lady

ther; and that these two herbs, put with barley or oats in broths made of fowls, or the flesh
of rein-deer, have an effect to recover the diseased most surprisingly in a short time, even
after having lost the use of their limbs.

The *Norway* cure affords the only one well-
attested instance, of this distemper being success-
fully removed by what would seem so diffe-

lady is here more sudden, and its progress more rapid, than any
where else. The patient has seldom any cure or alleviation till
the weather softens: for the month of *July* is very moderate,
which is almost the only pause of winter; and at this time the
scurvy-grass steps in, and performs incredible wonders. I have
been an eye-witness to many scorbutics who have recovered in
a few days, from what one would judge an irrecoverable state,
by a plentiful use of this *Greenland* salad. It is much coveted
by the sound as well as sick. Our field and garden scurvy-
grass are bitter and pungent; this is mild and esculent, resembling our sea scurvy-grass, or *cochlearia minima ex montibus Wal-
liæ*. It is said to acquire a pungency, if transplanted into
warmer countries; but this circumstance I much doubt. However, be that as it will, its efficacy in the scurvy is there an undoubted and daily experienced truth; and it may be justly
deemed one of the most powerful antiscorbutics in the world.
Vegetable food prevails over the sea-scurvy in all parts; but
this reinstates in as many hours, as any other course requires
days. I cannot dismiss these reflections, without observing
how kind and provident Nature has been in the plentiful supply of this sovereign plant every where in that country. *Ubi
morbus ibi remedium*, is an observation of antiquity; and no
where more justly verified than in the present case.

rent from the nature of vegetables, as a fossil
or earth. It is related by authors of undoubted credit (*n*), particularly by *Petræus* (*o*),
who practised at that place; and seems to have
been known before *Eugalenus* had confounded
most other diseases with the true scurvy; as it
is taken notice of in the year 1624 by *Sennertus*, when *Eugalenus*'s writings, in all probability, might not have reached *Norway*.   It is
a reddish or blackish earth, dug up nigh *Ber-
gen*; of which, from half a dram to a dram
is the dose; and operating by sweat, it is said
to cure the patient in a short time.

I mentioned two very bad scorbutic cases
which lately occurred in *Fife* (*p*).   The surgeon, upon seeing the patients, inquired what
had been their ordinary food, and whether
they commonly eat any green herbs or vegetables? One of them, a fisherman, replied,
That he lived upon bread, dried and salted fish,
which was all he could afford; and sometimes
salt beef, of which last he was very fond.   The
surgeon desired them to abstain from their former diet; in place of which, they were to

(*n*) *Vid. Wormii musæum; Bartholini epist. cent.* 1. *n.* 89.
(*o*) *Vid. Differt. harmonic.*
(*p*) *Vid.* Chap. 2. p. 174.

make

make two good meals a-day upon a vegetable
soop, prepared of coleworts and other green
garden-stuff; and to eat water-cresses by way
of salad. He besides prescribed a fomentation
for their legs, and gave them a dose or two of
very gentle physic. By which means they both
recovered; and one of them soon after, over-
joyed upon being restored to the use of his
limbs, walked several miles to return the gentleman thanks for his salutary advice.

I shall now conclude what I have to say on
this head, with the following cautions and observations.

1*st*, As to evacuations: It is to be observed,
that this disease, especially when advanced, by
no means bears bleeding; even although the
most acute pains upon the membranes, a
high degree of fever, and dangerous hæmorrhages, would seem to indicate it. The patient
generally dies soon after the operation. Nor
does it bear strong cathartics, which are often
injudiciously administered in its commence-
ment; many of which only farther promote
the colliquation and acrimony of the blood
and humours. The belly must at all times be
kept open, but chiefly by such laxative food,
when green vegetables cannot be obtained, as

may

may anfwer this purpofe, *viz.* barley and currants, ftewed prunes, *&c.*; or with a decoction
of tamarinds and *cremor tartar.* a morfel of
lenitive electuary, fea-water, and the like.
From blifters there is danger of a gangrene.
As to vomits; though I never have had any
great experience of their effects; yet, by the obfervation of others, fquill-vomits have been
found ferviceable.

2*dly*, Perfons in the advanced ftages of this
difeafe, are not, without great caution and pru-
dence, to be expofed to a fudden change of air;
or brought up from lying a-bed below in the
hold of a fhip, to the frefh air, in order to their
being landed. On this occafion, though feemingly pretty hearty, they are to be given a
glafs of generous wine, well acidulated with lemon or orange juice; which is likewife the
beft cordial in their fainting-fits. When they
drop down feemingly dead, it were to be wifhed, that fome methods were tried for their recovery; as putting them into a warm bed; u-
fing of ftrong ftimulants, and frictions; blow-
ing into the lungs, *anus, &c.*

3*dly*, After a long abftinence from greens
and fruits, fcorbutic perfons fhould be treated
like one almoft ftarved to death; that is, not
                                                    permitted

permitted for a few days to eat voracioufly, or
furfeit themfelves with them; otherwife they
are apt to fall into a dyfentery, which often
proves mortal.

Laftly, There are but few medicines carried
out in a fea-cheft, which are here of fervice.
Thofe of the foffil or mineral kind, fuch as
fteel, antimony, and efpecially mercury, do
manifeft harm.   Opiates occafion an unaccountable lownefs and dejection of fpirits, with
an oppreffion on the breaft.   When they are
abfolutely neceffary, as in fluxes, they muft
be given always of the warmeft kind; and a-
gree beft, when, before or during their operation, a ftool is procured: after which the patient is to be refrefhed with wine.   Where the
breaft was much affected, I always gave them
in a draught of fquill-mixture; or, in cafe the
ftools were not very frequent, I added a few
grains of vitriolated tartar to the opiate bolus,
in order to procure a difcharge that way.

After trial of many medicines in the fea-
invoice, there are but two I can principally
recommend.

The firft is the *cort. peruv.* infufed in wine.
I gave at the fame time a decoction of *lign.
guajac.* (of which there is great plenty in fhips),

with

with the addition of *rad. glycyrrh.* which prevented the heartburn that the decoction otherwise occasioned. The bark did not always a-
gree with the stomach; but where it did, I observed a more favourable appearance upon the
gums and ulcers, by its checking the putrefaction: and in two instances where a gangrenous
disposition was induced by too tight a roller,
the suppuration next day was more laudable.
It was of use in salivations and hæmorrhages,
but rather hurtful in fluxes. Warm draughts
of the decoction gave always relief, if the patient sweated; in which case the bark also a-
greed better.

But another, and more excellent medicine, is
the *oxym. scill.* from which I have experienced extreme good effects. It generally kept
the belly open, and promoted the secretion of
urine; by both evacuations discharging the a-
crimonious humours. It gave relief in many
of their complaints, particularly those of the
breast, which scorbutic people are seldom free
from. I had formerly gathered a great quantity of this root when at *Minorca*; and having
made the *oxym. scillit.* gave it to most of our
patients in the year 1747, at the rate of one
ounce, or an ounce and a half, in the space of
twenty-

twenty-four hours, with remarkable eafe of their complaints *(q).*

Conclufion of Dr Grainger's *letter (fee p.* 173.*), giving an account of fcurvies at* Fort-William.

——Warned by my former miftake, I never ufed the lancet, unlefs the patient was uncommonly plethoric; and then too a very fmall quantity of blood anfwered the purpofe. I have feen fellows who have often borne the lofs of twenty ounces, faint when only fix were drawn from them at this time.   Upon ftanding, it did not feparate, but appeared like the blood in malignant fevers, altogether diffolved, and of a livid colour.   Some of the fymptoms, vomits of *ipecacuan.* rather increafed, *viz.* pains, faintifhnefs, *dyfpnœa*, bleeding of the gums, *&c.*: they abated none of them.   Indeed it was lucky that the ftomach feldom required their adminiftration.

(q) The eminent antifcorbutic virtue of the fquill or fea-onion, at the fame time that it confutes the groundlefs opinion of the ill effects of acrid medicines in the moft putrid fcurvies, in fome meafure confirms the efficacy of what has been recommended in the foregoing chapter, and has been fo often experienced beneficial for prevention, *viz.* common onions, and even garlic, as in fome refpects they are all of fimilar virtues.

Purgatives,

Purgatives, however, were found highly beneficial, though repeated every third day,
They not only removed the troublefome fymptoms arifing from coftivenefs; but their operation, though fometimes pretty brifk, I never
obferved to impair the patient's ftrength, and
always remarkably abated their excruciating
tortures. Although I gave at firft an infufion
of jalap; yet, obferving bloody ftools to have
enfued on its ufe, I afterwards exchanged it for
a ptifan of *fenna*, with *cremor tartar.*; which
feemed to anfwer better. One man drank
falt water every other day, and found it a ferviceable purge. Would it cure the fcurvy?

But thefe, though ufeful, were not able a-
lone to cope with the diftemper. An atten-
tive confideration of its fymptoms feemed to
fhew it was putrid. On this I founded my
practice; and had foon the pleafure to find,
that fuccefs confirmed my conjecture.

The antifeptics I chiefly ufed, were, *el. vitriol.* to the quantity of half a dram twice a-day,
in water; or *fp. nitr. dul.* in a fmaller dofe. A
gentle *mador* was alfo folicited by a bolus of
camphire and nitre, of each half a fcruple, given every night. For this purpofe too they
were allowed to drink plentifully of warm fage
tea;

tea ; which, with the affiftance fometimes of
a glafs of mulled claret, feldom defeated our
intentions.   If they did not fweat, an increafe
of very fœtid urine fupplied happily that difcharge.   Greens were proper : but as they
could not be had, broths made of young flefh,
kid, *&c.* with barley, were indulged them ;
whilft camomile drank like tea, afforded a truly
medical breakfaft.   The good effect of this
management was foon vifible in all.

Ulcers of the gums, *&c.* not only required
the continuance of the prefcribed meafures,
but the bark, and detergent gargarifms, were
found indifpenfable auxiliaries.   I have applied
blifters to the pained members.   The practice
did not anfwer.   They brought on a gangrenous difpofition in one man ; which bark, and
the ftrongeft antifeptics, with difficulty put a
ftop to ; and in all rather increafed their tor-
ments.   The following epithems were found
highly anodyne.   ℞. *fp. è hordeo elicit.* (*vulgo*
whifky) *acet. acerr. ana lib.* i. *fp. tereb. lib.* fs. *fal.
tart. unc.* fs. *M.*   The milder was, whifky and
vinegar *p. æ.* camphire and foap *q. f.*   With one
or other of thefe the difcoloured and pained places were chafed.   Their gums at the fame time
were not neglected.   The pain of them made
the

the men extremely importunate for relief. Of
all the applications at that time ufed, I found
the greateft fervice from tobacco-juice and *tinct.
myrrh. et aloës*, rubbed on them feveral times a-
day. Alum-water, and oak-bark decoction,
reftored their ufual firmnefs.

In two weeks time, fometimes fooner,
the fymptoms began to abate, the *maculæ*
turned brown, and in four weeks they complained only of weaknefs. This, bathing in
the fea, and aromatic bitters with fteel, foon
removed. I had the good fortune not to lofe
a fingle man.

C H A P.   VI.

The theory of the difeafe.

IN order to underftand the true ftate and
condition of the body under this difeafe,
fome things muft neceffarily be premifed from
the known and eftablifhed laws of the animal
œconomy.

An animal body is compofed of folid and
fluid parts; and thefe confift of fuch various
and heterogeneous principles, as render it, of
all

all substances, the most liable to corruption and putrefaction.   Such indeed is the state and condition of every living animal, as to be threatened with this, from the mechanism of its own frame, and the necessary laws of circulation by which it subsists.   For by the uninterrupted circulation of its fluids, their violent attrition, and mutual actions on each other, and their containing vessels, the whole mass of humours is apt to degenerate from its sweet, mild, and healthful condition, into various degrees of acrimony and corruption.   Parts of the solids themselves, continually abraded by the repeated force of the circulating fluids, are again returned into their channels.   Hence the necessity of throwing out of the body, by different outlets, these acrimonious and putrescent juices, rendered thus unfit for the animal uses and functions, together with the abraded particles of the solids.   And a daily supply of food, or fresh nourishment, is required to recruit this constant waste, both of the solid and fluid parts. Thus the bodies of all animals are in a constant state of change and renovation, by which they are preserved from death and putrefaction.

There are two evacuations chiefly by which the blood is freed from these putrescent noxi-

ous

ous humours, *viz.* urine, and infensible perspiration. Not but that there are many other secretions necessary to health: yet they are rather
more properly adapted to other singular and
peculiar uses; except that of stool, which in
some cases may be substituted as a vent to these
corrupted humours, upon the defect of either
of the other two.

It would seem, that, by the urinary passages,
the rancescent oils and the acrid salts of the
blood, together with the earthy recrements
broke off from the solids, are daily washed a-
way, and expelled out of the body.

But the most considerable of all the evacuations, is that by infensible perspiration; which
Sanctorius found in *Italy* to be equal to five
eighths of the meat and drink taken into the
body. Most of the observations made by that
author will be found true; as they have been
confirmed by repeated experiments, by Dr
Keil in *England*, the learned *Degorter* in *Holland*, and others *(a)*; making a proper allowance for the different climates they lived in,
their different ages, ways of life, and constitutions. Upon which subject, I shall here ob-

(a) Dr *Lining* in *South-Carolina*, Mr *Rye* in *Ireland*, and Dr
Robinson.

serve,

serve, that, confidering how often animals, as well as plants, as appears by many experiments, are in an abforbing and bibulous condition, the exact quantity perfpired cannot at all times be juftly determined, without knowing the quantity imbibed. Upon this confideration, however, it will appear, that in many cafes it often exceeds the quantity affigned by *Sancto-rius*. It is indeed, beyond doubt, the moft copious evacuation of the whole body: and though it is fometimes in greater or leffer quan-tities, as influenced by various caufes ; yet it can never be partially fuppreffed long, much lefs can it be entirely obftructed, without the greateft detriment to health. For fhould its defect for a fhort time be fupplied by fome more copious and increafed evacuation, as it fometimes is by that of urine or ftool; yet towards perfect health, the integrity of all the animal functions, more efpecially the natural evacuations, are requifite: there being fomewhat thrown out of the body by each, which can-not fo conveniently pafs another way ; as *Sanctorius* rightly obferves, of any other eva-cuation fubftituted for this, " It diminifhes

" the

" the quantity, but leaves behind it the ill
" quality" *(b)*.

It may be proper farther to remark, that this
being the laſt and moſt elaborated action of a-
nimal digeſtion, the body is hereby freed from
what is conſequently the moſt ſubtile and putreſcent of the animal humours. And it is
certain theſe excrementitious humours naturally
deſtined for this evacuation, when retained
long in the body, are capable of acquiring the
moſt poiſonous and noxious qualities, and a
very high degree of putrefaction *(c)*; becoming
extremely acrid and corroſive: and do then give
riſe to various diſeaſes, according to the habit
or conſtitution of the perſon, *viz.* the ſtate of
the ſolids and fluids at that time, or the influence and determination of other cauſes.

Moreover, not only due and conſtant evacuations of what may be rendered thus ſo extremely pernicious to the body, are requiſite
towards the health and life of animals; but a
freſh and daily ſupply of a ſoft and mild liquor,
ſuch as the chyle, is farther neceſſary to correct and prevent the conſtant natural putreſcent
tendency of the humours, and to ſweeten and

(*b*) *Aph.* 19.
(*c*) *Vid. Hoffman. de venenis corporis humani. Sanctor. aph.* 43.

dilute the acrimony which they daily and hourly contract from the action of the body, and by life itself. It appears, that animals starved to death, do not perish from want of blood, or an insufficient quantity of other juices, but from the corrupt and putrid state of them.

It would be foreign to my purpose, to observe what various degrees and kinds of putrefaction may be induced in the human body by other means, *(viz.* by putrid ferments, or putrid substances of any kind, contagious poisons, and acrimony of different sorts, either taken inwardly, or outwardly applied); as the scorbutic putrefaction, it will appear, is purely the natural effect of animal heat and motion caused by the action of the body. How long life may be preserved during this putrefaction of the animal, or what degree of corruption in the humours may subsist during life, it is not easy to determine; though, beyond all doubt, such an alcalescent state or acrimony in the blood as is described by some authors, is not consistent with life. Alcaline and putrid substances are very different.

This being premised, I come now to observe the effects upon the human body of the several causes which are remarked to give rise to the
scurvy.

scurvy. *First*, An intense degree of cold, such as we have sometimes during severe winters in our own country, but especially such as the crews felt who wintered at *Spitzbergen* and *Greenland*, and is common in the winters in *Groenland* and *Iceland*, is experienced to be among the predisposing causes to this disease.

The obvious effect of cold on the human body is, to constringe the whole external habit, to dry and corrugate the skin; and all statical experiments prove, that cold obstructs or diminishes insensible perspiration. *Degorter* observed, that, *cæteris paribus*, the perspiration was always less, the greater degree of cold there appeared to be from the thermometer *(d)*. *Sanctorius*, who lived in a country where the winters are seldom long and severe, gives us a very just aphorism *(e)*, if rightly understood, on this subject. It is, That, during a cold constitution of air, the robust (or such as have strong elastic fibres, and a dense blood, by which a great degree of heat overcoming the force of the external cold, is soon generated in them, especially by muscular motion or exer-

(d) *Tract. de perspir. cap.* 12. § 34.

(e) *Frigus externum prohibet perspirationem in debili, in robusto vero auget, aph.* 68.

cise)

cise) may be made to perspire much more than at other times. But in weak persons, or those that use no exercise, and universally in all who cannot bring themselves into a degree of heat exceeding that of the atmosphere, perspiration will be lessened, according to the different degrees of cold to which their body is exposed; and which, when very intense, entirely stops this necessary evacuation. Hence such as use exercise, and keep warm, during cold winters, are not so subject to scorbutic complaints, as those who are weak, and use none.

But it must be remarked, that cold joined with driness and purity in the air, by keeping up a due degree of tension in the solids, is not naturally productive of this disease. It may indeed be supposed, that when the cold becomes very intense, as in the winter in *Greenland*, the vital or animal heat of the body may be so overcome by it, that the digestive faculties (as in a person starving with cold) are chilled and enervated; and the solids being overbraced by so high a degree of cold, may at last lose their tone or elasticity. In this case, the constitution becoming gradually habituated to an overcharge of what physicians call the *serosa colluvies*,

colluvies, by a long obstructed perspiration; instead of coughs, stitches, pleurisies, and the like disorders of the inflammatory kind, usual in such seasons from too tense fibres, the scorbutic *diathesis* may more naturally be contracted, especially if such food only is used as must contribute to form the disease. But this, though probable, cannot be ascertained from fact; because, as I observed elsewhere *(f)*, these northern countries, above all others, are continually pestered with fogs, even during their severest frosts. And by all faithful and accurate observations made on this disease, moisture is experienced to be the principal and main predisposing cause to it. This indeed of itself is sufficient to dispose the constitution to the scurvy in any climate, even the warmest. It is observable, that, in warm climates, the crews of ships at sea are liable to this malady, when the hot weather, by which the fibres of the body are much relaxed, is succeeded by great and incessant rains usual in these latitudes, or when the season proves very unconstant. The disease is there likewise much owing to the great length of these southern voyages. But, otherwise, it is not near so frequent a calamity as in

(f) P. 130.

colder

colder climates; the bad effects of moisture
being rendered much more pernicious when
combined with cold.   A cold and *moist* constitution of the atmosphere, together with wet
lodgings, damp beds, cloaths, and other inconveniencies which poor people necessarily
suffer at such seasons, is the most frequent and
strongest disposing cause to it.   And, upon the
whole, it is to be remarked, that whatever shuts
up the pores of the skin, and impedes or lessens perspiration, which moisture or dampness
effectually does, and that more strongly with
the addition of cold, is chiefly productive of
this disease.

Sanctorius, in several places, describes such
a scorbutic constitution of air, and its effects,
as is often met with at sea : " Too cold, windy,
" or wet air, lessens perspiration" *(g).* He
had before enumerated almost all the causes
which obstruct this evacuation, and occasion
the disease, *viz.* " *aër frigidus, cœnosus, et humi-*
" *dus, natatio in frigida,* grofs viscid food, and
" a neglect of exercise" *(h)*; and obferves
the confequence of perspiration being obstructed by such a moist grofs air : " It converts

" the matter of transpiration into an *ichor;*
" which being retained, induces a cachexy" *(i).*
He very justly afterwards paints out the scorbutic cachexy, when describing the effects of humidity, or of such an indisposition of air as
produces the scurvy: " Here perspiration is
" stopt, the passages of it clogged, the fibres
" are relaxed; and the transpiration retained,
" proves hurtful, and induces a sensible weight
" in the body" *(k).*

This he found by statical experiments to be
the fact. But, for the better understanding of
these excellent aphorisms, it may be proper to
observe, that, upon the state of the atmosphere, the strength and weakness of the fibres
of our body in a great measure depend. Too
moist an air not only stops up the pores of the
skin, but weakens and relaxes the whole system
of solids. Hence, during a rainy cloudy season, all the members of the body feel heavy,
the appetite is diminished, the pulse of the
heart and arteries is more feeble, and every
one is sensible of a languor of strength, and a
lowness of spirits. Farther, moisture, by weakening the spring and elasticity of the air, ren-

(i) Aph. 146.
(k) Aph. 148.

ders

ders it unfit for the many salutary purposes obtained by respiration. Such an air not being
able to overcome sufficiently the contractile
force of the pulmonary fibres resisting the di-
latation of the lungs, the blood is not here
sufficiently comminuted and broken, nor that
lentor removed which it had contracted in its
slow returning motion through the veins. From
the impaired action also of this *viscus*, the last
and most important office of animal digestion upon the chyle, that of sanguification, is not duly
performed. As we always find, that those who
have their lungs faulty, can never be properly
nourished; so indeed there can be no good
digestion without pure air. This is necessary;
as it mixes with the aliment in the mouth, has
free access to the stomach, and through the
whole intestinal tube, where it is a very active
cause of digestion; but chiefly as it assists the
lungs in performing that function of assimi-
lating and converting the crude chyle into
blood. Hence, during a moist constitution of
the air, improper food, or such as affords a
too viscous and tenacious chyle, can never
rightly be converted into this vital juice, for
the support and nourishment of the body.

But, further, persons in such situations where

they

they are continually expofed to moift air, in
damp lodgings, in wet cloaths, beddings, &c.
are found to abforb great quantities of the fur-
rounding moifture *(l)*. And thefe obftructed
and imbibed humours becoming more and more
acrid, this ferous *colluvies*, in length of time,
turns putrid in the human body *(m)*. All a-
nimal fubftances have naturally a tendency to
corruption in too moift an air.

(*l*) Dr *Keil (Med. Stat. Brit.)* feems to have been of opinion, that the diforders faid commonly to depend on retained
perfpirable matter, were owing to noxious particles abforbed. It
muft be owned there is fome difficulty in this matter: for though
the balance fhews the quantity of perfpiration to be equal to
five eighths (or whatever elfe different authors have affigned it)
of the *ingefta* more than what is abforbed ; yet the quantity perfpired may greatly exceed this, fince the quantity abforbed is
unknown. Moift air loaded with more heterogeneous particles
than dry air, may often produce bad effects, as much, or perhaps
more, by abforption of thefe particles, than by ftopping perfpiration. But it is fufficient to our purpofe, to take it for granted,
that moift air obftructs perfpiration, which is univerfally acknowledged. And we have no occafion to inveftigate the peculiar quality of the heterogeneous particles abforbed ; becaufe it appears
(fee chap. 1. p. 126.), that the perfpirable matter retained, as alfo
what is abforbed from moift or unwholfome air, is, though a general, only a remote caufe of the fcurvy ; and not what may be
called the *caufa proxima*, as the laft may in other epidemical and
contagious difeafes. Any perfon will be convinced of this who
confults the beft authors on that fubject, *viz. Hoffman de venenis
in aëre contentis, epidemicorum morborum caufis. Lancifius de noxiis
paludum effluviis. Ramazzini conftitutiones epidemicae.*
(*m*) *Vid. Sanctor. aph.* 43.

I

I come next to obferve the other concurring caufes which have fo great an influence in difpofing to this difeafe; fuch as lazinefs and indolence of difpofition, and from thence a neglect of ufing proper exercife, or a fedentary and inactive life.

Every one, from experience, muft be fenfible how much exercife contributes to the health of the body, as well as to chearfulnefs of mind. It is neceffary to keep up that due degree of firmnefs and tenfion in the folids, upon which the ftrength and foundnefs of a conftitution depend: and which is acquired by fuch motions as increafe the mutual action of the veffels on their contents, and each other. But the whole procefs of animal digeftion, as well as all the fecretions, depend upon this ftrength and firmnefs of the veffels and *vifcera*. Whenever the tone of thefe is relaxed and weakened, which is moft effectually done by keeping the body long at reft, or by neglect of due exercife, there muft follow a deficiency in the vigour and ftrength of the powers of digeftion; fo that they will not be fufficient to concoct and elaborate the aliment, efpecially if it is of a too crude and vifcid nature. And the whole fyftem of folids being thus relaxed,

by

by reason of a deficiency of their action and efficacy, the chyle cannot be properly assimilated, nor the heterogeneous mass of fluids intimately mixed and blended: so that the body here is not duly nourished, nor the secretions rightly performed; especially that of perspiration, which exercise powerfully promotes. Hence the scorbutic *diathesis*, want of proper digestion, weak and relaxed fibres, with a stoppage of perspiration.

The same state of things will likewise occur in those who have been much weakened by a preceeding fit of sickness; with this additional cause, that, besides the weakened tone of the solids, and of all the powers of digestion, there is often left in the constitution after fevers, an acrimonious state of the juices. Here such a diet is necessary to prevent the scurvy, as is adapted to the weakness of the organs, as requires the gentlest action of the *viscera* to concoct and assimilate it, and the smallest force to forward it in its passage, and is of a quality proper to correct the acrimonious disposition of the humours.

These being the predisposing causes of this disease, it plainly appears, that the effects produced by them, are, a relaxation of the tone of the

the animal fibres, a weakening of the powers of digeftion, together with a ftoppage of perfpiration. This laft particular may receive confirmation, by obferving, that fome of the paffions of the mind, as fear and forrow, which have been affigned as caufes of the fcurvy, and are almoft conftantly its effects, act with the fame remarkable influence on perfpiration, as they were found to have on this difeafe in Lord *Anfon's* crew *(n)*. But as the mechanical effects of thefe paffions upon the human body would require too long a difcuffion for this place, I fhall refer it to the authors who have exprefsly treated of them *(o)*.

I proceed to obferve what farther effects are produced by what has been affigned as the occafional caufe of this difeafe, *viz.* a grofs and vifcid diet in fuch circumftances as have been defcribed, and the want of frefh greens or vegetables, which are found fo effectually to check the fcorbutic virulence.

I imagine it would be unneceffary to infift

(n) Compare *Sanct. aph.* 456. 458. 460. 461. 462. 463. 469. 474. 478. with Lord *Anfon's* voyage, p. 101. edit. 5.
(o) Vid. A medical differtation on the paffions of the mind; and *Robinfon* on the food and difcharges of human bodies, p. 77.

long

long in fhewing how, in the unavoidable hardfhips that fometimes attend feamen in long
voyages, or the befieged fhut up in towns; as
likewife in times of fcarcity or famine, or when
people at any time ufe putrid flefh or fifh,
mouldy bread, or unwholfome waters; how,
I fay, from fuch corrupted fubftances, the
fcorbutic taint might probably be induced in the
body. The aliment is never fo far divefted of
its original qualities by digeftion, as not to
carry fome of them along with it into the
blood. I am indeed inclined to believe, that
where the predifpofing caufes already mentioned are wanting, fuch putrid and corrupt aliment would occafion other difeafes different
from the fcurvy. Though it may tend to
increafe it, and often concurs with other caufes
at fea to render it highly virulent; yet it is certain, the fcurvy appears moft frequently where
fuch food has no fhare in breeding it, however
generally it has been accufed; its moft common occafional caufe being the grofs vifcid diet
before defcribed *(p)*. In order to underftand
the effects of which, it may be proper to pre-
mife fome obfervations on the nature of digeftion in general, and the different changes

(p) Chap. 1. p. 119.

our

our aliment muft neceffarily undergo, in order to fit it for the various purpofes of life.

By the firft procefs of digeftion in the mouth,
ftomach, and inteftines, the food muft be rendered quite fluid; otherwife it can never pafs into
the blood, through the exceeding fine, and almoft
imperceptible lacteal veffels.   For which purpofe
it is broken and divided by the teeth ;   farther
fubdued, macerated, and diffolved, by the heat,
moifture, and various actions of the ftomach,
inteftines, *vifcera, &c.*; diluted by watery liquors, diffolved by others that are faponaceous,
till, in the nature of a fluid chyle, it is received
into the lacteals.   What is unconquerable by
thefe firft powers of digeftion, is thrown out
of the body by ftool.   After it has in this li-
quid form entered the blood, it feems but little
changed; retaining ftill a vegetable character,
and refembling the nature of milk, in colour as
well as other qualities ; all animals being thus
nourifhed, as it were, with their own milk.
It therefore requires a ftill farther and more
perfect elaboration, in order to animalife it, and
fit it for the important ufes of nutrition and
perfpiration.

To nourifh the fluids, is to replace a liquor
of the fame kind and quality with that which

O o   is

is gone. And as they are the thinneſt parts of the fluids which are continually loſt, ſo the aliment muſt be reduced extremely thin and fine to reſtore them. It muſt likewiſe be greatly attenuated, ſo as to paſs through the moſt minute canals of the body, in order to adhere to, and repair the waſted ſolids. *Laſtly*, It muſt ſtill be more ſubtiliſed, before it can paſs off, in the form of a volatile and inſenſible ſteam, by perſpiration.

Thus, the nouriſhment both of the ſolids and fluids, and the matter of inſenſible perſpiration, are all furniſhed from the aliment; that is, from the fineſt parts of the chyle, elaborated to an extreme degree of ſubtilty and perfection, and converted into the peculiar nature of the juices of our body, by the action which is called the *ſecond concoction*. What cannot, by the powers of this action, be thus duly digeſted and aſſimilated, as in the former concoction the recrements were thrown off by ſtool, muſt here paſs by urine. It requires a much ſtronger force of digeſtion, and a much longer time, to convert the chyle into nouriſhment, or into perſpirable matter, than to paſs it off crude by urine. In this way great quantities of liquor are ſoon paſſed. But for ſome
time

time after eating, the perspiration is always lessened, and is very small, whilst the white chyle
is circulating, unsubdued, in the blood *(q)*.
It is certain, that many sorts of gross and viscid
aliment, though they may pass the first concoction, are yet unconquerable by the subsequent
powers, so as to furnish proper matter either
for nourishment or perspiration.

From what has been said, the nature of aliment proper for these purposes may be understood; as likewise how it is fitted and prepared
for these uses, both without and within the
body.   Thus, whatever method of art or
cookery, by macerating, boiling, stewing, fer-
menting, *&c.* destroys the viscidity and cohe-
sion of its parts, or renders it thinner and more
fluid, performs part of that digestion which it
necessarily must undergo in the body.   By these
means, in many cases an aliment may be furnished, ready prepared, of suitable and similar
qualities to the chyle or humours of our body,
and which requires but a small force to convert it into nourishment; being at once miscible
with the blood, and all the rest of our humours.
Of this nature are light thin broths, fermented
bread, tender herbs and roots boiled, *&c.*

(q) Vid. Lower de corde, p. 243.

O o 2   Such

Such food is most proper for children, valetudinarians, and those who have any where a defect in their digestion. Hence likewise we
may know how the concoction of aliment is
promoted in the first passages, by diluting, saponaceous, and attenuating liquors; and by a-
romatic, bitter, and bilious medicines; and
what is particularly requisite for its farther elaboration afterwards, *viz.* muscular motion,
exercise of the whole body, strong fibres, the
action of the lungs, and a good air.

I observed elsewhere *(r)*, and it will appear
to follow from what has been said, that all
general rules or precepts which can be given
for diet, are to be understood only as relative
to the constitution or state of the body at the
time. In particular, the viscidity and tenacity, or the solidity and hardness of food, in all
animals, ought to be proportioned to the
strength of their vital powers of digestion.   I
mean by these, the whole collected powers or
faculties of the body, by which it assimilates into
its own animal nature, various sorts of aliment.
Such aliment as is too hard for these powers,
can never be sufficiently broken or dissolved,
and when its tenacity exceeds this force of

(r) P. 116.

digestion,

digeſtion, it can never be rightly converted into nouriſhment.

I proceed to apply this doctrine, and to conſider more particularly the nature and qualities of ſuch food as is truly the occaſional cauſe of the ſcurvy, *viz.* a diet of dried or ſalt fleſh or fiſh, together with the groſſer farinaceous ſubſtances unfermented.

It is obſervable, that the tenderer or ſofter fleſh is made by keeping for ſome time without ſalt, it is found to be the eaſier of digeſtion: but by being long hardened and dried with ſalt, its moſt fine, ſubtile, and nutritious parts, either fly off, or are fixed. Experience ſhews, that fleſh long ſalted is of very difficult digeſtion. It requires perfect health, together with exerciſe, plenty of diluting liquors, vinegar, and many other correctors, to ſubdue it in the firſt paſſages. And, after all, it will afford a too groſs and unconquerable chyle, where there is a defect in the organs of ſanguification, or thoſe of the ſecond concoction. The nouriſhment we receive from animal ſubſtances, or what paſſes into our blood, ſeems chiefly to be the gelatinous or lymphatic part; the fibres being indiſſolvable, even in the firſt paſſages, and from thence are paſſed by ſtool. Together with which,

which, part of the animal oil, or the fat of the
meat, likewife enters the lacteals.   This laft,
when long kept, even falted, is almoft always
rancefcent, efpecially that of pork. And as all the
nutritious particles are here intimately intangled
with fea-falt, this falt cannot, without difficulty, be extricated from them by the powers of
the body.   Hence fuch grofs, fharp, and faline
food, is rendered improper, in many cafes,
for that thin, foft, mild nourifhment required,

   The next part of diet to be confidered, is,
the farinaceous fubftances unfermented, *viz.*
fea bifcuit, pudding, *&c.*   It is certain nothing can be more wholfome than the mealy
feeds of feveral plants, as wheat, barley, rice,
&c.; as alfo feveral of the *legumina:* and for
this reafon, becaufe an oil feems neceffary to
the compofition of the animal emulfion; and
thefe in particular contain a vegetable one, of
mild and friendly qualities to-the human body,
They afford fo wholfome a nourifhment, that
they are ufed by the generality of mankind for
the greateft part of their food.   But fome of
thefe fubftances, in particular wheat-flour,
(which is moft commonly eat by the *Europeans*), requires a previous fermentation, in order to break the glutinous vifcidity which it
                              acquires

acquires by being mixed with water, and thus to subdue, out of the body, the mucous tenacity of its oils, and make them more miscible with the different humours; which, otherwise, people in the best health, and with the strongest force of digestion, find a difficulty in doing. Few can live altogether on ship puddings, dumplings, or the like, without being sensible of an oppression and uneasiness. But especially weak and exhausted people cannot well receive the necessary nourishment from such species of the mealy substances, until their *lentor* or mucosity is subdued by fermentation, or by some other method, by which they become lighter food. It is plain, that such a glutinous and viscid chyle as is afforded by hard sea biscuit, dumplings, ship-puddings, &c. requires the most perfect state of organs in the subsequent concoction for its farther elaboration *(f)*.

Hence

(f) It may be said, That as fresh flesh and fish are much more apt to become putrid out of the body than dried and salt flesh and fish, the latter ought not to produce the scurvy; and the farines do not putrify so soon as animal food does; and the less they are animalised, the less putrescent they become. This only proves how little we can learn of the effects of food and medicines in the body, by experiments made out of it. In a deep scurvy, there is the highest degree of putrefaction which a living animal can well subsist under : yet if we were so lucky as to find

out

Hence the effects of the above diet constantly used, are twofold.

1*st*, Chyle is by this means wanting of a
proper quality to dilute and sweeten the acrimonious animal juices, to correct the putrescent tendency of the humours, and to repair the decay of the body. We find, that
such a gross, ropy, and viscid chyle, cannot,
in scorbutic cases, be rightly incorporated with
the blood, or converted into nourishment.
And this weakness of digestion, or want of af-
similation of the aliment in such persons, (by
considering the effects produced by the predisposing causes of their malady), will appear to be
more owing to a fault in the organs of sanguification, than in the first concoction. These are
much weakened, commonly by want of exercise,
often by preceeding sickness, and always by the
universal lax state of their fibres. But especially, as the chief predisposing cause of this disease is a moist damp air, the action of the

out the most powerful antiseptic in nature, it is not probable the
scurvy could be thereby cured; although the body, after death,
might be preserved by it as long as an *Ægyptian* mummy. On
the contrary, the most putrid scurvies are daily cured by what
quickly becomes highly putrescent out of the body, *viz.* broth
made of coleworts and cabbage. However contradictory to
some modern theories these facts may be, the truth of them is
undeniable.

lungs,

lungs, the principal organ of sanguification, is thereby impaired and weakened. It is rendered imperspirable, as we shall more fully see afterwards. Gross viscid aliment, though it may be subdued in the first passages, and divided by diluting it, so as to enter the lacteals; yet, like starch passed through a sieve, it unites again; and its viscous tenacity and *lentor*, from a defect of energy in the solids and lungs, can never be broken to a sufficient degree of finenefs, to nourish the body; nor can it be perfectly assimilated with the other juices. Hence a tendency to a spontaneous putrefaction, from want of proper chyle and nourishment; and symptoms, as will appear afterwards, the same as in people starved.

But farther, this crude chyle not being either elaborated, or expelled the body, it muft, by repeated circulations, and continuing long there, become acrid and putrid, together with the other juices.

2*dly*, The tenacity of such aliment concurs in scorbutic cases; where the perspiration is already leffened, in a manner altogether to stop it. Indeed such a diet naturally leffens it, without the concurrence of other causes: for a laudable perspiration can only proceed from a du-

ly-

ly-prepared and well-concocted humour, obtained from such aliment as is thin, light, and easy of digestion. The matter of perspiration is the last and most elaborated humour of the body: the perfection of which depends upon its being reduced to the most imperceptible tenuity, by a compleat and thorough elaboration in all the different concoctions it undergoes. Hence all grofs indigestible aliment is found to be imperspirable. This all statical experiments confirm *(t)*. The effects of such viscid imperspirable food are particularly described by *Sanctorius*: " Imperspirable food begets obstruc-
" tions, corruption, lassitude, grief, and hea-
" vinefs of the body" *(u)*. These are the most remarkable scorbutic symptoms.

Upon the whole, the case of scorbutic people appears plainly to be a weakened and relaxed state of solids, with such a condition of the blood as naturally tends to that spontaneous putrefaction which proceeds from want of nourishment, (or a recruit of proper chyle to correct and sweeten the acrid putrescent juices), and from a remarkable stoppage of perspiration.

(t) Ubi est difficultas coctionis, ibi tarditas perspirationis. Sanct. aph. 250.
(u) Aph. 262.

This

This is evinced not only from the known and certain effects of the causes which give rise to their malady, but it hath the evidence also of ocular demonstration. Their swelled œdematous legs, and spungy gums, denote the state of their solids; their fœtid breath, stools, urine, ulcers, and blood, the condition of their fluids; and their spontaneous lassitude, but especially their dry, rough, or pellucid skins, prove a stoppage of perspiration.

Now, in such a state, it may be asked, What is proper to be done? Their perspiration cannot well be restored by diaphoretics or sudorifics. For though warm draughts of *decoct. lignor.* give a momentary relief to such people, and in some few cases a crude humour may thus be pushed through the skin in so relaxed a state of solids; yet such a humour goes off generally, and more naturally, by urine. And there being here no proper matter fitted for insensible perspiration, a change into a drier and purer air is not sufficient to recover them. Nor can the lax solids be braced up to advantage, while the juices are corrupt and unsound, and assimilation and nutrition wanting: so that exercise, stimulants, bark, steel, and astringents, will not cure them. Nor will a diet of even fresh flesh

broths

broths remove a high and virulent degree of this difeafe, without the affiftance of green vegetables.

We are upon this occafion told a very remarkable ftory by *Sinopæus (x)*.   " There are " whole nations in *Tartary* who live altoge- " ther on milk and flefh.   Thefe people are " never feized with the fmall pox; but, on the " other hand, are fubjeϗ to violent fcurvies, " which at times fweep off as great numbers as " the fmall pox does of other nations."   He had four of them (two men, and two women, who had been taken prifoners) in the hofpital at *Cronftadt*, in the year 1733.   The fcurvy being epidemic there that fpring, thefe poor people became afflicϗted with it, fell into profufe hæmorrhages, and every one of them died.

This leads me to inquire into the virtues of frefh green vegetables, which feem fo necef- fary to correϗt the bad qualities of other dry and hard food, and are experienced fo effeϗtu- ally to prevent, and often cure this diftemper.

Recent vegetables, frefh plants and fruits, are of a more tender texture than animals; and their parts being more eafily feparable, by rea- fon of the lefs force of their cohefion, and

(x) *Parerg. medic. p.* 311.

lefſer

lesser tenacity of their cementing *gluten,* they yield more easily to the dividing powers of our organs. They also contain less oil than either flesh or the farines. But gross oils (especially of the animal kind) seem not only to be the most unconquerable part of aliment; but, where there is already a corruption in the human body, may be apt, by becoming rancid, to acquire the highest and worst degree of it.

As these are the most necessary and requisite qualities in the present case, so perhaps by no other can all green fresh vegetables be characterised. There is no other particular virtue in which they all agree; a greater diversity of qualities being found in vegetable than in animal substances. But, besides what has been mentioned, vegetables have great and peculiar virtues in this disease, arising from a combination of various qualities; of which all vegetables possess one or more, in a higher or lesser degree; and do from thence accordingly become more or less antiscorbutic. The best remedies are furnished from a composition of different plants, most eminent for the properties required: and whatever simple possesses the most of these qualities, is, of all such, the most serviceable and

efficacious

efficacious for preventing and curing the malady.

It is to be remarked, that, in moft properties here requifite, vegetables differ from animal fubftances. That there is a confiderable difference in the conftituent principles of vegetables and animals, is plainly proved by their chemical analyfis. In the latter, the falts are found to be more volatile; and, by a great degree of fire, a volatile alcalefcent falt is obtained from them: whereas a fixed alcaline falt is found copioufly to abound in moft vegetables when burnt; and indeed this laft is properly of vegetable extraction.

But, without this chemical torture, which fhews fo great a diverfity in their component parts, many plants are of an acefcent quality; whereas animal fubftances, on the contrary, are almoft all of an alcalefcent, or perhaps rather a putrefcent nature. It would indeed appear, that man, both from the ftructure of his organs of digeftion and appetite, was defigned to feed both on animal and vegetable fubftances. But though we perceive a perfon in health, and of a found ftate of body, has a wonderful faculty of converting almoft all forts of alimentary fubftances into nourifhment at times; yet
experience

experience shews, that no man can long bear
a diet entirely of flesh and fish without nausea-
ting it, unless corrected by bread, salt, vinegar,
and acids; and that for the reason before observed, *viz.* because the intention of digestion
in the first passages is to draw from the aliment a
milky, sweet, white liquor, resembling in quality a vegetable emulsion; not indeed acid, but
acescent; contrary to the nature of animal substances, which are observed in like circumstances to become putrid. And for this and other
reasons *(y)*, a mixture of vegetable substances
seems requisite towards the composition of good
chyle, and to correct the continual putrescent
tendency of the animal humours.

(y) An. Cocchi, present Professor of anatomy at *Florence,* in
his elegant academical discourse on the *Pythagorean* diet, among
other things observes, *Ciò che deve pienamente persuadere ogni gi-
usto pensatore della salubrità e potenza del vitto vegetabile, si è il con-
siderare gli orrendi effeti dell' astinenza da un tal vitto, se ella non
è brevissima, i quali s'incontrano amplamente e sicuramente registrati
nelle narrazioni più interessanti e più autentiche degli affari umani.
Le guerre, e gli assedi delle piazze, e i lunghi castrensi soggiorni, le
lontane navigazioni, le popolazioni de' paesi incolti e marittimi, le
famose pestilenze, e le vite degli uomini illustri, somministrano a chi
intende le leggi della natura, incontrastabili evidenze della malvagia e
velenosa attività del vitto contrario al fresco vegetabile.* P. 65.

*Freschi vegetabili ho sempre detto, perchè i secchi anno quasi tutte
le incomode qualità de' cibi animali, massime essendo le loro particelle
troppo fortemente coerenti terrestri ed oleose.* P. 49.

Thus

Thus one quality entering the moſt perfect antiſcorbutic compoſition, is that of a vegetable aceſcency. Hence milk of all ſorts is experienced to be of great benefit in this diſeaſe, being a true vegetable emulſion of different herbs fed upon by the cattle. And acids of any kind are found uſeful; ſuch as vinegar, ſpirits of ſalt and vitriol; though far from being ſufficient either to prevent or cure the ſcurvy, as wanting ſome other properties much more neceſſary than acidity.

If it be ſaid, That ſcurvy-graſs, creſſes, and other acrid alcaleſcent plants, are found highly antiſcorbutic; it muſt likewiſe be remembered, that they are not perhaps altogether ſo efficacious as the aceſcent fruits; or at leaſt become much more ſo by the addition of lemon-juice, oranges, or a little ſorrel; which laſt the *Greenlanders (z)* are taught by experience to join with them for their cure: *the chief and moſt eſſentially requiſite quality* in the antiſcorbutic compoſition, *viz. a ſaponaceous, attenuating, and reſolving virtue,* poſſeſſed by ſuch acrid vegetables in the moſt eminent degree, being thereby heightened, improved, and exerted in its full force.

(z) See chap. 5.

Soap

Soap is a mixture of oil and falt; by means of which various fubftances are brought intimately to mix together, and to incorporate, which otherwife they would not do. And whether the falt be acid, alcaline, or neuter, it is found to have this property. Soap is likewife a powerful attenuant of vifcid fubftances; for which purpofe fomething faline is always required. Now, in this charadteriftic, all fucculent plants, roots, and fruits agree; and whether their falts be of an ammoniacal or nitrous quality, the compofition in all is truly faponaceous.

It has been obferved, that water alone may, by its intervention, dilute, and keep afunder for a while, the parts of vifcid and grofs food; and that in this manner they may even pafs the ladteals: but, upon coming again into contadt, they naturally will cohere. Now, this tenacity is beft deftroyed by vegetable foaps, and the juices of fuch herbs and fruits as are of an attenuating and refolving quality. We find, that, by the immoderate ufe of fummer-fruits, the whole humours of the body may be melted down. Hence *diarrhœas, cholera morbus,* &c. fo frequent at that feafon. But though the abufe of them proves fo hurtful, yet they were certainly defigned for the benefit of man-

Q q   kind

kind. And in the present case they become e-
minently serviceable, from their salutary composition. They consist of a great quantity of
water, whereby they dilute; of mucilaginous
parts, by which they obtund the stimulating
putrefactive acrimony; and of a fine penetrating
salt, antiseptic in the human body.

Moreover, as, by the scorbutic putrefaction,
the *crasis* of the blood was broken and dissolved, these give a homogeneous and saponaceous
quality to the whole mass. At the same time
they prove greatly aperient, in scouring and
cleansing the furred and obstructed passages of
the machine, especially the different emunctories. And thus the acrimony first blunted by
these soaps, is expelled the body *(a)*.

The chyle, by their means likewise, being
imbued with a saponaceous and diluting quality, is now rendered miscible with the other
humours, and fitted for the uses of nourishment and perspiration. Accordingly, we constantly experience good effects in this disease,
from whatever subdues the viscidity of the
chyle, and makes it more saponaceous; as e-

(a) They generally, upon first using, open the belly, promote
urine plentifully, and restore perspiration; but if voraciously
eat, induce a dangerous flux of the belly.

ven

ven foap itfelf, honey, but efpecially *oxym.
fcillit.* or pills made of foap and fquills; and
likewife whatever, as *Sanctorius* obferves, either
perfpires itfelf, or affifts the perfpiration of o-
ther food; as moft of the acrid antifcorbutics.
And for this purpofe he recommends fome of
the beft of them, *viz.* onions and garlic *(b)*,
ale *(c)*, wine moderately ufed *(d)*; and in
particular well-baked bread *(e)*. Thefe, according to his remarks, not only perfpiring
freely themfelves, but by promoting the concoction and affimilation of groffer foods, fit
them alfo for this fecretion.

Laftly, There is another property peculiar
to many green vegetables, and efpecially to the
riper fruits, which are found fo beneficial here;
and it is, that fermentative quality, by which
they are preferved longer from corruption, both
without and within the body. For whereas flefh
and animal fubftances, without any other intermediate ftate, tend directly to putrefaction;
vegetables are preferved longer from it by a
fermentative tendency, which many vegetable
juices naturally have, or may acquire by the
addition of a proper ferment. We evidently

(b) *Aph.* 283.   (d) *Aph.* 369.
(c) *Aph.* 282.   (e) *Aph.* 210.

Q q 2   fee

fee in this difeafe the good effects of fpruce beer, cyder, ale, wine, and other vinous liquors, prone to fall into this ftate in the ftomach; on the contrary, the pernicious effects of diftilled fpirits, which check fuch a fermentation. And I am of opinion, for feveral reafons, that this is fome how neceffary to the perfection of animal digeftion.

In a fituation fimilar to that of the ftomach, with regard to heat, moifture, and air, many fubftances muft naturally fall into a fermentation. We are certain by their effects, that ripe fruits and fome vegetables cannot well be prevented from it, and actually do often ferment in the ftomach: and obferving, that, in the fcurvy *(f)*, and fome other difeafes, food of this tendency is requifite, and that abftinence from it is prejudicial; hence we conclude, that this operation, and food which tends to promote it, is neceffary to digeftion, and to prevent the fcorbutic corruption.

(f) Kramer obferved, that in a thoufand patients he had cured by the juices of fcurvy-grafs and creffes, each dofe of the juices occafioned prodigious belchings and wind. It was fo uncommon, that he imagined it proceeded from the active and volatile falts of the herbs fet loofe in the ftomach; to which he afcribed their cure. He therefore ftrictly injoined his patients, to prevent as much as poffible thefe falts from making their efcape.

The

The fermentation here is certainly never completed: but the effects of a beginning fermentation are still very powerful, though soon stopt; as will appear to those who are acquainted with the surprising effects of the subtile imperceptible *gas,* which is set free from such substances in this act.

As animal digestion is a process *sui generis,* which no chemical operation has been found to imitate; none being able to convert food into chyle, or that into blood; all we can infer from experience, is, that in certain cases, as in the scurvy, vegetable juices and fruits of this tendency are found necessary to preserve health and life. If flesh, or animal substances, promote this process in the stomach, as would seem by some late experiments *(g)* ; we may from thence fairly conclude, flesh-soops stuffed with vegetables to be eminently antiscorbutic, which daily and incontestable experience sufficiently confirms.

Upon the whole, it follows, and will be found true in fact, that the more any food, drink, herbs, or medicine, partake of any of the aforesaid qualities, the more antiscorbutic they become ; but that the most perfect and

(g) Pringle's experiment 35.

effectual

effectual remedies are found in a compofition
of different ingredients, each poffeffing in a
high degree one or other of thofe virtues,
from the combination of which, a vegetable,
faponaceous, fermentable acid may refult.
Such an acid, ready prepared, is to be had in
a certain degree in oranges, and moft ripening
fub-acid fruits; from whence they become the
moft effectual prefervatives againft this diftemper.

C H A P.   VII.

Diffections.

THE appearances in fcorbutic dead bodies, are here diftinguifhed under different numbers, for the convenience of making
proper references to them in the following
chapter.

N° 1. contains the obfervations made by Lord
Anfon's furgeons upon the blood of their patients, and upon the diffection of dead bodies, in
the feveral ftages of this diftemper at fea. N° 2.
a diffection made upon one of *Jaques Cartier*'s crew *(a)*. N° 3. to 21. *inclufive*, is

(a) See Part 3. chap. 1.

Mr

Mr *Poupart*'s account of many, and very accurate diffections of fcorbutic bodies, in the hofpital of *St Lewis* at *Paris*, in the year 1699 *(b)*. It will admit of no doubt, that this laft was a true fcurvy, as it proceeded from the fame caufes, *viz.* long want, improper food, grief, melancholy, cold, *&c.*; and the fymptoms were entirely alike with thofe in Lord *Anfon*'s crew; fuch as gums monftroufly putrid, fwelled legs, livid blue fpots and hardnefs on the body, contracted limbs, the fcorbutic *deliquium*, often ending in the moft fudden and unexpected death, fluxes and hæmorrhages of all forts, *&c.*

Nᵒ 1. In the beginning of the difeafe, the blood, as it flowed out of the orifice of the wound, might be feen to run in different fhades of light and dark ftreaks. When the malady was increafed, it ran thin, and feemingly very black; and after ftanding fome time in the porringer, turned thick, of a dark muddy colour; the furface in many places of a greenifh hue, without any regular feparation of its parts. In the third degree of the difeafe, it came out as black as ink; and though kept ftirring in the veffel many hours, its fibrous parts had

(b) *Etranges effets du fcorbut arrivez à Paris, par M. Poupart.* Memoires de l'academie des fciences 1699, p. 237.

only

only the appearance of a quantity of wool or hair, floating in a muddy fubftance. In dif- fected bodies, the blood in the veins was fo entirely broken, that, by cutting any confider- able branch, you might empty the part to which it belonged of its black and yellow li- quor; and when found extravafated, it was all of the fame kind. *Laftly*, As all other kinds of hæmorrhages were frequent at the latter end of the calamity, the fluid had the fame appear- ance as to colour and confiftence, whether it was difcharged from the mouth, nofe, ftomach, inteftines, or any other part.

2. The heart was found white and putrid; its cavities were quite full of corrupted blood. The lungs were blackifh and putrid; more than a quart of reddifh water was found in the *thorax*. The liver was pretty found; but the fpleen fomewhat corrupted, and rough as if it had been rubbed againft a ftone.

3. All thofe who had any difficulty of brea- thing, or their breafts ftuffed or ftopped up, had there a quantity of ferofity; and we found more or lefs of it according as they were op- preffed.

4. The breaft, belly, and feveral other parts of the body, were filled with this lymph or
ferum ;

ſerum; which was of different colours; and ſo corroſive, that having put our hands into it, the ſkin of them came off, attended with heat and inflammation.

5. We have ſeen ſome whoſe breaſt was ſo oppreſſed, that they died all of a ſudden.   In the mean time, we found no ſeroſity, neither in their breaſts nor in their lungs.   But the *pericardium* was entirely faſtened to the lungs; and the lungs were glued to the *pleura* and *diaphragm.*   All the parts were ſo mixed and blended with each other, that they made up but one maſs or lump, ſo confounded that one could ſcarce diſtinguiſh one from another.   As the lungs were ſqueezed together in the midſt of this maſs, they were deprived of their motion, and the ſick perſon was choked for want of breath.

6. All they who died ſuddenly, without any viſible cauſe of their death, had the auricles of their heart as big as one's fiſt, and full of coagulated blood.

7. We have ſeen ſeveral, who without pain dropped down dead.   They had no apparent ſickneſs; only their gums were ulcerated, without any ſpots or hardneſs on their ſkin: yet we found their muſcles were gangrened, and

R r   ſtuffed

ftuffed with a black corrupted blood; and upon handling them, they fell to pieces.

8. A youth of ten years had his gums much
fwelled, and deeply ulcerated; his breath intolerably ftinking. The furgeon was obliged to
pull out all his teeth, for the better dreffing of
his mouth. There appeared afterwards ulcers
upon his tongue and cheek. He died all of a
fudden, and his bowels were found corrupted.

9. Some with no other fymptoms but flight
ulcerations of their gums, had afterwards fmall
red hard tumours on their hands, feet, and o-
ther parts of their body: after which there appeared impofthumes in their groin, and under
their arm-pits, together with blue fpots on
their body. We found the glands under their
arm-pits very big, and furrounded with matter;
as well as the mufcles of their arms and thighs,
whofe interftices were all filled with it.

10. We obferved fome whofe arms, legs,
and thighs, were of a reddifh black. This proceeded from that black and coagulated blood
which we always found under the fkin of
thofe perfons.

11. We alfo found their mufcles fwelled and
hard. This was occafioned by blood fixed in the
body of the mufcles, which were fometimes fo
full

full of it, that their legs remained bent, without being able to extend or ftretch them out.

12. The blue, red, yellow, and black fpots, which appeared on the body, proceeded purely from extravafated blood under the fkin. As long as the blood kept its red colour, the fpot was red; if the blood was black and coagulated, the fpot was alfo black, *&c.*

13. We fometimes obferved certain fmall tumours, which, upon breaking, formed fcorbutic ulcers. They proceeded from the blood, with which the tumour was filled: for as often as we took off the plaifter, we ftill found under it a great deal of coagulated blood.

14. Some old perfons had fuch large bleedings from the nofe and mouth, that they died of them. The coats of the veffels were corroded and eat through by the fharp and corrofive humour.

15. In fome, when moved, we heard a fmall grating of the bones. Upon opening thofe bodies, the *epiphyfes* were found entirely feparated from the bones; which, by rubbing againft each other, occafioned this noife. In fome we perceived a fmall low noife when they breathed. In thofe the cartilages of the *fter-*

num were found feparated from the bony part of the ribs.

16. All thofe in whofe breaft any matter or ferofity was found, had their ribs thus feparated from the cartilages, and the bony part of the rib next the *fternum* carious for four fingers breadth.

17. There were fome dead bodies, in which, if we fqueezed, betwixt two fingers, the end of the ribs which began to be feparated from the cartilages, there came abundance of corrupted matter. This was the fpungy part of the bone: fo that, after fqueezing, there remained nothing of the rib but the two bony plates.

18. The ligaments of the joints were corroded and loofe. Inftead of finding in the cavities of the joints the ufual fweet oily mucilage, there was only a greenifh liquor; which, by its cauftic quality, had corroded the ligaments.

19. All the young perfons under eighteen had in fome degree their *epiphyfes* feparated from the body of the bone; this water having penetrated into the very fubftance of it.

20. In fcorbutic people the glands of the mefentery are generally obftructed and fwelled. Some of thefe were found partly corrupted and impofthumated. In the liver of fome few, the

matter

matter or corruption was hardened, and, as it were, petrified. Their spleen was three times bigger than natural; and fell to pieces, as if composed of coagulated blood. Sometimes the kidneys and breast were full of imposthumes.

21. What was very surprising, the brains of those poor creatures were always found and entire, and they preserved their appetite to the last.

C H A P.   VIII.

The nature of the symptoms, deduced and explained from the foregoing theory and dissections.

THE symptom most commonly preceeding the others in this disease, is a preternatural change of colour in the face. To explain this, it must be understood, that the solids in the human body are extremely small in proportion to the fluid parts; as appears plainly in cases of inanition and atrophies. But the colour of the whole body, especially the face, principally depends upon the nature and condition of the latter. We observe, a

small

318 Of the nature of the symptoms. Part II.

small quantity of bile mixed with the blood, tinges the whole surface of a living body; and a lucky anatomical injection will give any designed colour to that of a dead one. A natural and lively colour in the face denotes a well-conditioned, healthful, and homogeneous state of blood; such as is produced by the integrity of all the digestive powers, by the action of such good lungs, and elastic solids, as perfectly digest and assimilate the chyle into an animal nature. Paleness of the face, and a bloated complexion, are, on the contrary, signs of weakly fibres, and of a degeneracy of the humours, from the aforesaid sound and healthy condition, into a crude and morbid state.

The chyle is white when it enters the blood: but if (as in scorbutic cases) it remains there unsubdued, by reason of its viscidity, and the weakness of the concoctive faculties, it undergoes different changes of colour, and from white becomes yellow, greenish, livid, &c. This will be visibly discovered in the countenance through the translucent vessels of the skin; where the least alteration of colour in the fluids is easily perceptible; especially where these vessels lie most exposed, in the lips, gums, caruncles of the eye, &c.

But

But this crude heterogeneous humour dif-
tending the veffels in an inert ftate of folids,
will naturally either ftagnate in the lateral ca-
pillaries, where with difficulty it can be pro-
pelled forwards; or be extravafated in the *tunica adipofa*, at the greateft diftance from the
heart, where the circulation is moft languid,
and a *nifus*, contrary to its own gravity, required to pufh it on ; as in the legs, when in an e-
rect pofture. Hence fuch perfons are obferved
to have œdematous fwellings at firft about their
ancles, and on their legs. As the body becomes overloaded with a greater quantity of
fuch crudities, thefe tumours increafe; and o-
ther parts likewife, efpecially the face, becomes
pale, fwelled, and bloated.

Where the chyle is not affimilated, fo as to
nourifh the body, the *moles movenda* is increafed, (or a quantity of fuch humours is daily accumulated); mean while the *vires moventes*
are diminifhed : the ftrength and vigour of
our bodies being fupported chiefly by well-di-
gefted food Hence a laffitude, heavinefs, and
an averfion to exercife.

A fudden and remarkable proftration of
ftrength is indeed obferved conftantly to attend
all

all putrid difeafes *(a)*; of which this is the higheft degree of the chronic kind. But in the cafe of fcorbutic people, it is fomewhat fingular, and peculiar to them, that though when at reft they find themfelves quite well; yet, upon the leaft exercife, they are fubjeft, at firft, to a panting and breathleffnefs; which, as the difeafe increafes, degenerates into a pronenefs to faint; and, laftly, in the height of the malady, upon ufing exercife, or an exertion of their ftrength, or upon being expofed to a fudden change of air, they are apt to drop down dead.

In order to fet this in a clear light, it muft be obferved, that although the fcorbutic laffitude in general is owing to an obftrufted perfpiration; yet it does not fo much proceed from the weight of four or five pounds retained in the body, (which might eafily be carried about by any perfon, without uneafinefs, or being felt), as from the *vires imminutæ*, or the relaxed ftate of their fibres. In like manner, the more peculiar fymptoms mentioned, are produced by the effefts of this obftruftion, particularly in the lungs.

Perhaps it may be difficult to afcertain the

(a) Vid. Hoffman. de putredine.

exaft

exact quantity of perspirable matter sent off
from thence *(b)*. But it will appear to be a
very great proportion, if we consider the vast
extent of the perspirable surface of that organ,
the watery vapour constantly emitted from it so
visible in a cold air, and the just observation
of *Sanctorius*, " That it is a sign of health,
" when, after ascending a steep place, the bo-
" dy feels lighter" *(c)*; which would seem best
explained, by allowing a freer circulation of the
blood at this time through the lungs, when
freed from perspirable matter.

But such a moist air as is productive of the
scurvy, is already replete with humidity: so
that the moisture continually issuing from the
lungs, cannot be absorbed by it. On the contrary, the wet external air is continually
drawn into the vesicles; by which this bowel is
oppressed, not only with its own natural moisture, but is kept as it were in a continual watery bath of external air. Hence it becomes
surcharged with a serous *colluvies*; its tone is
consequently weakened, and some of its small-

(b) *Sanctorius* attempted it by breathing upon a glass: but Dr
Hales has made more accurate experiments.
(c) Aph. 17.

S f   er

er capillary veffels are neceffarily compreffed and obftructed.

When the body is at reft, the circulation is languid and flow: the blood then, in a fmall quantity, glides gently through the lungs, notwithftanding the obftruction in them. But when, upon ufing exercife, or an exertion of ftrength, the velocity of the blood is accelerated, and a much greater quantity, *viz.* that which, when at reft, was almoft ftagnating in the veins, is at once returned into the right cavities of the heart, and from thence into the lungs; the weakened and obftructed veffels of the lungs not being able fo quickly to tranfmit fo great a quantity, the blood is neceffarily accumulated in the *finus venofus*, right auricle and ventricle of the heart: which caufes a breathleffnefs and panting; that is, an effort is made by all the powers fubfervient to refpiration, to dilate the breaft fuller and more frequently, for the paffage of this increafed quantity of blood.

This will receive confirmation by feveral confiderations; as, that upon exerting a degree of ftrength, we hold in our breath; as alfo that the right ventricle of the heart is larger than the left ventricle, the *fyftole* of both is fynchronous,

chronous, and yet, what is fingular, the pulmonary vein is lefs than the pulmonary artery.

But when the perfpiration has been long obftructed by this damp air, which, as *Sanctorius*
fays, turns the perfpirable matter into ferofity,
or an *ichor*, as he calls it *(d)*, which is found
to be truly the cafe in fcorbutic people upon diffection (fee chap. 7. N° 2. and 3.), the paffage of
the blood through the lungs muft ftill be more
ftraitened. Hence, upon the leaft motion of the
body, by which the circulation is quickened, and
a greater quantity of blood fent at once into the
heart, the heart becomes in fuch cafes not able
to overcome the refiftance it meets with in forcing the blood through the lungs, as well as
the weakened unclaftic arteries. Whence,
as before obferved, the blood being accumulated, and ftagnating as it were, in the
cavities of the heart, there muft follow an almoft entire ftoppage of the circulation for fome
time, a paufe and ceffation of the vital motions for a little; that is, the patient muft
faint away, till, by the exertion of the vital prin-
ciple, and the heart being evacuated by the

(d) Aph. 146.

perfon's

person's lying at rest, the circulation is again quickened, and he recovers *(e)*.

Lastly, It appears by the weakness and fee‑bleness of the pulse, and many other symptoms in this disease, as likewise from the known effect of putrefaction on animal bodies, by which the fibres are always rendered softer and tenderer, that the whole system of solids is in the most relaxed and weakened condition. E‑ven the heart itself was found putrid, (N° 2.), whose force to circulate the blood is not inde‑finite, more than its cavities, which can con‑tain only a proportioned quantity. The first is certainly here greatly impaired; while the lat‑ter, or its cavities, were found preternaturally weakened and dilated, (N° 6.). In this state, such people are apt to drop down dead upon an exertion of their strength, or from ex‑ercise, but especially upon being exposed to a sudden change of air; that is, by removing them at once from the warm and moist air in the hold of a ship *(f)*, into a colder, drier, and

(e) The swoonings of scorbutic persons are different from what happen to very weak and exhausted people in other diseases, upon being raised up. When they sit, they are quite hearty, and have a considerable degree of strength.

(f) The air in the hold of a ship is always moister than even
upon

and purer air. For the effect of this is, to
conftringe the whole external habit of the body,
and to drive the blood at once with great force
from thence towards the heart; at which time
the velocity, as well as quantity of it, is increafed in the internal parts. So that the heart is
not able to overcome the refiftance it meets with
in the weak and unfound lungs, (whofe veffels
are alfo ftraitened by the contact of fuch frefh
air); nor in the arteries, which will be in proportion to the quantity of blood with which they
remain diftended. But the weak unelaftic ar-
terial fyftem is not here able to contract and
propel the blood in their canals. On the contrary, the cutaneous veffels being thus conftrin-
ged by the external air, the blood may perhaps have, as it were for an inftant, a retro-
grade motion towards the heart, which this
debilitated mufcle (N° 2.) cannot overcome.
Hence fuch people drop down dead fuddenly,

upon the upper deck. This is owing to the cables, and the o-
ther contents of the hold, not having a free circulation of air or
wind, to dry up the water, either of the fea or rains, poured
down upon them. Places below become alfo extremely moift,
by the frefh water and beer fpilt in pumping them from the
cafks, by the bilge-water, and by the cutaneous and pulmonary perfpiration of a number of people pent up in the fick-
apartment.

without

without any other vifible caufe of their death found upon diffection, (N° 6.), than the weakened auricles of their heart aneurifmatic, and diftended with blood. They are obferved to have a panting or breathleffnefs for about half a minute before they expire *(g)*.

In Lord *Anfon's* crew it was remarked, that a ftraitnefs of the breaft, with an obftinate coftivenefs, was one of the moft dangerous and fatal fymptoms. Now, in this cafe, there was no relief to the breaft, no evacuation to free it from the load of obftructed perfpiration; part of which, no doubt, may be carried off by ftool. Accordingly, where a derivation is made of the humours in fcorbutic people by an open belly, their breafts are generally found much eafier.

Of the fame kind perhaps with the perfpiration from the lungs, and external furface of the fkin, is that moifture continually exhaling from all parts within the cavities of the body. It is at leaft fupplied by the like means, *viz.*

(g) Why only the auricles of the heart in this cafe become aneurifmatic, *vid. Lancif. de aneurifmatibus in genere, prop.* 52. This fpecies of fudden death is called by the great *Harvey, fuffocatio ob copiam*; and is beautifully illuftrated by his experiment, *Exercitat.* 1. *de motu cordis.*

from

from proper aliment *(h)*. By it the bowels, and their cavities, are kept separate, and prevented from adhering to each other. This being wanting in some, proved likewise the occasion of their death, (N° 5.); while in others the corrupted and putrified state of their body put an end to their lives, (N° 7. 8. 9.).

I come now to account for the pathognomonic signs of this disease, *viz.* the putrid gums, &c. I shall upon this occasion observe, that although it is no easy matter to say why, in several general and universal disorders of the body, some particular parts are only or principally affected, while others, in such a state of almost universal corruption and putrefaction, as in the scurvy, continue to perform their functions as in health (see N° 21.); yet we may hereby perceive the goodness of Providence, who, by certain signs peculiar to each disease, points out the malady, and gives us a medical and demonstrative certainty of its existence. But as this reasoning may appear too unphilosophical, I shall endeavour to account for these symptoms in the mechanical way.

The pathognomonic signs of the scurvy, which are putrid gums, a stinking breath, and

(h) Vid. p. 290

loosening

loosening of the teeth, we find also in persons who, by long fasting, are deprived of a supply of fresh chyle. This confirms what I observed before, that the scorbutic corruption is of that species which is the natural effect of heat and motion ; the humours of the body, from want of a proper chyle to dilute and sweeten them, becoming rank and putrescent. In several orders of different religions, those who are obliged, by way of penance, to abstain a considerable time from food, perceive their breath become fœtid, their teeth loose, their gums spungy and soft *(i)*. The same symptoms are also observed in those who are starved to death *(k)*. In all those, as well as in scorbutic cases, these symptoms seem principally owing to the *saliva*; which, upon such occasions, becomes acrid. Every one's experience must convince him it is more so after ten or twelve hours abstinence from food, than at other times.

But to understand more particularly why the

(i) I have always observed men of the rigorous orders in the church of *Rome* greatly scorbutic. They are remarkable for rotten gums, (part of which is commonly eat away), want of teeth, and a most offensive breath.

(k) Vid. Tschirnhauf. medicin. corporis, p. 23. Lister de humoribus, cap. 12.

gums

gums are principally, and often first, affected by this acrimony, it must be observed, that the vessels here lie very much expofed to the external air; which has a great effect in haftening corruption, to which the *reliquiæ ciborum* may contribute. At the same time their fubftance is the moft tenfe and hard of any part of the mouth *(l)*, and perhaps of the whole body. Now, by the acrimony of the blood, *faliva*, or other juices, we may be fuppofed to underftand a change of figure in their particles; from being foft, blunt, and obtufe, to somewhat fharp, angular, and pointed. Hence the effect of acrimony on the human body is, to ftimulate and irritate the parts.

Thus, in the gums, thefe acrimonious particles occafion at firft an uneafy itching. But they are the moft tenfe, and confequently the moft elaftic, of any other parts of the mouth. The ofcillations or contractions of the very numerous veffels, therefore, will here proportionably be greatly increafed; and thence action and reaction become in this place greater than in any other. The blood is confequently more moved, broken, and protruded even into the dilated lateral veffels, (according to the *Boer-*

(l) See *Winflow expof. anatom. de la ftructure du corps humain.*

T. t   *haavian*

haavian system); which in such a case will admit larger globules than can pass through their extremities. They therefore appear swelled, and distended with a livid blood; and in this state are apt to bleed upon the least friction of their tender dilated vessels. But the resistance of the solids being at last quite overcome, and their elasticity destroyed, the blood must stagnate in all the vessels; and, by stagnation and rest, of course becoming more acrid, corrode their coats, and bring on a general state of corruption and putrefaction on these parts.

The effects indeed of such acrimonious juices are felt universally in the body upon any increase of motion, and consequently of their force against the containing vessels; scorbutic people being most sensible of their pains upon motion or exercise of any sort, according to the known axiom, *Acria nulla agunt si non moveantur.*

It was observed before, that the depending situation of the legs in an erect or sitting posture, particularly determined the humours to stagnation there, in the very beginning of the disease; which in the increase of it often become monstrously swelled. But such stagnating corrupt blood and humours are, upon the least rupture of the skin, apt to form into

scorbutic

scorbutic ulcers. These generally occur upon the shin; where the least accidental squeeze makes a considerable bruise of the thin skin, against the hard and sharp spine of the *tibia*. Their appearance is truly described N° 13. and accounted for N° 10. and 11.

In such a state of blood (N° 1.) as appeared both in living and dead bodies, we have no reason to be surprised at the frequent hæmorrhages from all parts of the body, fluxes, dysenteries, &c. to which such people are subject; nor at its bursting out from the scars of old wounds in Lord *Anson*'s crew. These are, for many reasons, liable to such accidents; not only from the hard and imperspirable *cicatrix* with which they are generally covered, but from a want here of the *tunica adiposa*, into whose cells the extravasated blood is poured, when it appears in spots on the body (N° 12.).

Putrefaction is found to be the most subtile of all dissolvents, powerfully separating and resolving the component parts of putrifying bodies; and in particular, breaking and dissolving the *crasis* of the blood. So that both here and in the plague, the spots appear altogether alike, as observed by *Diemerbroeck de peste*.

There is somewhat indeed singular in the

effects

effects of the scorbutic acrimony upon the
bones, (see N° 15. 16. but particularly 17.);
whereby it appears to affect chiefly the internal cellular part, which is known to be of a
different texture from the outward bony *laminæ.*
And from thence it is easy to account for those
remarkable cases which occurred likewise in
Lord *Anson*'s squadron, where the *callus* of
broken bones, which had been compleatly
formed for a long time, was found dissolved,
and the fracture seemed as if it had never been
consolidated. It must be remembered, that the
bones, like all the other parts of the body, are
daily nourished and repaired by the aliment.
There are many instances of entire bones being generated in the body anew. And it appears, that a *callus* is not (as has been vulgarly
supposed) a rude glutinous mass, spued out
from the extremities of the bones, by which
they are glued together: but is really, like new
flesh generated in wounds with loss of substance, a true organised part restored, of the
same cellular texture with the other parts of
the bone; with this difference, that it wants
the outward bony *lamella (m)* : so that, from
this defect, it becomes, of all other parts of

(m) *Vid. Rusch thesaur. anatom. n.* 8.

the

the bone, most liable to be affected by the scorbutic taint.

Now, if the humours of the body, in the advanced stages of this malady, are capable of acquiring so corrosive a degree of acrimony, that, like a *menstruum*, they work upon and dissolve the cellular texture of the very bones, it is natural to suppose, that the nutritious particles are here so much depraved in the very beginning, or where there is only a scorbutic habit of body, that no *callus* can be formed; of which Dr *Mead* furnishes us with a remarkable proof *(n)*. However, it is almost universally the case in the scurvy, as observed elsewhere *(o)*, that as long as any bone is sufficiently defended by its external thick plates, it will not be found carious in this disease until broken and separated, (as in N° 16. and 17.); so that the humour has access into the internal cellular substance of it. For this reason, it is rare to find a carious jaw, after the most virulent ulcers in the gums, unless by some accident, as the pulling out of a tooth, part of the *laminæ* of that bone has been broken. In the same manner, the teeth will likewise be

(n) Discourse on the scurvy, p. 107.
(o) Chap 2. p. 164.

preserved

preserved found, if their outer coats are entire.

There is a reason assigned N° 18. for the loss of motion which happens commonly to the joint of the knee in this disease. To which it may be added, that the lubricating liniment of the joints is said to be partly composed of the perspirable matter *(p)*; which being here either deficient, or degenerated into a morbid state, may induce this symptom.

It likewise appears, that the oily mucilage that lubricates the hard tendons, and their sheaths, and which fits them for motion, is of a similar nature with the liquor found in the cavities of the joints *(q)*. We have a proof of its extreme depravity in N° 18; so that they must necessarily become hard, contracted, and unfit for motion.

It is indeed the universal perspiring humour, exhaling from all parts, both external and internal, of the body, which gives softness, pliancy, and suppleness, to the whole machine. And it is a deficiency of this which occasions hardness of the flesh, contraction of limbs, want of motion, and indurated tendons, in scorbutic cases.

(p) Vid. Van Swieten comment. in Boerhaave aph. 556.
(q) Vid. Kaau de perspiratione, n. 854.

Lastly,

Lastly, If we confider the other appearances obferved upon diffection, *viz.* the fwelled, obftructed, and putrid ftate of the *vifcera*, (N° 20.); the rottennefs of the heart itfelf, (N° 2.); in fome the univerfal putrefaction of the body *(r)*, (N° 7. 8. and 9.); the cauftic acrimony of the lymph found in its different cavities, (N° 4.); with the condition of that vital fluid the blood, even when alive, (N° 1.), where its dark and livid colour, but efpecially the greenifh hue, denoted the higheft degree of putrefaction *(f)*; we will have no reafon to be furprifed at the moft extraordinary and anomalous fymptoms, which fometimes have occurred in this difeafe.

The following letter from Dr *John Cook*, phyfician at *Hamilton*, was received too late to be inferted in its proper place.

I Here fend you fome brief remarks I made in general upon the fcurvy in *Ruffia*, *Tartary*, &c. in all which countries it is an endemic and dreadful difeafe.

Taverhoff lies in 52 deg. of N. Lat. where the

(r) Bachftrom, p. 20. obferves, that the dead bodies of fcorbutic people corrupt much fooner than others, and are attended with a remarkable *fœtor*.

(f) See Dr *Pringle's* experiments, exper. 45. on putrified blood.

ftream of the *Verona* is received into the *Don.* It is
fituated, as moſt towns on the banks of that river, on
a low fandy foil, and furrounded with lakes, marſhes,
and woods. The winter commonly begins in the
month of *October.* In *November,* all the rivers, lakes,
and marſhes, are quite frozen over, and the whole
country is covered with ſnow; which continues until
about the beginning of *April,* O. S. At this time the
ſnow ſuddenly melts away, leaving the earth covered with graſs, and many wholſome vegetables. The
ſpring is ſo very ſhort, that the inhabitants are ſcarcely
ſenſible of it : for in leſs than fifteen days the weather becomes exceſſive hot; and the cold froſty winter is ſuddenly expelled by a very warm ſummer,
that continues until the month of *September*: during
which time the weather is very hot and moiſt. When
I was there in the years 1738 and 1739, 27,000
boors were employed in cutting wood, and preparing
it for building of ſhips for the uſe of the army; as
alſo about 5 or 600 ſailors, who were their overſeers,
and between 2 and 3000 ſoldiers, who guarded the
boors to prevent their making an eſcape. In the
month of *February* 1738, the ſcurvy made its appearance. The boors were not ſo much afflicted with it
as the ſailors, nor the ſailors ſo much as the ſoldiers.
Many, both ſailors and ſoldiers, were ſent to our hoſpital this month; but their numbers were greatly increaſed in *March.* Towards the latter end of *April*
they were moſtly recovered, and many were diſcharged from the hoſpital. In *June* none remained except

cept the moſt inveterate caſes. In *July* an intermitting, and an obſtinate remitting fever, prevailed. From the 1ſt to the 20th of *Auguſt* we had but few patients. From that time to the 1ſt of *October*, agues raged with more violence than ever; and fluxes ſucceeded in *October*. This month the firſt ſnow fell; and at that time children were univerſally affected with ſore throats. We had afterwards ſettled froſty weather, and but little ſickneſs, except a few inflammatory fevers; until about the beginning of the year 1739, when the ſcurvy began to ſhew itſelf, much about the ſame time as in the preceeding year, and continued its uſual length of time.

Aſtracan is ſituated in 46¼ deg. N. Lat. on a ſmall iſland waſhed by the *Volga*. Here are many ſalt lakes, both upon the iſlands and deſart. The garriſon-ſoldiers are much more ſubject to the ſcurvy than the boors, and theſe laſt than the ſailors. The ſoldiers live a very indolent life, having but little duty to perform. They eat hardly any thing elſe, even in their hoſpitals, beſides rye bread and meal, with fiſh; and have nothing but water for drink, except the decoctions preſcribed for them by the ſurgeons. Their hoſpitals are very damp and rotten. This poor garriſon of five regiments, conſiſting of about 6000 men when compleat, is yearly recruited with between 600 and 1000 men. The boors live alſo but a lazy indolent life; being employed either in fiſhing, or in navigating great boats, from *Aſtracan* ſometimes as far as *Tweer*. On the contrary, the ſailors work hard,

at

at all times of the year, both in the docks and at fea; and live much better, having good provifions of all forts. The winter begins commonly in *October*, and continues till *March*. It is extremely fevere during the months of *January* and *February*. The fcurvy generally breaks out in the latter end of *February*. I found it here often complicated with other difeafes, *viz.* the *lues venerea*, agues, dropfies, *phthifis*, &c. The violence of the diftemper (except in complicated cafes) feldom continues after *June*, or to the middle of *July*.

Riga, the metropolis of *Livonia*, is the laft place I fhall mention. The winters are here very long. The foil for many miles about it is fandy, and covered with many lakes, moffes, and moraffes. The boors living better than they do in *Ruffia* and *Tartary*, are not fo fubject here to the fcurvy as the foldiers in the army, nor thefe fo much as the proper garrifon; for by their labour they gain money, and can purchafe flefh in winter. The garrifon-foldiers, confifting of between 6 and 7000 men, are moft miferably lodged. The walls of their ill-contrived barracks are continually moift and warm. At *Riga*, in the years 1749 and 1750, but efpecially in the year 1751, the fcurvy raged with the utmoft violence. It broke out in the month of *February* that year. Here I faw the moft dreadful fpectacles that ever I beheld. Their rotten gums gangrened, as alfo their lips, which dropped off; the *fphacelus* fpread to their cheeks, and mufcles of their lower jaw; and the jaw-bone in fome

fell

fell down upon the *sternum.* When the mortification first began, we tried the bark, to no purpose. Nothing but death rid the unhappy wretches of their frightful misery.

Dr *Nitzsch*'s method of cure *(t)* corresponds with, and is agreeable to the method practised in *Russia,* especially by the *German* physicians and surgeons. What he terms the *hot* or *painful scurvy,* is generally a complication of this disease with the pox. Although some may die in the state he describes, without having any outward swelling upon the body; yet such persons have always scirrhous swellings of the glands in the *abdomen,* particularly of the mesenteric glands, and of the liver, which are perceptible to the touch, even before death. My method of cure was in general as follows, unless some particular symptoms or cases required me to deviate from it. I commonly began with a very gentle purge or two, and then gave the *decoct. antiscorb. (u)*, and *essent antiscorb.* At *Astracan,* we gave the juice of *rad. raphan.* mixed with a very little brandy, twice a-day. The patients had fresh flesh-meat every day, and what greens or salads we could procure them. They used the warm bath once or twice a-week. Before they eat, drank, or swallowed any medicines, their mouths were well gargarised with solutions of nitre, &c. Their gums were dressed with *ung. Ægyptiac. tinct. myrrh. tinct.*

(t) Vid. Part 3.

(u) I presume the Doctor means the *decoct. sum. pin.* &c described by *Nitzsch.*

lact.

lacc. &c. I obliged them to ufe exercife, and to walk about both forenoon and afternoon, when the weather would permit. I allowed them to fleep moderately; and forbid them all dried, falt, and fat meats. Fumigating the wards, is common in all the hofpitals in *Ruffia.*

When I came home to this country, I found the denomination of *nervous diforders* univerfally applied to moft chronic and cachectic ailments. Upon examining thofe complaints in the lower fort of people, who live entirely on the farines and a grofs diet, I obferved, they had a univerfal laffitude, pains which they termed *rheumatic* flying through their body, and a breathleffnefs upon ufing exercife. The legs were fometimes fwelled, and the *abdomen* almoft always tenfe and tumified. But, whether they had fwellings or not, they had generally an ill-coloured fcorbutic complexion, and were liftlefs and inactive to a great degree, with complaints of pains in their jaws, teeth, &c. I made no fcruple to pronounce fuch cafes fcorbutic; and by proper antifcorbutic regimen, medicines, diet, and exercife, feldom failed to give very fenfible relief. I have difobliged many patients, by faying they had the fcurvy; a difeafe as hateful as it is unknown in this part of the world: but the relief they obtained from antifcorbutics, foon convinced both them and myfelf, that their cafes were not miftaken.

A

A
TREATISE
OF THE
SCURVY.

PART III.

CHAP. I.

Paſſages in ancient authors, ſuppoſed to refer to the ſcurvy; together with the firſt accounts of it.

THIS diſtemper, barbarouſly in the *Latin* denominated *ſcorbutus*, is ſaid to derive its appellation from *ſchorbeſt* in the *Daniſh* language; or the old *Dutch* word *ſcorbeck*: both which ſignify a tearing or ulcers of the mouth. Moſt authors have deduced the term from the *Saxon* word *ſchorbok*, a griping or tearing of the belly; which is by no means ſo uſual a ſymptom of this diſeaſe; though, from a miſtake in the etymology of the name, it has been accounted ſo by theſe authors. The word ſeems to me moſt naturally to be made out from *ſcorb* in the *Sclavonic* language, which ſignifies a *diſeaſe*; this being the endemic evil in *Ruſſia*, and thoſe northern countries, from whence we borrowed the name (*a*).

(*a*) Vid. Hiſt. natural. Ruſſiæ. Commerc. literar. Norimb. ann. 1733. p. 274.

It

It is faid to have been known and defcribed by the ancient writers in phyfic under other denominations; and particularly by *Hippocrates,* as the ιλιὸς αιματάδης, or third fpecies of *volvulus (b).* He fays, thofe who labour under that difeafe, have a foetid breath, lax gums, and an hæmorrhage from the nofe; ulcers fometimes on their legs, which heal up, while others break out anew. Their colour is black, their fkin fine and thin; they are chearful, and prompt to action. He afterwards adds, that it required a tedious cure, was with difficulty removed, and often accompanied the patient to his death. *Langius* was of opinion, that this contained a defcription of our modern fcurvy. He imagined alfo the *lues venerea* to be nothing more than a complication of fymptoms and difeafes which had been before defcribed by the ancients; to prove which he wrote two of his epiftles *(c).* *Foëfius, Dodonæus,* and fome others, would here willingly fupply a defect, by putting in the particle ὁ. This would indeed quite alter the fenfe of *Hippocrates,* making the difeafe attended with an averfion to all fort of exercife, more agreeable to the true genius of the fcurvy.

But the moft prevailing opinion is, that, in different parts of his writings, *Hippocrates* has defcribed the fcurvy under the name of Σπλῆν μέγας, *a fwelling and obftruction of the fpleen.* After having told us *(d),* that an hæmorrhage from the nofe, in people otherwife feemingly healthy, prefaged either a fwelling of the fpleen, pain in the head, or floating images before the eyes, he defcribes thofe with the fwelling of their fpleen, as having unfound gums, and a ftinking breath. If thefe fymptoms did not appear, they then had ulcers on the *tibia,* and black *cicatrices.* After mentioning fome fymptoms

(b) *Lib. de intern. affectionibus. Edit. Foëfii, p. 557.*
(c) *Epift. 13. et 14.*
(d) *Prorrhetic. lib. 2. p. 111.*

which

which give reaſon to expect an eruption of blood from
the noſe, he adds another diagnoſtic, *viz.* a ſwelling
under the eye-lids; to which if there be joined a ſwelling of the feet, they would ſeem to labour under a
dropſy. He treats of this diſeaſe in another place *(e)*;
where he takes no notice of the gums being affected, but
only of the breath being offenſive; the patient's loſing
colour, being lean, and having bad ulcers. The ſpleen
felt hard, and always of an equal bigneſs, in thoſe of
a bilious habit; but in a pituitous conſtitution, it was
ſometimes bigger, and ſometimes leſs. Several received ſmall benefit from medicine, by which the ſwelling
of their ſpleen was uſually but little abated: and the
diſeaſe not yielding to any remedies, ſome in progreſs
of time fell into dropſies; but in others the hardneſs
and ſwelling continued to old age. If it ſuppurated,
they were cured by burning the part. He is elſewhere *(f)* ſtill more particular in his deſcription of
that diſeaſe. In thoſe who labour under it, the belly
is firſt ſwelled, then the ſpleen is enlarged, and feels
hard, with acute pain. They loſe their colour; become black, or pale, of the hue of a pomegranate rind;
emit a diſagreeable ſmell from their ears and gums, (the
latter of which ſeparate from the teeth); have ulcers on
the *tibia*, extenuated limbs, and a coſtive belly. He
attributes theſe ſwellings *(g)* to the drinking of ſtagnating, raw, and unwholſome waters; where he deſcribes
the *lienoſi* as thin, meagre, and extenuated by the diſeaſe.

The reader will hereby be enabled to judge, or better by conſulting the original itſelf, how far *Hippocrates*
has deſcribed the modern ſcurvy under the appellation of
a ſwelling of the ſpleen. It appears by ſeveral paſſages

(e) Lib. de affectionibus, p. 521.
(f) Lib. de intern. affectionibus, p. 549.
(g) Lib. de acre, aquis, et locis, p. 283.

in

in his works, that he imagined the yellow jaundice owing to an obftruction of the liver, and the black to that of the fpleen, efpecially to a *fcirrhus* of it. An obftruction or hardnefs of that *vifcus*, as well as fome parts contiguous to it, which he might eafily miftake for it, often occurs in practice; and is owing chiefly to fuch caufes as he affigns (*h*), *viz.* ill-conditioned fevers, particularly of the intermittent kind; and, as he juftly adds, is a difeafe not in itfelf mortal, though of tedious cure (*i*). But diffections have fufficiently proved, that in the fcurvy the fpleen is but feldom affected, or at leaft is not the caufe or feat of the difeafe. Dr *Mead* gives us an inftance (*k*) of a preternatural fwelling of the fpleen found after death in a countryman of the ifland of *Sheppey*, who had fcorbutic fymptoms. But it is to be remarked, the patient laboured under a complicated difeafe, efpecially a violent intermitting fever, which is often attended with obftructed *vifcera*. That this difeafe was not known or defcribed by *Hippocrates*, farther appears from his making no mention of fpots, an ufual fymptom in the fcurvy, nor of many others which almoft conftantly attend it. Upon the whole, we may be perfuaded, that had this divine author feen the diftemper, he, who ftudied nature with fo much care, and copied her with fo great exactnefs, would have left us a more accurate defcription of it. But the truth is, the warm fouthern climate in which he lived, was not then, nor is at this day, productive of it: and the nature of the coafting voyages of the ancients gave him no opportunity of being acquainted with it at fea. So that there

(*h*) *Lib. de intern. affection. p.* 521.
(*i*) This diftemper is obferved by my ingenious friend Mr *Cleghorn* to be one of thofe to which the inhabitants of *Minorca* are fubject, from their fcarcity of well-water, and the frequency of tertian fevers in that ifland. *Obfervations on the epidemic difeafes of Minorca, Introduction; p.* 67.
(*k*) *Monit. et præcept. medic. cap.* 16. *de fcorbuto.*

feems

feems no occafion for paying him a compliment here; as it is not to be expected he fhould have hinted at, much lefs have defcribed a difeafe, which in all proba- bility he never faw nor heard of. It muft indeed have been a frequent malady, if it was the fame as the en- larged fpleen, which he fo often and fully defcribes in his writings. If we might have expected it any where, it would have been in his account of the inhabitants of *Phafis (l)*; where he compares the nature and make of the *Afiatics* with the *Europeans*, and accounts for the various conftitutions, manners, &c. of different nations, from their particular foil, climate, and air. He de- fcribes the *Phafians* inhabiting a low, damp, marfhy foil; living in wooden houfes built upon the waters; preferving a communication with each other by means of ditches, upon which they were continually paffing in boats made of hollowed trees. Their air was thick, moift, and impure; the waters they drank, ftagnant and warm, corrupted by the fun, and fupplied by the rains; which were there inceffant and violent. Upon account of which fituation, they differed from other men in their make; being in ftature taller, and fo corpulent, that their veins and joints hardly appeared; their colour was pale, inclining to yellow; they had a harfher voice than other nations, and were naturally flower to action. Thefe are all the remarks he makes upon them, without adding any one fcorbutic appearance, to which we would naturally have fuppofed them fubject.

The fucceeding *Greek* and *Roman* authors, are like- wife upon this difeafe entirely filent. They copy from *Hippocrates* pretty nearly the account they give of the *lienofi*; without adding any one fymptom which

---

(l) Lib. de aëre, aquis, et locis.
Phafis was a city in the ancient kingdom of *Colchis*, upon the eaft- ermoft fide of the *Black fea*, between *Georgia* and *Circaffia*, not far from the ancient *Sauromatæ*.

would

would induce us to believe, that either he meant, or they underſtood it to be the ſcurvy (*m*).

It alſo ſeems to have been a diſeaſe altogether unknown to the *Arabian* writers. They have made no mention of ſuch a diſtemper in any part of their works; though *Avicenna* (*n*), the moſt conſiderable amongſt them, has deſcribed the ſpleen-malady at great length, with the ſame ſymptoms as done by the *Greeks*.

Some who are extremely fond of attributing much to the knowledge of the ſage ancients, would have it to be the ſame with the *oſcedo* deſcribed by *Marcellus* (*o*). Dr *Poupart* thought the malignant ſcurvy obſerved at *Paris*, had a reſemblance to the *Athenian* plague, as deſcribed by *Lucretius* (*p*). *Moellenbroek* imagined the ſervant of the centurion at *Capernaum* (*q*) to have had this diſtemper. But ſuch opinions deſerve no ſerious confutation.

It has, laſtly, and with greater ſhew of reaſon, been eſteemed the ſame malady which afflicted the *Roman* army under the command of *Cæſar Germanicus.* In order to judge of which, it may be proper to tranſcribe the narration as it is in *Pliny* (*r*).

(*m*) *Celſus*, in his elegant manner, almoſt literally tranſlates *Hippocrates*.

Quibus ſæpe ex naribus fluit ſanguis, his aut lien tumet, aut capitis dolores ſunt: quos ſequitur, ut quædam ante oculos tanquam imagines obverſentur. At quibus magni ſunt lienes, his gingivæ malæ ſunt, et os olet, aut ſanguis aliquâ parte prorumpit. Quorum ſi nihil evenit, neceſſe eſt in cruribus mala ulcera, et ex his nigræ cicatrices fiant. Lib. 2. cap. 7.

Ætius, tetrab. 3. *ſerm.* 3.
Paulus Ægineta, lib. 3. *cap.* 49.
Aretæus de cauſis et ſignis morborum, lib. 1. *cap.* 14.
Cæl. Aurelian. chronic. ſive tardar. paſſion. lib. 3. *cap.* 4.
(*n*) *Can.* 3. *ſen.* 15. *tract.* 2. *cap.* 5. *de ſignis apoſtematum ſplenis.*
(*o*) *Lib. de medicamentis, cap.* 2.
(*p*) *Lib.* 6. *Vid. Thucydid.*
(*q*) See *Matth.* viii. 5.
(*r*) *Hiſtor. natural. lib.* 25. *cap.* 3.

" The

" The *Roman* army under the command of *Cæſar*
" *Germanicus* having incamped in *Germany*, beyond the
" *Rhine*, near the ſea-coaſt, they met with a fountain
" of ſweet water; by the drinking of which, in the
" ſpace of two years, the teeth dropt out, and the joints
" of the knees became paralytic (ſ). The phyſicians
" called the malady *ſtomacace* and *ſceletyrbe*. They
" diſcovered a remedy againſt it, *viz. herba Britannica,*
" a ſalutary medicine not only in diſorders of the mouth
" and nerves, but for the quinſey, bite of ſerpents, &c."
The whole ſeems pretty extraordinary. And I cannot
help remarking, that the loſs of their teeth, and the uſe
of their limbs, in two years after drinking this water;
the extraordinary virtues aſcribed to *herba Britannica*;
and the romantic directions afterwards added of gathering
it before thunder, ſavour much of that fabulous credu-
lity for which this author is ſo juſtly blamed. But had
a more credible hiſtorian given us this relation, it would
ſtill ſeem exceptionable, upon many accounts, as referring
to the ſcurvy.

Thoſe places beyond the *Rhine*, *viz.* the northern
parts of the *Netherlands*, are now well known, and no
ſuch fountain has ever been diſcovered. No mention
is made of ſcorbutic ſpots, which are more frequently
obſerved than what has been here interpreted the *ſceletyrbe*. This is ſuppoſed to refer to the rigid tendons in
the ham. But his delineation by no means ſeems to ex-
preſs this peculiar ſymptom in the ſcurvy. It is underſtood by *Galen* (t), the only author who uſes the appellation, to mean a ſpecies of palſy very different from
the ſcorbutic contraction.

Strabo (u) mentions a like malady occaſioned by the uſe

(ſ) *Compages in genubus ſolverentur.*
(t) *In definition. medic. p. 265, tom. 2. Ed. Charterii.*
(u) Στομακάκκη τί καὶ σκιλοτύρβη πιιραζομίνης τῆς ρατιᾶς ἰπιχωρίοις πάθισι, τῶν μίν πιρὶ τὸ ρόμα, τῶν δὶ πιρὶ τὰ σκίλη παραλυτίν τινα δηλώϛαν, ἰκ τι τῶν ὑ- δριίων, καὶ τῶν βοτανῶν. Strabon. geograph. lib. 16. ſub finem.

of

of certain fruits, &c. to have afflicted the army under the command of *Ælius Gallus* in *Arabia.* But *ſtomacace* may juſtly be underſtood to mean various other diſorders of the mouth, (aphthous, and other kinds), without ſuppoſing it to be the ſcurvy; as this calamity, when general in an army, occaſioning the *ſceletyrbe,* or depriving the ſoldiers of the uſe of their limbs, muſt needs have been attended with other concomitant ſymptoms, equally conſtant and remarkable in the diſeaſe *(x).* Theſe would no doubt have been particularly deſcribed by the ſucceeding writers in phyſic, who had opportunity of ſeeing both *Pliny*'s and *Strabo*'s writings.

There would have been no occaſion to have dwelt ſo long upon this inquiry, (as it may appear a matter of no great importance, to be rightly informed whether this diſeaſe was known to the ancients or not), if a miſplaced eſteem for their works had not been productive of ill conſequences on practice, and in the cure of this diſeaſe. Many, believing the ſpleen the ſeat of it, have adapted their medicinal intentions to the relief of that bowel; while others have wrote whole volumes to diſcover the true *herba Britannica,* endued with ſuch ſuppoſed miraculous virtues.

But as people are apt to run from one extreme to another, ſuch has been here the caſe. Many not finding the diſeaſe in any deſcription of the ancients, have ſuppoſed it a new calamity, making its appearance in the world, like the *lues venerea,* at a certain period of time *(y)*; an opinion equally, if not more cenſurable than

---

(x) Not that I would be underſtood to mean, that the ſcurvy never afflicted armies of old; but only that the accounts we have of it are dubious and imperfect. The firſt deſcription of a true ſcurvy that I have met with, is what occurred in the Chriſtian army in *Ægypt,* about the year 1260, under *Lewis* IX. But there mention is made, not only of the legs being affected, but alſo of the ſpots. The fungous and putrid gums are particularly deſcribed, &c. *Vid. Hiſtoire de Lewis IX. par le Sieur Joinville.*
(y) Vid. *Freind*'s hiſtory of phyſic.

the former. For as there ſeem to have been two reaſons principally why it is ſo imperfectly, if at all, deſcribed by the ancients, *viz.* their little knowledge of the
northern countries, where it is peculiarly endemic, and
their ſhort coaſting-voyages; ſo we find, that as ſoon
as arts and ſciences began to be cultivated among thoſe
northern nations, (about the beginning of the ſixteenth
century, a period remarkable for the advancement of
learning over all *Europe*), this diſeaſe is mentioned by
their hiſtorians and other authors. We could not have
expected it ſooner from their phyſicians, if we reflect upon their extreme ignorance, and the little eſteem this
ſcience was held in by them (*z*). But when, after the
taking of *Conſtantinople*, the *Greek* writings were di-
ſperſed over the weſtern parts of the world, and in the
beginning of the next century were made general and
public by the late invention of printing, the art of
phyſic began to flouriſh in the northern parts of *Europe*;
and we ſoon after find this diſeaſe accurately deſcribed
there by phyſicians.

In like manner, no ſooner were long voyages performed to diſtant parts of the world, by the great improvement of navigation, and by the diſcovery of the
Indies, which happened much about the ſame period of
time, but the ſeamen were afflicted with it; as appears by
the voyage of *Vaſco de Gama*, who firſt found out a paſſage by the Cape of *Good Hope* to the *Eaſt Indies*, in the
year 1497; above a hundred of his men, out of the
number of a hundred and ſixty, dying in this diſtemper.
In the relation of which voyage, the firſt account of this
diſeaſe at ſea is to be met with (*a*). At that time, and
for a conſiderable time afterwards, it was a diſeaſe little
known; as appears by the following narration.

(*z*) *Vid. Olaum Magnum de medicina et medicis ſeptentrionalibus*
(*a*) See the hiſtory of the *Portugueſe* diſcoveries, &c. by *Her-*
man Lopes de Caſtanneda.

The

The second voyage of James Cartier *to* Newfoundland, *by the grand bay up the river of* Canada, ann. 1535 (*b*).

" In the month of *December*, we underſtood that the
" peſtilence was come upon the people of *Stadacona*;
" and in ſuch ſort, that before we knew of it, above
" fifty of them died.   Whereupon we charged them
" neither to come near our forts, nor about our ſhips.
" Notwithſtanding which, the ſaid unknown ſickneſs
" began to ſpread itſelf amongſt us, after the ſtrangeſt
" ſort that ever was either heard of or ſeen; inſomuch
" that ſome-did loſe all their ſtrength, and could not
" ſtand upon their feet; then did their legs ſwell, their
" ſinews ſhrunk, and became as black as a coal.   Others
" had alſo their ſkin ſpotted with ſpots of blood, of a
" purple colour.   It aſcended up their ancles, knees,
" thighs, ſhoulders, arms, and neck.   Their mouth
" became ſtinking; their gums ſo rotten, that all the
" fleſh came away, even to the roots of their teeth:
" which laſt did alſo almoſt all fall out.   This infection
" ſpread ſo about the middle of *February*, that of a
" hundred and ten people, there were not ten whole:
" ſo that one could not help the other; a moſt horrible
" and pitiful caſe! Eight were already dead; and more
" than fifty ſick, ſeemingly paſt all hopes of recovery.
" This malady being unknown to us, the body of one
" of our men was opened (*c*), to ſee if by any means
" poſſible the occaſion of it might be diſcovered, and
" the reſt of us preſerved.   But in ſuch ſort did the cala-
" mity increaſe, that there were not now above three ſound
" men left.   Twenty-five of our beſt men died; and all
" the reſt were ſo ill, that we thought they would never
" recover again: when it pleaſed God to caſt his pitiful
" eye upon us, and ſend us the knowledge of a remedy
" for our health and recovery.

(*b*) *Hakluit*'s collection of voyages, vol. 3. p. 225.
(*c*) See the diſſection, Part 2. chap. 7. N° 2.

" Our

" Our Captain conſidering the deplorable condition
" of his people, one day went out of the fort, and
" walking upon the ice, he ſaw a troop of people co-
" ming from *Stadacona.* Among thoſe was *Domagaia,*
" who not above ten or twelve days before laboured
" under this diſeaſe; having his knees ſwelled as big as
" a child's head of two years old, his ſinews ſhrunk,
" his teeth ſpoiled, and his gums rotten and ſtinking.
" The Captain, upon ſeeing him now whole and ſound,
" was thereat marvellous glad, hoping to know of him
" how he had cured himſelf. He acquainted him, that
" he had taken the juice of the leaves of a certain tree,
" a ſingular remedy in this diſeaſe. The tree in their
" language is called *ameda* or *hanneda (d)*; by a decoc-
" tion of the bark and leaves of which, they were all
" perfectly recovered in a ſhort time."
Of the colony ſent over from *France,* under the Lord
of *Roberval,* there died in the winter fifty in this diſeaſe (e). We have ſome time afterwards the following
farther account of it.

Nova Francia; *or, A deſcription of that part of* New
France *which is one continent with* Virginia; *in three
late voyages and plantations, made by Meſſieurs* de
Monts, du Pontgrave, *and* de Poutrincourt (f), *publiſhed by* L'Eſcabot, ann. 1604.

" Briefly, the unknown ſickneſſes like to thoſe de-
" ſcribed by *James Carrier,* aſſailed us. As to remedies,
" there were none to be found. In the mean while, the
" poor creatures did languiſh, pining away by little for
" want of meats to ſuſtain their ſtomach; which could
" not receive hard food, by reaſon of a rotten fleſh

(d) See Part 2. chap. 4. p. 222.
(e) Ann. 1542. See *Hakluit,* vol. 3. p. 240.
(f) Collection of voyages and travels, compiled from the libra-
ſy of the late Lord *Oxford,* vol. 2. p. 808.
" which

" which grew and over-abounded within their mouths;
" and when one thought to root it out, it grew again in
" one night's ſpace, more abundantly than before. As
" to the tree called *ameda*, mentioned by the ſaid *Car-*
" *tier*, the ſavages of theſe lands know it not *(g)*. It
" was moſt pitiful to behold every one (very few ex-
" cepted) in this great miſery, and the miſerable wretches
" dying, as it were, full of life, without any poſſibility
" of being ſuccoured. Thirty-ſix died; and thirty-ſix
" or forty more ſtricken with it, recovered themſelves
" by the help of the ſpring, ſo ſoon as that comfort-
" able ſeaſon appeared. The deadly ſeaſon is the end
" of *January*, the months of *February* and *March*;
" wherein the ſick die moſt commonly, every one in
" his turn, according to the time they begin to be ill;
" in ſuch ſort, that he who is taken ill in *February* and
" *March*, may eſcape; but thoſe who betake themſelves
" to bed in *December* and *January*, are in danger of
" dying in *February*, *March*, or the beginning of *April*.
" Which time being paſt, there are hopes and aſſurance
" of ſafety. Monſ. *de Monts* being returned into
" *France*, conſulted the Doctors of phyſic upon this
" ſickneſs; which, in my opinion, they found very new,
" and altogether unknown to them; for I do not find,
" that when we went away, our apothecary was char-
" ged with any order or directions for the cure thereof."
The author afterwards obſerves it to be the ſcurvy, a
malady to which the northern nations, the *Dutch*, &c.
are very ſubject; and upon this occaſion, quoting a paſſage from *Olaus Magnus*, ſays, " I have delighted my-
" ſelf to recite the words of this author, becauſe he
" ſpeaketh thereof as being ſkilled, and has well de-
" ſcribed the diſeaſe; only he maketh no mention of
" the ſtiffening of the hams, nor of the ſuperfluous fleſh
" which groweth in the mouth." He further obſerves,

(g) The *Indian* nation at *Stadacona* by this time had been cut off.

that

that the favages ufe frequent fweatings for cure of this malady; and that a fingular prefervative againft it is content, or mirth, and a chearful humour; as it common-ly attacked the difcontented, idle, and repining.   But the laft and moft fovereign remedy, was the *ameda* men-tioned by *Cartier*, which he calls the *tree of life*.   This Monfieur *Champlein*, who was then up the country, had orders to fearch for among the *Indians*, and to make provifion of it for the prefervation of their colony.

THE name of the difeafe is faid to be in the hiftory of *Saxony*, written by *Albert Krantz*; and if fo, I be-lieve he will be found the firft author now extant who calls it the fcurvy *(h)*.   It is next taken notice of by *Euri-tius Cordus*, in his *Botanologicon*, publifhed *ann.* 1534.   It is obferved by one of the fpeakers in that dialogue, that the herb *chelidonium minus* is called by the *Saxons fchorbock rout*, being an excellent remedy for that difeafe. Being afked, what difeafe this is? it is replied, It would feem to be the *ftomacace* of *Pliny*; as it occafions the teeth to drop out, and all the mouth is affected by it. In the year 1539, it is mentioned in the fame manner by *Jo. Agricola*, in his *Medicina herbaria*.   *Olaus Ma-gnus*, in his hiftory of the northern nations, publifhed *ann.* 1555, obferving what difeafes are peculiar to them, gives us a long defcription of the fcurvy *(i)*.

Soon

(h) He brings down his hiftory to the year 1501.   According to *Melchior Adams*, and *Chevreau* in his hiftory of the world, he died *ann.* 1517.   I own I could not find it in the edition which I perufed: but it is faid fo by *Wierus*, *Schenkius* in his obfervations, and others; unlefs they have miftaken him (which could not be *Wierus*'s cafe) for *Geo. Fabritius*, an author who flourifhed about the year 1570, and mentions, in his *Annales urbis Mifnæ*, a difeafe breaking out in the year 1486, *viz.* the fcurvy; which he very imperfectly defcribes.

(i) *Eft et alius morbus caftrenfis, qui vexat obfeffos et inclufos, talis, viz. ut membra carnofa, ftupiditate quadam denfata, et fubcutaneo tabo, quafi cera liquefcens, digitorum impreffioni cedant; dentefque, veluti ca-furos, ftupefacit; colores cutium candidos reddit cæruleos, torporemque*

Y y   *inducit*

Soon after we find three eminent phyſicians, all cotemporary, treating expreſsly of this diſtemper, *viz.*
Ronſſeus, *Echthius*, and *Wierus*. To whom *Langius* may
be added as a fourth, having wrote two epiſtles upon
this ſubject. What is called *Echthius's Epitome*, was
the firſt wrote, though the laſt publiſhed. It would appear from *Forreſtus (k)* to be a letter ſent, in the year 1541,
to *Blienburchius*, a phyſician at *Utrecht*; whoſe anſwer
is now loſt. The firſt book publiſhed expreſsly upon
the ſcurvy was by *Ronſſeus*, in the form of an epiſtle.
The year is uncertain, as he afterwards corrected, and reprinted it in a different form. He is ſo modeſt as to
ſay, that had he firſt ſeen *Wierus's* accurate obſervations, he would not have publiſhed any thing upon
the ſubject. There is an edition of *Ronſſeus* put down
by *Mercklin (l)* and *Lipenius (m)*, in the year 1564; and
of *Wierus's* obſervations in 1567. The learned Dr *A-
ſtruc (n)* is of opinion, that theſe laſt were not publiſhed
till 1580. It is thus far certain, that thoſe authors corre-
ſponded together; and upon *Wierus* ſending to *Ronſſeus*,
Echthius's letter, now called his *Epitome*, he publiſhed

inducit, cum medicinarum capiendarum nauſea; vocaturque vulgari
gentis lingua ſcorbock; *Græce,* cachexia, *forſitan à ſubcutanea mol-
litie putreſcente: quæ videtur eſu ſalſorum ciborum, nec digeſtorum,
naſci, et frigidâ murorum exhalatione foveri. Sed vim tantam non ha-
bebit, ubi muri interiùs tabulis quorumcunque lignorum ſunt cooperti.
Inſuper, ſi diutiùs graſſetur iſie morbus, abſinthiaco potu continuato illum
arcere ſolent.* Lib. 16. cap 51. *Viribus, primis annis, demum (mi-
lite ſtragibus continuis diminuto) artibus, dolis, et inſidiis, obſidentium
ſurripiunt commeatum, præſertim pecudes; quas ſecum abductas, in her-
boſis domorum tectis paſcendas imponunt; ne, defectu carnium recentiorum,
morbum incurrant, quibuſvis ægritudinibus triſtiorem, patriâ linguâ
ſcorbock nuncupatum; hoc eſt, ſaucium ſtomachum, diris cruciatibus et
diuturno dolore tabefactum. Frigidi enim et indigeſti cibi avidiùs ſumpti,
morbum hujuſmodi cauſare videntur, qualem medici cachexiam univer-
ſalem appellant.* Lib. 9. cap. 38.
  (k) Obſerv. medic. lib. 20. obſ. 11.
  (l) Linden. renovat.
  (m) Bibliotheca real. medic.
  (n) Lib. de morbis venereis.

it, together with his own work, *Wierus*'s obfervations, and two of *Langius*'s epiſtles, in the year 1583.

C H A P.   II.

Bibliotheca ſcorbutica. or, *A chronological view of what has hitherto been publiſhed on the ſcurvy.*

J Oan. Echthii de ſcorbuto, vel ſcorbutica paſſione, epi-   A. D.
     tome.   1541.

He propoſes it as a queſtion, Whethei the blood here may not be corrupted, without the ſpleen or any other of the *viſcera* being affected ? but is inclined to think the ſpleen often is. He aſſigns as cauſes of this diſeaſe, groſs unwholſome food, of ſalt, dried, or putrid fleſh and fiſh, pork, ſpoiled bread, ſtinking water, &c. He diſtinguiſhes the ſymptoms into two claſſes. The firſt contains ſuch as appear at the beginning, and are common to it with other diſeaſes; the ſecond, the ſucceeding and more certain ſigns of the malady. Under the firſt, he comprehends a heavineſs of the body, with a ſpontaneous laſſitude, generally moſt ſenſibly felt after exerciſe; a tightneſs of the breaſt, and a weakneſs of the legs; an itching, redneſs, and pain of the gums; a change of colour in the face to a darkiſh hue : and obſerves, that where all theſe concur, we may foretel an approaching ſcurvy.

But the more immediate and certain ſigns he enumerates under the ſecond claſs, *viz.* a fœtid breath, a ſpungy ſwelling of the gums, which are apt to bleed, with a looſening of the teeth; an eruption of leaden-coloured, purple, or livid ſpots, on the legs; or of ſomewhat broader ſpeckled or dark-coloured *maculæ*, ſometimes on the face, at other times on the legs. As the diſeaſe advances, the patients loſe the uſe of their legs, and are fubject to a difficulty of breathing, particularly when moved, or when they fit erect; at which times they are apt to faint: but upon being laid down again, they recover, and breathe freely; nay, when lying, they affirm that nothing ails them. But as they cannot always thus continue without fome motion, they are fubject to thefe perpetual fwoons. The appetite is feldom bad; on the contrary, they generally have a good one. There is fometimes obferved an aggravation of the fymptoms; with fome on the fourth or fifth day, in others on the third. Some few have it every day, but without any fever: others become feverifh. Preceeding fevers may terminate critically, as it were, in the fcurvy: and with fuch fcurvies whole families and monafteries are together infected; which generally end either in a deadly dyfentery, or, at other times, in a fudden and mortal faint. During the courfe of this difeafe, fome are apt to be very coftive; while others have a continual *diarrhœa.* Sometimes their fpotted legs fwell fo monftroufly, as to refemble the *elephantiafis* of the *Arabians*; while others have them fo extenuated, that the bones feem only covered with fkin. The fpots of fome feparate into black and dufkifh fcales, like the *morphæa* and leprofy of the *Greeks*; while in others they remain foft, fmooth, and fhining; and the impreffion of the finger continues for fome time upon the part. In thofe who die, the fpots fometimes difappear; at other times, they break out afrefh. Laftly, There have been obferved varicofe fwellings of the veins, as in thofe under the tongue, and of the lower lip.

He afterwards delivers the indications of cure, without giving us any remedies. And it may not be amifs to remark, that this is the firft defcription now extant of the fcurvy by a phyfician.

1560. *Jo. Langii medicinalium epiftolar. mifcellan. lib. 3.*
epift.

epiſt. 13. *de novis morbis* ; *epiſt.* 14. *de veterum ſtoma-
cacia et ſceletyrbe, et morbi Gallici tuberibus.*

These two epiſtles were reprinted by *Ronſſeus,* as
ſerving to prove the ſcurvy to have been a diſeaſe known
to the ancients.

Balduini Ronſſei de magnis Hippocratis lienibus, Pli-   1564.
niique ſtomacace ac ſceletyrbe, ſeu vulgò diƈto ſcorbuto,
*commentarius.   Ejuſdem epiſtolæ quinque ejuſdem argu-
menti.*

He aſcribes the frequency of the ſcurvy in *Holland*
to their diet and air; to their eating great quantities of
water-fowl ; but principally to their living on fleſh, firſt
ſalted, then ſmoked and dried.   The weather, he ſays,
had a very great influence upon this diſtemper.   For
though it was met with in the country at all ſeaſons ;
yet, by long obſervation and experience, he had found,
that a moiſt air, and ſoutherly winds, contributed greatly to increaſe it : and inſtances in the year 1556, when,
during that whole year, they had almoſt continual rains,
with ſoutherly and weſterly winds ; which were followed by a great frequency of this diſeaſe ; and to ſuch
a height, that many were brought in danger of their
lives by it.   In 1562, after a very rainy ſeaſon, there
likewiſe enſued frequent and very troubleſome ſcurvies.
So that although this malady was at all times endemic
with them, from the peculiar air of the country, and
their bad waters ; yet, upon very ſlight occaſions, it
often became more general or epidemical during a moiſt
ſeaſon.   It uſually prevailed moſt in ſpring and autumn ;
was milder in the ſpring, and ſhorter : but in the autumn, it was of longer continuance, and more obſtinate,
ſo as ſometimes to endanger the life of the patient.   No
age was exempted from its attack ; which, though ſevereſt with old people, yet was more incident to thoſe
of a middle age.

From a miſtaken theory in judging it a diſeaſe of the
ſpleen,

ſpleen, he begins the cure by bleeding. He afterwards preſcribes an aperient and attenuating decoction of a number of antiſcorbutics, with the addition of *ſenna*, and ſome other purgative ingredients : but obſerving, that the more ſimple compoſitions were generally the moſt efficacious, he thinks, that the uſe of ſcurvygraſs, wormwood, and germander, is alone ſufficient ; the vulgar curing themſelves by ſcurvygraſs, brooklime, and water creſſes. At the end of the cure, he gives gentle phyſic ; forbidding all violent and acrid medicines, eſpecially draſtic purgatives ; till towards the decline of the malady, when the patient is able to bear them. For twelve years paſt, he had uſed with great ſucceſs, both for prevention and cure, a tincture, in ſpirit of wine, of *fumaria, cochlearia, abſinthium*, and *chamædrys*, or herbs of the like virtue. The ſpirit was extremely well ſaturated by repeated infuſions of the freſh plants, and the belly kept moderately open during the courſe.

As to diet, upon which much depends ; he orders it ſhould be inciding and attenuating. They muſt abſtain from all kind of ſea and water fowls ; from pork, and ſalt meats. Their drink ſhould be a wormwood and germander wine by turns. He preſcribes a gargariſm with alum and honey for the mouth ; and orders the rigid tendons in the ham, after friction, to be anointed with cowfeet jelly. He has ſeveral remedies for the ulcers on the legs. To prevent the diſeaſe, he recommends gentle phyſic in the autumn ; but eſpecially the uſe of a light wormwood ale or wine : by which (with the help of a diet of eaſy digeſtion, the benefit of good air, and dry lodgings) he has known it often not only prevented, but cured.

In his firſt epiſtle, he accounts for the frequency of this diſtemper in ſome places more than in others ; from their different ſoils, climates, and weather, and eſpecially from the quality of the waters they uſed : and obſerves, that, univerſally, in marſhy and boggy countries, people were

moſt

moft afflicted with the fcurvy; though their diet and o-
ther circumftances were alike with others. In his fecond epiftle, he maintains, that this diftemper was known
to the ancients, againft the opinion of *Wierus*; and remarks, that feamen in long voyages cure themfelves of
it by the ufe of oranges. In his third epiftle, he recommends the fteel and mineral waters.

Jo. Wieri medicarum obfervationum hactenus incogni- 1567.
tarum lib. 1. *de fcorbuto.*

He tranfcribes all the fymptoms out of *Echthius* at
great length, with the following additions. The weaknefs in the legs felt upon the approach of the difeafe, is
attended with a ftiffnefs there, and a fmall pain. The
flefh of the gums is often deftroyed to the roots of the
teeth. Smaller fpots, refembling blood fprinkled upon
the part, (or flea-bites, but larger), appear on the legs,
thighs, and on the whole body; but the very large, livid, and purple fpots, chiefly on the legs. Sometimes
this livid colour will fhew itfelf in the *fauces* of thofe
who are near death. In the progrefs of the difeafe, the
tendons of the legs become ftiff and contracted. Some
are feized with a flow erratic fever. After ardent malignant fevers, and double tertians, ill cured, he has
known the fcurvy to follow; upon which a malignant
quartan has enfued. This ftill left the fcurvy behind
it; which was at laft cured by the proper method. When
the legs are greatly fwelled, they are fometimes altogether of a livid colour. The pulfe, as in a quartan
fever, varies: fo that at different times, and according
to the ftate of the difeafe, it is fmall, hard, quick, and
weak. The urine is reddifh, turbid, thick, and fæculent, like new red wine, refembling that which is ufual
in the fit of a quartan when fweating; and of a bad
fmell. He adds afterwards, in his prognoftics, that if
ulcers break out on the *tibia*, they are with great difficulty healed up; being extremely fœtid, of a gangrenous

nous difpofition, and fo putrid, as not to feel the application of a hot iron.

He affigns as caufes of this diftemper, unwholfome
air, fuch bad and corrupt food as was ufed in the northern countries, and by their fhipping, *viz.* ftinking pork,
fmoked rancid bacon, mouldy bread, thick fæculent
ale, bad water, melancholy and grief of mind, preceeding fevers, the ftoppage of ufual evacuations, *&c.*

Though he fometimes bleeds in the cure, yet he forbids it when the difeafe is advanced. In this cafe,
after evacuating the *primæ viæ* by a lenient of *fenna,* or
the like, (obferving that it does not bear violent purgatives), the patient is to be fweated twice a-day, *viz.*
in the morning, and at four after noon, with a draught
of four ounces of the expreffed juices of the antifcorbutic herbs; which are, *cochlearia, nafturtium aq. et
nafturtium hyber.* of each equal parts, with but half the
quantity of *becabunga;* adding a little cinnamon and fugar. The proportion of the different ingredients may
be diminifhed or increafed, according to the conftitution of the patient, ftate of the difeafe, and heat of the
body. He would have the herbs always frefh and green
when ufed; and they may fometimes be boiled in goats
or cows milk, or rather in whey: but their expreffed
juice mixed with whey, is preferable to their decoction.
He fometimes adds *abfinth vulgare, fumaria, chamædrys,* and, in certain cafes, *nummularia.* To people
who are fond of a *farrago* of medicines, he gives a long
lift of all the antifcorbutic and aperient herbs, roots,
feeds, *&c.* to which later authors have made but a fmall
addition; and remarks, that he generally made fuccefsful cures by a proper ufe of a few of thefe plants. The
following remedy he underftood had cured many. ℞ *abfinth. vulg. ficc. bacc. juniper. contuf. ana manip. i. lact.
caprin. lib.* iv. *Coq. ad tertiæ partis confumptionem.* A
dram of faffron is to be infufed in the ftrained decoction,
and a warm draught taken three times a-day. After giving

ving some other cures usual in his time for this distemper, he observes, that there is nothing specific in the common antiscorbutic herbs, as they are called; but that all acrid plants which incide and attenuate, as also many aperient roots, and warm seeds, are highly serviceable. At the same time, a diet of easy digestion, and similar intention, must be used, with good sound ale or wine with wormwood infused, or milk and whey. Care must be taken to procure dry chearful lodgings, and to banish grief, cares, &c.

He afterwards subjoins various topical applications for the different symptoms. For the putrid gums, R *sal. mar alum ana ar.* ii. *aq. font. lib.* i. M. *Bulliant simul.* The people of *Friesland* use the following. R *acet. cerevis. lib.* ii. *bol. armen. unc.* ss. *alumin. dr.* ii. *mellis unc.* iii. M. *Bulliant simul.* The *Saxons* add to the former, *herba sabina.* If the putrefaction is very great, *ung. Ægyptiac.* or *alum. ust.* mixed with honey, may be used; or it is to be stopped by touching with *ol. vitriol.* In his appendix, he particularly recommends whey for the cure of this disease; and gives a description, at great length, of the *cochlearia*, and some other antiscorbutic herbs.

Remberti Dodonæi praxeos medic. lib. 2. *cap.* 62. E- 1581 *jusdem medicinalium observationum exempl. rar. cap.* 33. *de scorbuto.*

He ascribes the scurvy chiefly to bad diet. He relates, that it was occasioned in *Brabant, ann.* 1556, by the use of some corrupted rye brought from *Prussia* during a scarcity of corn. At this time many had not the spots; but their gums were chiefly affected. He gives an instance, however, of its being contracted in a prison, where confinement alone was the occasion; the place being well aired, and the diet such as he thought could give no suspicion of its proceeding from thence. He never bled any patient in this disease, but the per-

Z 2 son

fon in the prifon, who had figns of a *plethora.* He generally performed a cure by the ufe of a few herbs, *viz.*
nafturt. hortenf. et aquatic. cochlearia, and *becabunga* ;
which laft he efteems of inferior virtues to the others.
Thefe he thinks fufficient to remove the fcurvy, if, at
the fame time, proper diet is ufed, efpecially well-baked
wheat-bread. He fometimes gives a gentle purgative at
firft, and repeats it occafionally : but if the difeafe is
far gone, caution here muft be had. When only the
gums were affected, he has cured thefe often by topical
applications. The large livid fcorbutic fpots like bruifes, are oftener feen on the lower extremities than on the
arms. If the difeafe is very virulent, and not removed,
the *hypochondria* will alfo become livid ; and the patient
in this cafe be feized with violent gripes, and die.

1589. *De fcorbuto propofitiones de quibus difputatum eft pu-*
blicè Roftochii, fub Henrico Brucæo.
The fcurvy is endemic in particular countries, from
their fituation, air, water, and food. In thefe countries,
fcorbutic mothers bear fcorbutic children, often mifcar-
ry, at other times bring forth dead fœtufes. He mentions no other fymptom, but what is taken notice of by
Wierus ; except a pain fometimes in the right, at other
times in the left *hypochondrium,* attended with a fenfe of
weight. Upon the malady's increafing, the belly fwells,
and grows alfo painful ; with an entire lofs of appetite.
In his theory of the difeafe, he fuppofes, that either the
liver, or fpleen, fometimes both, but oftener the fpleen,
was obftructed ; although it was feldom found fcirrhous.
He afterwards fays, there is often no fwelling or obftruction in any of thefe parts ; though, from the quality
of the fcorbutic humour, produced by improper and
grofs food, it was natural to expect the fpleen might be
affected. When the difeafe is very inveterate, it degenerates into the *affectio hypochondriaca* ; a diftemper frequent among the inhabitants on the fhores of the *Baltic.*
It

It is fometimes complicated with other difeafes, *viz.* the dropfy, atrophy, and bilious diarrhœa; at other times there is a flow continual fever, and fometimes a tertian intermittent.

His cure confifts in diet and medicines. For the firft he directs well-baked wheat-bread; broth of flefh or fowls, with radifh, hyffop, thyme, favory, or the like herbs. He allows all forts of flefh or fowl (except water-fowls) that are of eafy digeftion, and afford good nourifhment. Whatever is dried, falted, fmoked, long kept, and rancid, or of grofs and difficult digeftion, is to be avoided. Milk is proper for thofe who are far gone in fcorbutic atrophies. At table the antifcorbutic herbs are to be ufed by way of falad; and for drink, ripe *Rhenifh* wine, or good found beer, with wormwood infufed. After a gentle bleeding, if indicated by a *plethora*, and clearing the firft paffages with a lenient purgative; *cochlearia, nafturtium, becabunga,* and *rad. raphani,* are to be given boiled in milk; or their expreffed juices, mixed with whey; adding *abfinthium* or *mentha,* if the ftomach is weak; *acetofa* and *fumaria,* where the conftitution is hot, and a fever apprehended; or *rad. helenii,* and *herb. hyffopi,* when the breathing is affected. If the patient is of a cold habit, has œdematous legs, and the fpots are black, the juices are beft given in wine, with cinnamon or ginger: or he may take an infufion of *rad. raphani* in *Rhenifh.* The author likewife recommends the fweating courfe from *Wierus,* particularly the laconic or dry bath, when the fcurvy appears on the external habit or fkin. The belly is to be kept open by gentle phyfic, given in goat-whey, repeated every day, or every other day, during cure, as the patient bears it. This method, together with the diet before recommended, will effectually remove the fcurvy. For lax and bleeding gums he orders the pickle of olives; but in his other receipts tranfcribes from *Wierus.*

De scorbuto tractatus duo ; *auctore Balthazaro Brunero.*

He has copied *Wierus* in most things; but is more
explicit and full in describing the air productive of the
malady. Thus, if the atmosphere of any place is impure, and polluted with exhalations that are grofs, moift,
putrid, or liable to putrefaction, it begets this infection;
as in marfhy, damp, and maritime countries; or places
where ftagnating waters are left after inundations. To
which alfo rainy feafons contribute a great deal, efpecially where the fun has not influence fufficient to raife
and diffipate the vapours of fuch waters ftagnating in the
country and marfhes. To the diet obferved by other
writers to occafion the fcurvy, he adds black coarfe
bread; and obferves, that the pernicious effects of fuch
diet and air are confiderably augmented, by immoderate watchings, the forrowful paffions of the mind, and
ftoppage of the natural and ufual evacuations. People,
by way of prevention from this difeafe, when in the
air of *Saxony*, take plenty of muftard-feed, finding the
good effects of it by experience, together with gentle
aftringents.

He defcribes the fymptoms and cure in the fame manner as *Wierus* ; only, by a typographical error, the *deliquium animi* is faid to occur when the patient fweats;
having *fudat* inftead of *fedet*, (when he fits up). The
whole is taken from *Wierus* ; who immediately adds,
decumbens refpirat facilius, reficiturque. It may be proper to note another miftake which he and many other
authors have fallen into, in tranfcribing a medicine from
Wierus for phagedenic ulcers of the gums. It is the
following. ℞ *mercur. fublimat. fcr.* ii. *alum. uft. dr.* ii. fs.
aq plantagin. lib. i *M.* But as this author, in his obfervations, wrote in *Dutch*, had called the firft medicine
fimply *fublimate*, after the manner of the chemifts, by
which he meant mercury; his tranflator into *Latin* unluckily here put in arfenic, making it to be *arfenici fublimat.*

limat. fcr. ii.; in which dangerous miftake many have followed him.

Brunerus has but one fingular obfervation, *viz.* He has often remarked, that violent pains in the legs preceeded the fcurvy, and that the fpots and putrefaction of the gums followed upon them. Thefe are chiefly about the ancles and joints; on the *tibia*, and foles of the feet; fometimes in other parts of the body; attended with a fenfe of heat and pricking betwixt the fkin and flefh. If they continue long, and efpecially if they become moft fevere in the night, and do not yield to medicines, and are exafperated by oily and greafy applications, it is a certain fign of a future fcurvy. The pains ceafe upon an eruption of the fpots, which are here generally very large. In this cafe, warm fteams, difcutient fomentations and cataplafms, muft only be ufed, and, if poffible, a fweat procured upon the parts. He concludes with the cafe of a fcorbutic patient; whom he firft purged, then ordered the juice of water-creffes in goat-whey; of which fix ounces were taken twice a-day; and, by fweating him, a number of fcorbutic fpots appeared, by which a violent pain in the thigh was allayed.

Scorbuti hiftoria propofita in publicum; *à Solomone Alberto, &c.*   1593.

He is of opinion, that the difeafe may be hereditary, or got from an infected nurfe, and that it is contagious; but adds nothing to the defcription or fymptoms of it as delivered by *Wierus*, unlefs it be a ftiffnefs or *rigor* of the lower jaw, feemingly from a contraction of the temporal mufcle; in the fame manner as the tendons in the ham become ftiff and contracted in the progrefs of this malady, as had been obferved by all authors. He fays, it is moft ufual in children, and in either a hereditary fcurvy, or that which is got from the nurfe.

He treats of the diet proper in this difeafe at great length :

length : recommends the juices of acid and auftere
fruits, *viz.* oranges, and the like; with which roaft
meats when on the fpit are to be fprinkled. Thefe are
likewife to be put in foops, and vinegar and wine in the
gruels and barley-water. Exercife is neceffary.

In his pharmaceutical directions, he orders bleeding at
firft, but only if there be a *plethora*; obferving, that
when the difeafe is advanced, efpecially if the fpots
have appeared, it is extremely improper. In this cafe,
if there is an obftruction of the *menfes* or *hæmorrhoids,*
thefe evacuations are by all means to be promoted; which
will be of great fervice, though they may not prove a
cure; having feen women regular after childbed, yet o-
ver-run with the fcurvy. He prefcribes very gentle
phyfic, obferving the mifchief done by violent purgatives; then gives a numerous catalogue of aperient and
deobftruent medicines. Whatever incides, deterges, and
attenuates grofs, vifcid, and fæculent humours, is proper, in order to their being prepared and fitted for evacuation by any of the outlets of the body. For this purpofe, in a particular manner, the common antifcorbutics, *viz, cochlearia, nafturtium,* and *becabunga,* are adapted; being fuch whofe virtues have been approved by
long experience. To thefe he afterwards adds other
herbs under the denomination of *hepatic, fplenetic,* and
thoracic; from an imagined property in them to remove
obftructions, and relieve and ftrengthen particular parts
and bowels. When by thefe means all obftructions are
removed, and the morbid humour, the immediate caufe
of the difeafe, is fufficiently attenuated and prepared,
he obferves nature itfelf will throw it out of the body,
either by the kidneys or fkin. It is the bufinefs only of
art, to farther her intention, by giving diuretics if it tends
to the kidneys; having particularly remarked, that, by
a flow of urine, the diforders of the breaft in this difeafe
were moft effectually relieved : or by taking diaphoretics and fudorifics internally, at the fame time fweating

ing in ftoves and in baths moift and dry; as it is often
diffipated by infenfible perfpiration, at other times by
profufe fweats. The dregs of the difeafe evacuated this
way, have been obferved to foul the very fkin. He remarked, that fcurvies were very frequent in that and
the preceeding year, from the unconftant weather and
very rainy feafons they had after warm fummers.

Petri Forefti obfervationum et curationum medicinali-   1595.
um lib. 20. *obf.* 11. *de fcorbuto malo cognofcendo et cu-*
rando; *obf.* 12. *ibid. de quinque ægris à fcorbuto curatis.*

This is a long letter which the author wrote firft to
his brother in the year 1558, and afterwards fent to his
two nephews ftudents of phyfic, *ann.* 1590. He feems
to have been acquainted with no other authors upon this
fubjeƈt but *Ronffeus* and *Ecbthius.* The laft he copies
in defcribing the fymptoms; all which he confirms and
illuftrates by various cafes of patients. He makes it a
difeafe unknown to the ancients, though, according to
his theory, a diforder of the fpleen. It was indeed fo
little known in his time, that many died of it, (particularly one *Martin Dorpius* a clergyman at *Louvain*), to
the great furprife of the phyficians, who were entirely
unacquainted with the very name of the difeafe, its nature, or method of cure. He mentions likewife one
Safbotus, a counfellor at the *Hague,* who laboured under a virulent fcurvy; and was given over by his phyficians, when an *Amfteraam* phyfician difcovered his cafe,
and cured him; obferving, that the *Hague* doƈtors did
not know this diftemper fo well as thofe who refided at
Amfterdam, or as he did at *Alcmaer,* where they became
well acquainted with it by feeing it among the feamen.
This laft patient being fubjeƈt to a relapfe at times, our
author prefcribed him the juices of brooklime and fcurvygrafs boiled into a fyrup with fugar; which effeƈtual-
ly prevented the diftemper. And this medicine, going
under the name of *fyr. fceletyrb. Forefti,* became afterwards

wards univerfally famous, and continued in repute for a confiderable time, over all *Flanders*, *Brabant*, and *Holland*, for the cure of the fcurvy. It was principally ufed in the winter-feafon, when the green plants could not be procured. He indeed very ingenuoufly owns, that phyficians were firft made acquainted with thofe remedies by the vulgar; they having only contrived the exhibition of them in more elegant forms.

He illuftrates the feveral intentions of cure at great length in the cafe of a failor at *Alkmaer*, who fell into the fcurvy after an autumnal quartan, which had continued with him feven months. This perfon told him, he had formerly the fame difeafe at fea, in a voyage to *Spain*; and that it was very common among the *Dutch* failors, who generally recovered by change of air, and the ufe of a wormwood-ale. But he had been quite cured of it before having had the ague. Upon this occafion, the author obferves, he has known many fall into the fcurvy after fuch intermitting fevers. The patient was troubled with a great difficulty of breathing, had loft the ufe of his limbs; his left knee, and whole leg, being fwelled, fcirrhous, fpotted, and fo ftiff, that he could not walk, or even move himfelf: his gums were fwelled and bled. The phyficians and furgeons faid, he was poxed; but when the author faw him, he found it to be the fcurvy. It was indeed a complicated cafe; the fever having left behind it a hectic difpofition, with obftructed bowels.

Foreftus, who has had great practice in this difeafe, fays, the pathognomonic figns of it are, a ftraitnefs of the *præcordia*; weaknefs and pain of the legs; rednefs, pain, and itching in the gums; with an alteration of colour in the face. However, in the beginning it is not fo eafily known; being fometimes flow in its progrefs, and having the above fymptoms, together with a laffitude after exercife, common to it with other difeafes. But where all fuch figns appear together, he thinks it the

beginning

beginning of the diſtemper, or at leaſt there is ſome certainty of an approaching ſcurvy : though he ſometimes
heſitates here for ſome little time; till, in the progreſs
of the diſtemper, the violence of thoſe ſymptoms is
increaſed; and the fœtid breath, ſpungy bleeding gums,
looſe teeth, and purple and livid ſpots upon the legs,
&c. confirm his former judgment of the diſeaſe. He
proceeds to recite the ſymptoms from *Echthius*'s epitome; adding, almoſt after each, inſtances of patients in
whom they occurred. In particular, after the remarkable proneneſs to ſwoon in the height of the malady,
he adds, that he has known ſeveral drop down dead in-
ſtantly; as happened to a magiſtrate he mentions, who
had a *Haerlem* phyſician to attend him, who ſaid he was
poxed ; the ignorant in thoſe days pronouncing all extraordinary and unknown diſeaſes to be the *lues venerea.*
However, this gentleman's ſon, labouring under the
ſame diſtemper, was cured by our author. He recommends butter-milk when the patient is inclinable to be
hectic : but where there was no fever, he cured many
by milk alone, in which *cochlearia* and *becabunga* were
boiled. Theſe obſervations, although extremely tedious,
are valuable for the many truly ſcorbutic caſes they
contain.

Hieronymi Reuſneri diexodicarum exercitationum liber 1600.
de ſcorbuto.

This voluminous author, remarkable only for his
theory, deſcribes the ſcurvy, in its different ſtages, altogether in the ſame manner as the authors before him;
with the addition of the following ſymptoms. A hæmorrhage from the noſe, which he ſays is uſual even in
the beginning of the diſeaſe; as likewiſe a continual ſpit-
ting. Some have a pain at the mouth of the ſtomach,
and there is a want of appetite ; or at leaſt if they long
for food, it is rather hurtful to them. He obſerves, that
ſcorbutical women are ſubject to the *fluor albus,* and

menfes difcolores. The urine is for the moft part thin, pale, and watery, without any fediment, and of a fœtid fmell. The pulfe is low, weak, flow, and inordinate. He is extremely prolix on the cure. But it were to be wifhed, that the many chemical and galenical remedies recommended, had been proved ferviceable by experience, rather than by being agreeable to his theory.

1604. *De morbo fcorbuto liber; cum obfervationibus quibufdam, brevique et fuccincta cujufque curationis indicatione. Auctore Severino Eugaleno.*

This book muft have been publifhed by the author in a very loofe immethodical drefs; as it has undergone feveral corrections by different editors; and the order of the whole is ftill very inaccurate. *Geo. Stubendorphius* publifhed it in the year 1615, with great alterations: and *Brendel*, Profeffor of Medicine at *Jena, ann.* 1623, again corrected it; and with great labour has claffed the different fymptoms, or rather fpecies of this difeafe, into different fections, making in all forty-nine in number. They will admit of feveral fubdivifions; and comprehend a pretty round catalogue of almoft all diftempers, acute or chronic, incident to the human body. There are here alfo fifty prognoftics, with thirty general diagnoftics of the fcurvy; befides the fpecial diagnoftics of each fymptom, or rather difeafe, by which it is known to be fcorbutic. But as I have elfewhere animadverted at great length upon this book, it may be fufficient here only to repeat, that the merit of the author has always been fuppofed to confift in his great fagacity in detecting this deceitful difeafe lurking under fo many different forms. This he tells us was his profeffed defign in writing. So that the defcription of the fymptoms makes up the greateft part of his performance. In the beginning of it, he affigns the fame occafional caufes of the fcurvy as *Wierus* had done much more accurately before him; and to this author likewife he recommends us for

the

the cure. The firft five pages (as far as § 4.) contain
what he has copied from other authors: but the reft of
the treatife may, with great propriety, be deemed entirely new, and his own.

The fymptoms are as follow.   I. Putrid gums.   II.
Blackifh, purple, and livid fpots.   III. Malignant ulcers. Acquainting us, that thefe are obvious figns, known
even to the vulgar, he obferves, that the difeafe often
proves fatal before they appear; and therefore he proceeds,
without ftopping longer here, to other fymptoms equally
charaᵃeriftical and demonftrative of the fcurvy. But
before we go any farther, it will be neceffary to tranfcribe that peculiar ftate of urine and pulfe which he
fo often refers to in his account of the following fymptoms, and which was with him the pathognomonic figns
of the difeafe.

The urine of thofe who labour under this malady,
varies extremely, according to the habit of the body,
the different nature of the difeafe, and of the putrefcent
humour. If there be only a flight putrefaction, and
the difeafe but beginning, the urine is fometimes of a
citron colour, and thin; at other times thick and white.
But fuch urines difcover nothing certain concerning
the fcurvy. As the diftemper increafes, it becomes
fometimes thin, and of an intenfe red colour, inclining
to a livid hue. If the patient paffes this urine when
feemingly in perfeᵃ health, having little or no drought,
it is a certain fign of the fcurvy. Frequently the
urine appears thick, red, and manifeftly livid; it either
remains thus thick, or drops a thick red heavy fediment
like bran or fand, befides having for the moft part a
thick turbid matter fufpended a-top: fuch likewife is a
demonftrative fign of the difeafe, provided the patient
languifhes, without any thirft or fever. Of fome the u-
rine is thick, white, and turbid; and drops feveral
roundifh whitifh particles like fand, without becoming
any clearer. The urine of thofe who live irregularly,

is in fome thick, black, and turbid; in others blackifh, with an obfcure palenefs; and thefe perfons have a violent thirft while they pafs fuch urine. After thofe long accounts, he adds in another place, that where there is no fever, nor putrefaction of the humours, thick, white, and turbid urine, having a white roundifh heavy fediment, like fand or brick-duft, is the moft undoubted fign of the fcurvy. The pulfe peculiar to this malady, is quick and fmall, but particularly unequal.

We now proceed to tranfcribe the other fymptoms. And the IV. is a difficulty of breathing; known to be fcorbutic, 1*ft*, By the part affected; which is under the diaphragm, at the orifice of the ftomach. 2*dly*, By the complaint. It is a great and uneafy ftraitnefs and oppreffion upon the *præcordia*, not eafily expreffed. 3*dly*, By its remiffion and intermiffion; though fometimes it is almoft continual. 4*thly*, By its having none of the fymptoms which ufually follow diforders of the breaft, *viz.* cough, pain, *orthopnœa*, &c.

V. Vomitings, retchings; and even the *cholera morbus.* A vomiting is known to be fcorbutic, 1*ft*, By not yielding to the common medicines, and thofe prefcribed by the ancients in this diforder; on the contrary, the patient becomes worfe after ufing them. 2*dly*, Its fudden unaccountable remiffion, and equally unexpected return. 3*dly*, Its feizing without any previous pain, diforder of the ftomach, or a diftemper defcribed by the ancients. The retchings are here very violent, without bringing up much from the ftomach. But the moft certain proofs are had from the urine and pulfe. VI. A loofenefs, or coftivenefs of the belly. VII. A baftard dyfentery; known to be fcorbutic by want of gripes, the blood not being mixed with the excrement; but chiefly by the pulfe and urine.

VIII. Irregular fevers. IX. Intermitting fevers. X. Continual fevers. Under thefe he comprehends moft fpecies of fevers, *viz.* flow, putrid, remitting, and intermitting,

termitting, of all kinds. They are all afcertained to be fcorbutic, by the anxiety upon the *præcordia*, not agreeing in type with thofe of the ancients, *&c.* but more infallibly by the pulfe and urine. The firft, though ftrong and hard during the fever, upon its remiffion returns again to its peculiar, fmall, and unequal ftate.

XI. Fainting-fits. XII. Pains of the legs. XIII. A pain in the hands, and ends of the fingers. This is known to proceed from the fcurvy by the pulfe. XIV. A pain in the neck. XV. Pains in almoft every part of the body, *viz.* the teeth, jaws, back, *&c.*; burning pains in the kidneys, head, arms, *&c.* XVI. The baftard pleurify; difcovered in a girl to be fcorbutic, by the fmallnefs and inequality of the pulfe ; the intermiffion of the pain ; and being free from cough but at times; by the urine, and her having no thirft, and breathing without pain. But the intermiffion of the pain, and its returning at intervals, are fufficient to diftinguifh this from the true pleurify. XVII. Violent colic pains; eafily known when fcorbutic, by their intermiffion, the urine, and pulfe. He gives two inftances of ruptures occafioned by the acutenefs of thefe pains. XVIII. Hard tumours fimilar to thofe in the pox, *viz.* in the groin, and other glandular parts of the body; or in any other part, as in the interftices of the mufcles, *&c.* They are often varicofe. Thefe give no pain while the patient is at reft, and the part kept eafy; but upon walking, or hanging the legs, they become fo very painful as to occafion fainting. Sometimes the whole body is covered with fuch tubercles. XIX. Weaknefs of the legs upon walking. XX. Retraction of the heel backwards towards the ham ; known when occafioned by the fcurvy, from the pulfe alone. XXI. Troublefome prickings in the foles of the feet, next day followed with a palfy of the lower extremities. XXII. A palfy of the legs ; diftinguifhed from palfies defcribed in ancient authors, by differences very equivocal, and too long here to mention. XXIII.

A

A *hemiplegia.* XXIV. Weakneſs of the whole nervous ſyſtem. XXV. A colic ending in a palſy. XXVI. A convulſion or contraction of the members, gradually approaching. XXVII. The epilepſy is known when ſcorbutic, by the pulſe and urine; as likewiſe, 1*ſt*, By its attack accompanied with a fever. 2*dly,* Its ſudden attack, and equally ſudden remiſſion. 3*dly,* Its proceeding from no cauſe aſſigned by the ancients. XXVIII. An apoplexy. XXIX. Convulſion of a particular part. XXX. The gout; known to proceed from the ſcurvy, by not being fixed, but ſhifting from one joint to another; and its being quickly cured by antiſcorbutics. XXXI. The dropſy; requiring quite a different method of cure from that deſcribed by the ancients; and is eaſily diſtinguiſhed from it, by the *dyſpnœa* becoming much worſe after purgatives. The difficulty of breathing is at all times greater, even in the beginning; with extreme anxiety under the diaphragm. XXXII. The encyſted dropſy. Before this is fixed in any particular place, it cauſes a momentaneous ſwelling as it were, in different parts of the body; which moſt commonly happens upon change from a finer to a thicker air, or to thoſe who uſe groſs food; otherwiſe the legs ſwell firſt, then the whole body is covered with a hard and unequal ſwelling, and with various indolent tubercles, &*c.* XXXIII. The ſcorbutic atrophy; which can be cured only by antiſcorbutics. It is known by the patient's languiſhing, without having any diſeaſe deſcribed by the ancients; by the pulſe, urine, and recurring anxieties; but eſpecially by ſpots on the body. XXXIV. Ulcers and gangrene of the toes. XXXV. Ulcers on different parts of the body, cancers, &*c.* XXXVI. Peſtilential fevers, and their tumours; diſtinguiſhed from the true plague, generally by the mildneſs of the ſymptoms, but more eaſily by the pulſe, and ſometimes by the urine. XXXVII. A mortification, either with or without ulceration. XXXVIII. The ſcorbutic *eryſipelas;* known by the pulſe, urine, and ſhifting

ing its place. XXXIX. Madnefs, and the memory impaired. Thefe two more rarely occur, being not fo demonftrative fymptoms of the fcurvy as many of the preceding. XL. *Carus*, and a profound fleeping. XLI. A falivation. XLII. A *languor*, without any evident caufe. XLIII. A diforder like to a *languor*. XLIV. Copious fweats, the forerunner of an atrophy. XLV. A cutting or tearing pain in the acceffion of fevers. XLVI. A toffing or concuffion of the limbs, being a mixture of a paralytic and convulfive diforder. XLVII. *Tremor* of the limbs. It is known to be fcorbutic by the pulfe alone. XLVIII. Ulcer of the *penis*. XLIX. Dry ulcers. The book is concluded with feventy-two obfervations, containing a variety of cafes in thefe difeafes.

Felicis Plateri praxeos medicæ lib. 3. *cap.* 4. *de defæ-* 1608.
datione. Under which title, he treats of the *lues venerea, fcorbutica*, and *elephantica*.

He feems not to have feen *Eugalenus*'s book, or at leaft has copied nothing from it : for he ftill delivers the fame defcription of the fcurvy, as *Wierus*, and all other authors preceding *Eugalenus*, have done. He, however, takes notice of one fymptom not mentioned by them, *viz.* tumours, fometimes indolent, at other times more painful, refembling a fcrophulous gland. Thefe are feated either on the glandular parts of the body, or in the interftices of the mufcles. The fweat of fcorbutic perfons is fœtid ; their urine red and turbid ; their pulfe feeble ; as had been obferved by all others before *Eugalenus.* He feems inclined to believe, that, like the *lues venerea,* the fcurvy might have been brought from abroad, efpecially by failors. It fometimes produces convulfions and palfies ; and may end in an atrophy, confumption, dropfy, or dyfentery. He recommends for prevention, as alfo cure, a confection of muftard-feed and honey ; likewife the juice of oranges.
This

This laſt is to be uſed for gargariſing the putrid gums; as alſo *ſal. prunell.* diſſolved in a proper liquor. The patient may be ſweated with *decoƈt. lignorum.*

1609.	*Gregor. Horſtii traƈtatus de ſcorbuto.*

This author is in many places ſeemingly inconſiſtent with himſelf; having firſt followed *Foreſtus,* then *Eugalenus,* in his deſcription of the diſeaſe; concluding with a diet, regimen, and cure, tranſcribed chiefly out of *Albertus.* The remote cauſes are, thick foul air, and groſs viſcid food; both which, as productive of the ſcurvy, he pretty well deſcribes. He obſerves, that though in the *Lower Saxony,* and *Old Marche* of *Brandenburg,* it was a diſeaſe generally very well known; yet in ſome places it was a much rarer and ſlighter malady than in others; being moſt frequent and dangerous where they uſed thick unwholſome new ale, and where the ſoil was marſhy and damp. So that the year before, when he practiſed in the *Old Marche,* he found it extremely frequent at *Soltquell*; but much leſs ſo in the neighbouring country. In that place, beſides uſing the ſame groſs food as other northern countries, their ſituation was very marſhy; and they drank thick new ale hardly cold, without hops, which had undergone no fermentation or depuration. He recommends *ſp. vitriol.* given along with antiſcorbutics; and has perhaps nothing elſe new on the diſeaſe; but theory.

Matthæi Martini de ſcorbuto commentatio.

He copies entirely from *Eugalenus* his deſcription of the ſcurvy, adding ſome new ſymptoms firſt mentioned by himſelf; ſuch as, ſwelling of the eyes, recurring darkneſs over them; virulent ulcers upon the *uvula* and *fauces*; ſuch variety of pains in all parts of the body as cannot be expreſſed, *viz.* tenſive, pulling, pricking, biting, eroding, gnawing, *&c.* on the muſcles, membranes, and nerves. Theſe are not only ſevereſt in the
night-

night-time, (as is moſt commonly the caſe), but afflict likewiſe in the evening, morning, and through the day. They
may all with great certainty be known to proceed from
the ſcurvy, by the ſmallneſs and inequality of the pulſe.
Even pains peculiar to each part, are rendered wonder-
fully anomalous by the ſcurvy. This diſeaſe is nearly
allied to the plague; as it occaſions carbuncles, buboes,
cancers, &c. Moſt tertian vernal fevers are ſcorbutic.
A ſudden and unaccountable looſening and faſtening of
the teeth; large fiſſures in the lips, cloſing in a moſt ſurpriſing manner after drinking, are ſymptoms of the
ſcurvy. Here *Eugalenus* is every where an oracle; his
whole book being tranſcribed, and digeſted into a much
more methodical order, with the addition of ſome things
from *Wierus*, *Albertus*, &c.

Dan. Sennerti tractatus de ſcorbuto. Ejuſdem practi- 1624.
ea medicinæ lib. 3. pars 5.

He has tranſcribed from *Eugalenus* and *Martini* all
that they have ſaid on the diſeaſe. This, together with
his theory, makes up the greateſt part of his book.
What he calls his own new and rare obſervations, are
as follow. One is the caſe of a ſtudent, who, upon the
ſtriking in of an itch, was ſeized with a *gutta ſerena*,
difficulty of breathing, and tightneſs of the breaſt. He
recovered his ſight by the uſe of ſome purgative medicines, and diuretics of the antiſcorbutic kind. The
other, a boy of twelve years of age, who had alſo the
itch; and it being repelled by an improper unction, he
loſt his ſight, and afterwards died epileptic. The author having often remarked, after an itch in ſuch manner injudiciouſly treated, pains and prickings in the
breaſt to enſue, with baſtard pleuriſies; and likewiſe
tertian and quartan fevers, which were removed upon
the appearance of the eruption, but returned again upon
its diſappearing; from thence he concludes the ſcorbutic

3 B   humour

humour combined with the *scabies,* to have produced those surprising symptoms.

He then proceeds to still more uncommon and remarkable symptoms of the scurvy; and, upon the testimony of *Doringius,* relates cases of a jaundice ending in a *hydrops ascites;* an asthma; a *tinea,* covering not only the whole scalp, but the forehead; a *herpes* of the left arm; a gangrene in the fore-finger; a hæmorrhage from the lips, no conspicuous orifice of a vein being discovered; palpitations of the heart; burning and intolerable pain in the soles of the feet, with livid spots on the legs; and a running of putrid and purulent matter from the *uterus.* *Timoth. Ulricus* observed not only the knees, but the whole body, as it were, contracted; with an excrescence of flesh from the eyes under the *palpebræ;* the *tunica adnata* of the eye being yellow, but the *palpebræ* of the same colour with the *iris.* In some, though more rarely, upon each motion of their joints, a noise was plainly heard as from broken bones, or like the crackling of nuts. Where there was a dropsy, in a night's time the whole teeth became loose, so that the patient was in danger of losing them all; but next day they were found firm in their sockets. In a patient where no spots could be made to appear, even by the help of medicines, upon forcing a sweat, the muscular part of the arm was seized with a sense of heat and burning, as if drops of boiling water had been thrown upon it; mean while nothing was to be seen appearing outwardly. A widow in a continual fever, had her whole body covered with large black spots; her face resembling in colour the skin of smoked bacon boiled. Upon which he concludes, such is the strange variety of diseases and symptoms occasioned by the scurvy, that not only the vulgar, but even a physician unacquainted with the distemper, would be greatly amazed, and might believe the person to have died of poison. He very ingeniously, however, accounts for them all, according

to

to his own *hypothesis*; making up sixty-two symptoms, by adding several to what are mentioned by *Eugalenus, viz.* blindness; a stench of the body; a stoppage of the courses in women; in place of which they have a white acrid saltish running, apt to infect men: and men from this disease are rendered unfit for generation, by having a watery vitiated *semen.* He is very prolix on the cure; copies from his predecessor *Albertus* the therapeutic intentions; and abounds with almost all the *recipe's* given by preceding authors, together with what he learned from other hands. Where there is a heat of the body, or fever, he uses the cooling antiscorbutics, *viz. cichoreum, endivia, acetosa, acetosella, succ. citri, aurantior. limon. sp. salis, vitriol. vel sulphur.* He recommends steel where there is not the convenience of mineral waters; but forbids the use of vinegar in this disease.

Arnoldi Weickardi thesaur pharmaceutic. galeno-che- 1626. *mic. sive tractat. practic. &c. lib. 3. cap. 5. de stomacace, seu scorbuto.*

This author, although usually ranked among the number of writers on the scurvy, has nothing new upon it. He makes no mention of the symptoms. His cure consists in bleeding, purging, and afterwards sweating the patient, and in administering the common antiscorbutics in very improper forms; all transcribed out of other authors.

Gul. Fabricii Hildani observ. et curationum chirurgic. 1627. *cent. 5. obs. 5.*

There is here a short letter to the author from *Ludov. Schmid*, giving an account of the Prince of *Baden*'s youngest son, a child of fourteen months, afflicted with the scurvy; who was cured with antiscorbutics. *Hildanus*, in his answer, mentions an obstinate scorbutic ulcer cured likewise by antiscorbutics; which is all that is to

be

be met with on this difeafe in the works of that celebrated practitioner.

1633.   *Joannis Hartmanni praxeos chymiatricæ p.* 345. *de
fcorbuto. Ed. Genev. Opus poftbumum.*

He is the firft who obferves the pernicious effects of
mercury in the fcurvy; for the cure of which he relies
much upon fome chemical preparatioms, *viz. tartar.
vitriolat. fp. vim tartarifat. &c.*

1640.   *Lazari Riverii praxeos medicæ lib.* 12. *cap.* 6. *de
fcorbutica affectione.*

As the fcurvy was hitherto fo little known in the
fouthern parts of *Europe,* that it had not been fo much
as mentioned by any author there, he likewife would
have omitted treating of it; the difeafe never appearing
in *France,* attended with all the fymptoms defcribed by
northern writers. However, as difeafes were obferved
accompanied with fome of its fymptoms, and as
thofe authors inform us, that one fymptom peculiar
to the diftemper was fufficient to difcover it, he would
therefore defcribe it. But as it was a malady by no
means common in his country, where moft phyficians
believed they had no fuch difeafe, he does not pretend to defcribe the true fcurvy; therefore calls it the
affectio fcorbutica, as approaching near to it. He thinks
the fcurvy nothing elfe but the *affectio hypochondriaca,*
attended with fuch extraordinary and unufual fymptoms
as denote a degree of malignity; and imagines the *pancreas* is often affected.

1645.   *Confilium medicæ facultatis Hafnienfis de fcorbuto.*

This was publifhed for the benefit of the poor in the
country; and is divided into four fections. The 1ft re-
cites the caufe of the difeafe, and the figns by which it
is known; the 2d, how it may be prevented; the 3d,
how

how it ought to be cured; the 4th, what is proper for the removal of its primary fymptoms.

Sect. 1. They obferve, that it is an endemic evil with them and other northern nations. It attacks the patient in various fhapes, according to his habit and conftitution, or other difeafes with which it may be complicated. The immediate caufe, is a bad concoction, from a crude, melancholy, corrupted humour, oppreffing the organs, both of the firft digeftion in the ftomach, and of fanguification. Hence enfue for the moft part difficulty of breathing; fwelling, putrefaction, and bleeding of the gums; loofe teeth; a weaknefs, fwelling, and ftiffnefs of the legs; fpots, and the like. The external caufes are, 1. The impure, grofs, moift, and cold air, of their country; thofe perfons being moft fubject-to it who live in the northern parts near the fea, or where they are furrounded with lakes. 2. Grofs and corrupted food, *viz.* bad bread, not fufficiently baked, made of fpoiled flour; falt and dried flefh and fifh; old cheefe; rancid butter; peafe, and other grains, when fpoiled; together with unwholfome malt-liquors. 3. Thofe of a fedentary inactive way of life are moft afflicted with it; together with thofe, 4. who are apt to be coftive, or labour under a fuppreffion of any natural evacuation; as alfo the dejected and forrowful. 5. This difeafe often fucceeds others; as obftructions of the liver and fpleen, and particularly quartan agues. It is likewife hereditary and infectious. From thefe external caufes proceeds the internal or immediate caufe of the difeafe before mentioned. Although the malady may not eafily be difcovered in the beginning, by reafon of its appearing under the form of other difeafes; as alfo from its unexpected and flow attacks, (fo that, in countries in which it is endemic, we are to fufpect anomalous difeafes not yielding to the ufual remedies, efpecially if the patient is of a melancholy difpofition, to be fcorbutic); yet when the diftemper is violent, it is eafily known. It is ufually preceded

ceded by a laffitude of the whole body, weaknefs of the
legs, breathleffnefs upon walking, a livid colour of the
face, and by a greater corpulency. In its progrefs,
flying heats become troublefome; the gums itch, with a
great flow of *faliva*; the urine is fometimes turbid, at
other times quite watery. When farther advanced, the
difficulty of breathing is fo great, that the patient cannot walk or move himfelf, but he falls into a fwoon; of
which he recovers when laid in bed. It is attended
with colic-pains; the gums are fwelled, and bleed upon
the leaft touch; the teeth are loofe, and fall out without pain, the flefh at their roots being quite putrid; the
breath is fœtid; and the legs fwell, and grow ftiff, fo
that the patients cannot walk. Sometimes on the legs,
and over the whole body, there appear various red, purple, or azure fpots. Now and then they are afflicted
with the *cryfipelas*, malignant ulcers, and nocturnal
pains; and fometimes the body waftes away. Different
fevers, and various fymptoms, almoft of every kind
that can be mentioned, often accompany this difeafe.
The urine is turbid, thick, and clayifh, of a purple colour; but it does not long retain the fame appearance.
The pulfe is variable; fometimes weak, at other times
ftrong, when the patient feems very weak; and now
and then it is altogether obfcure. This evil is eafily
removed by proper remedies in the beginning; but
when advanced, it is not fo eafy to prevent relapfes.
Where proper diet and medicines are neglected, health
is feldom reftored. It commonly ends in a dropfy or
atrophy. A difficulty of breathing, and black fpots on
the legs, are dangerous fymptoms; as alfo continual
pains and *borborygmi* about the navel. A hereditary fcurvy is feldom cured. It is a more dangerous difeafe in old people than in young. Where the mouth
is affected, remedies are fpeedily to be ufed; otherwife
the malady fpreads farther, and may infect the whole
throat.

throat. Fevers and ulcers accompanying this difeafe, cannot be cured without antifcorbutics.

Sect. 2. Prevention is propofed, by living in dry lodgings; fumigating apartments, with the fteam of aromatic woods and gums; and by avoiding fuch food as has been obferved productive of the difeafe. There is likewife recommended the ufe of a wine medicated with wormwood; and feveral other warm, bitter, aromatic ingredients. The belly is at all times to be kept open, and the other evacuations (efpecially when fuppreffed) are duly to be promoted. Exercife, baths, phyfic in the fpring and autumn, are alfo neceffary. They who are very fubject to it, are to take now and then two or three fpoonfuls of the following antifcorbutic water; which may be made more pleafant and ftronger, by adding fome of their fcorbutic fyrup, which is the fame with *Foreftus*'s. R rad. raphan. ruft. lib. iii. fcorzon. unc. ii. cort. rad. cappar. tamarifc. ana unc. fs. fol. cochlear. nafturt. aq. petrofel. becabung. recent. ana manip. iii. fem. cochlear. cardui bened. aquileg. fœnicul. ana dr. iii. crem. tartar. dr. ii. gran. paradif. cardamom. ana dr. i. Affunde vini Rhenan. lib. xii. aq. cochlear. fumar. ana lib. i. Stent in digeftione 24 horis, dein per cineres deftillentur. Or they may take the juice of fcurvygrafs mixed with wine; or their elect fcorbuticum, which is the conferves of feveral antifcorbutic herbs, with the addition of a very fmall quantity of fpir. vitriol.

Sect. 3. and 4. containing the indications of cure, and the treatment of the fymptoms, have nothing new; the medicinal intentions being pretty much the fame as directed by *Albertus*. The whole is concluded with a number of long prefcriptions, adapted to the various intentions of prevention and cure delivered in the *confilium*. Here the prices of the feveral medicines are marked for the fake of the poor.

Bericht und unterricht von der kranckheit des fchmertz-machenden 1647.

machenden fcorboëts : -or, An account and information concerning that painful difeafe the fcurvy. By *John Drawitzs.*

This book has undergone no lefs than four editions, being efteemed the beft written upon the fubjeët in the *German* language. The difeafes treated of as proceeding from the fcurvy, are as follow. 1. The gout. 2. A fpafmodic affeëtion. 3. The palfy. 4. Pains in other parts of the extremities, though not in the joints. 5. The headach. 6. The toothach. 7. The pleurify. 8. The belly-ach; or the fcorbutic colic, and iliac paffion. 9. A pain about the *os facrum,* back, and *perinæum,* refembling a true fit of the ftone. He had been certainly informed from the *Eaft Indies,* that the failors there were fpeedily and effeëtually cured of the fcurvy, by eating oranges; which he finds great difficulty to reconcile to his theory of the difeafe. He had heard from *Dantzick,* that fome mafters of fhips carried out with them an acid water, got in the preparation of *antimon. diaphoret.* which prevented the fcurvy at fea.

1662.   *Baldaffaris Timæi opera medico-praëtica.*

This author gives us many hiftories in his writings, of fuch cafes as he deemed fcorbutic; *viz.* Book 1. of praëtical cafes and obfervations; cafe 3. a fcorbutic headach; cafe 7. a fcorbutic delirium; and cafe 15. the hypochondriac melancholy, beginning with the fcurvy. In his 3d book, cafe 24. an *hydrops afcites,* joined with the fcurvy; and cafe 32. the *affeëtio hypochondriaca,* with this difeafe alfo; cafe 35. a fcurvy and atrophy, of which the patient died; cafe 36. the *arthritis vaga fcorbutica.* Book 6. cafe 15. *fcabies pruriginofa fcorbutica.* Book 8. cafe 15. a fcorbutic tertian; and cafe 18. a fcorbutic quartan.

In his epiftles, book 3. epiftle 10. 11. and 12. the *cashexia fcorbutica*; epiftle 20. and 28. the *affeëtio hypochondriaca fcorbutica*; and book 5. epiftle 9. the *arthritis*

tis vaga. His method of cure, which has nothing new in it, is to be found in the 34th cafe of his 3d book; by which he fays he generally fucceeded, unlefs the fcurvy was hereditary, or very deeply rooted: as likewife in the 29th and 30th epiftles of his 3d book; where we have the treatment of the Queen of *Sweden*, when labouring under this difeafe, by the celebrated *Hermannus Conringius.* And there (epiftle 29,) we have mention made of a new fcorbutic fymptom, by *Otto Œflerus, viz.* a burning internal pain, feated in the mefentery, attended with violent drought, and colics moft violent in the night.

Valentini Andreæ Moellenbrocii, de varis, feu arthritide 1663. vaga fcorbutica, tractatus.

He makes the fcurvy a moft univerfal difeafe, a calamity common almoft to all mankind. Its immediate caufe is, a volatile falt in the blood, endued with great acrimony and malignity. The laft of thefe properties he thinks demonftrable, from the fudden weaknefs and proftration of ftrength, anxiety, and difficult refpiration, that occur even in the beginning of the difeafe, as if the patient had fwallowed poifon; as alfo from an eruption of livid fpots, which is often feen after death.

Thomæ Willis tractatus de fcorbuto. 1667.

He fets out with telling us, that a great variety of fymptoms, and diforders of the moft oppofite kinds, are fuppofed to proceed from the fcurvy; which, like a condemned and infamous name, has the fcandal of moft difeafes charged to its account. How far he clears up this confufion, or has abridged the number, will appear by the following detail he gives of fcorbutic fymptoms. He obferves, that no fingle defcription or definition of this diftemper can be given; and, confequently, that the beft method of defcribing it, is according to the different

3 C   parts

parts affected of the body; in all which it produces
manifold fymptoms.

He begins with the head : where the fcurvy caufes
headachs, violent, and habitual ; and fometimes vague,
or periodical; oftentimes fleepinefs, and dulnefs of the
fpirits, at other times obftinate watchings ; frequent *ver-
tigines, fcotomiæ,* convulfions, palfies, falivations, ulcers
of the gums, loofe teeth, and fœtid breath.

The breaft is affected with pains in different parts of
its membranes, chiefly on the *fternum,* where they are
very violent, acute, and darting ; frequent afthma's; difficult and unequal refpiration; ftraitnefs of the breaft; violent cough ; inordinate pulfe ; palpitation of the heart;
frequent faintings, and the continual dread of them.

In the *abdomen,* where this difeafe has its principal
feat, it begets a multitude of evils, *viz. naufea,* vomiting, *cardialgia,* inflations and murmurings of the
hypochondria, frequent colics, and moft troublefome
fhifting pains; an almoft conftant *diarrhœa,* fometimes
the dyfentery, or *tenefmus*; the *atrophia,* and now and
then the *afcites.* The urine is very often reddifh and
lixivial, having a cake fufpended in it, or adhering to
the fides of the glafs : and fometimes, though feldom,
a great quantity of pale watery urine is difcharged.

In the limbs, or even over the whole body, there are
wandering pains, often very acute, and becoming worfe
at night ; a fpontaneous laffitude ; wafting of the flefh ;
lumbago, a weaknefs of the other joints; fpots of various
colours on the fkin ; tumours, tubercles, and often *ca-
coethic* ulcers ; a *ftupor* or ftinging pain about the mufcles;
a fenfe of cold as it were in the parts; contractions and
fubfultus of the tendons. Befides thefe, fcorbutic people
are fubject to irregular effervefcencies of the blood, erratic fevers, and profufe hæmorrhages. He concludes
this long detail with obferving, that thefe are the moft
common and ufual fymptoms of the fcurvy, fometimes
more, fometimes fewer, of this or that kind, afflicting
the

the difeafed : but befides what have been already mentioned, there occur in it more uncommon and prodigious appearances.

The principal caufes are, unwholfome air, and a vitiated *crafis* of the blood by preceding ficknefs.   In
this diftemper, either the blood, nervous juice, or both,
are affected.   The *dyfcrafy* of the blood is here twofold;
either *fulphureo-faline*, or *falino-fulphureous*.   If the firft
be the cafe, and the fulphurs fuperabound, then repeated bleedings, a cooling regimen, and the moft temperate remedies, are proper ; avoiding above all things the
hot and acrid antifcorbutics.   But, on the contrary, where
there is the *falino-fulphureous diathefis*, and the falts of
the blood are predominant, then the warmer medicines
are proper, and fuch as are poffeffed of a volatile falt,
together with fteel and the like.   The dyfcrafy in the
nervous juice is threefold.   It is, *1ft*, Either too thin
and poor ; or, *2dly*, It has degenerated from its fpirituous faline conftitution into a fharpnefs ; or, *3dly*, It may
abound with heterogeneous and morbid particles.   And,
according to thefe imagined dyfcrafies of the blood and
nervous juice, he makes a fecond diftribution of the
fymptoms ; and accounts for the whole number he enumerates in this difeafe, which he fuppofes to be hereditary and infectious.

The therapeutic intentions are divided into three
claffes. 1. The prefervatory ; under which he lays
down the procefs of cure, or rather the method in general of removing the caufes of the difeafe. 2. The
curatory, or means of alleviating and relieving the moft
urgent fymptoms.   The 3d comprehends what he calls
the vital indications, or the means of preferving and reftoring the ftrength and health of the patient.

The prefervatory intentions, or cure, confift in cathartic, digeftive, and antifcorbutic medicines ; with blood-
letting occafionally repeated. If the ftomach is much
difordered, or oppreffed with phlegm, he gives a vomit,

weaker

weaker or stronger, according to the strength or habit of the patient. This in some he repeats every month, where it is indicated : otherwise he begins the cure with a purgative, which he repeats occasionally, and of a different kind, suited to the warmer or colder constitution of the patient ; or, to use his own terms, according as the *dyscrasy* of the blood is *sulphureo-saline,* or *nitro-sulphureous.* In both cases he furnishes us with variety of *formulæ* ; observing, that they should be repeated no oftener than at an interval of five or six days ; as too violent and frequent cathartics serve only to weaken the tone of the *viscera,* and strength of the patient, without removing the disease. After once or twice purging, if a fulness of blood, and its viscidity, make it necessary, the patient is to be bled in the arm, or with leeches in the hæmorrhoidal veins ; rather repeating the operation, than taking away too much at a time. Those evacuations being premised, according as they are severally indicated ; provided there be no urgency from any particular symptom, he proceeds to the general method of cure, *viz.* removing the cause, and extirpating the disease. For these purposes, the digestive and specific antiscorbutic medicines (divided into two classes, *viz.* hot and cold) are to be given every day, unless when under physic ; to which, if needful, diaphoretics and sudorifics may be joined. He calls these *digestive medicines,* which assist or restore the functions of the stomach, and other chylopoietic *viscera ;* and *antiscorbutics* or *specifics,* such as remove the scorbutic dyscrasy of the blood : both which are to be joined together, or at least given the same day. *Cremor, sal,* or *tinctura tartari, tartar. vitriol. chalybeat. el. propr. &c.* are proper digestives. They are to be administered in a small dose, evening and morning.

For the cold scurvy, he abounds with an ample variety of antiscorbutic compositions, of *cochlearia, nasturtium aq. becabungæ, cort. winteran. bacc. juniper. rad. raphani, ni*, and other acrid aromatic herbs and roots, together with their conferves, the candied spices, *pulv. ari comp.* steel, *&c.* He has often succesfully prescribed the following remedy. R *sum. geniftæ manip.* iii. *minutim incif. Coquant. in cerevif. fort. lib.* iii. *ad medietatem.* Two or three ounces to be given twice a-day.

In the hot scurvy, the more cooling and temperate antiscorbutics are neceffary. Of these he gives the same variety; making use, in most prescriptions, of the *tefta- ceous* powders, the abforbents, *fal. abfinth. &c.* He re- commends wines made of gooseberries, and other fum- mer-fruits, but especially cyder: obferves *rad. lapathi acuti* to be among the best of our antiscorbutics. This infufed in ale, with brooklime, water-creffes, sliced o- ranges, citrons, pine-tops, *&c.* makes a noble remedy.

After having thus delivered the cure of the difeafe in general, he proceeds to the curatory indications for re- lief and removal of the most urgent symptoms. For a difficulty of breathing, and asthmatic fits, he recom- mends cardiacs and antifpafmodics, *viz. fp. cornu cervi, tinct. caftor. flor. benzoin. el. propr. &c.* given in any an- tifcorbutic liquor. If the *dyfpnœa* be entirely fpafmo- dic, opiates afford the greatest relief: acrid glyfters, fudorifics, and diuretics, are likewife ferviceable. In fcorbutic diforders of the ftomach, vomits, purges of rhubarb, *el. propr. &c.* with fomentations to the part, are neceffary: opiates fometimes give eafe. In fcor- butic colics, glyfters are to be given; fomentations, li- niments, and cataplafms, ufed externally; and opiates internally, efpecially when joined with purgatives: the *teftaceous* powders are proper; likewife the ufe of fome purging mineral water, as *Epfom.* An inveterate *di- arrhœa,* fuch as fcorbutic perfons are fubject to, is not to be ftopt by aftringents: the mineral waters impreg- nated with fteel and vitriol, are in this cafe the beft me- dicines; and next to thefe, preparations of fteel, efpe- cially its *crocus.* A *vertigo,* faintings, palfy, and convulfions,

vulfions, require a mixture of cephalic and antifcorbutic
remedies.   The other fymptoms are to be treated likewife with fuch medicines as are proper for the original
difeafes compounded with antifcorbutics.

He afterwards relates a fymptom which he had obferved three or four times, *viz.* a crackling of the bones
upon moving the joints.   Even upon turning in bed, by
rubbing of the *vertebræ* on each other, a confiderable
noife was perceived, like to the rough handling of a fke-
leton;   which he remarks is an almoft incurable fymptom.

Laftly, We have what he calls the *vital indications.*
He here directs the ufe of cardiacs, reftoratives,
opiates, &c. together with a proper diet.   He blames
the immoderate ufe of fugar in this prefent age, for the
frequency and violence of the fcurvy; and concludes
with fome hiftories of cafes.

1668.   *Morbus polyrhizos et polymorphæus.*   A treatife of the
fcurvy.   By *Everard Maynwaringe.*

To the caufes of this diftemper ufually affigned by
others, he adds the ufe of tobacco, and immoderate ve-
nery;   particularly the firft, which he inveighs againft at
great length.   He runs down all former theories and
methods of cure recommended by authors;   pretending
to be poffeffed of moft effectual remedies;   which, however, he does not make public.

1669.   *Praxeos Barbettianæ, cum notis Frederici Deckers, l:b.* 4.
cap. 3. *de fcorbuto, et affectione hypochondriaca malè vul-*
gò dicta hyfterica.

Barbette gives a defcription of the fcurvy, and its
fymptoms, pretty much from *Eugalenus:* cautions a-
gainft bleeding, and violent purgatives, in the cure;
but thinks gentle phyfic proper at times, and that the
peccant humour fhould be prepared by inciding remedies;   the moft proper for this purpofe being volatile
salts.

falts. After a long lift of the common antifcorbutic medicines, (to which *Deckers* fubjoins many more, adapted to the particular fymptoms of the difeafe), he obferves, the *fp. fal. d. ammoniaci, et cochleariæ,* are the principal remedies. He concludes with two cafes: one a young man not able to walk through his chamber, who recovered in feven days by a decoction of *rad. raphani* in whey; another, a merchant, having fcorbutic fpots, who was cured by the ufe of *fpir. fal. ammoniac.* and proper diet. *Deckers* adds another cafe, and feemingly a very genuine fcurvy, which was removed by fourteen drops, for a dofe, of the *fp. fal. ammoniac.* given in an infufion of *rad. raphani* in wine.

De fcorbuto liber fingularis; auctore Gualtero Charleton. 1672.

Obferving it might be a tafk fit only for *Jove* himfelf to give an accurate account of the fcurvy, and all its fymptoms, he thinks it neceffary to give only a catalogue of thofe which moft frequently occur, and are the moft afflicting. In this number he ranks almoft all the fymptoms enumerated by *Eugalenus, Sennertus,* and *Willis*; and afterwards diftinguifhes the difeafe itfelf into three kinds, from its different caufes. The firft is denominated a *rancid fcurvy,* from the predominancy of the fulphurs in the blood combined with fome of its falts; the fecond, a *fcurvy from fixed falt,* where the tartareous or terreftrial faline particles prevail; and the third, an *acid fcurvy,* owing to a fharpnefs and acidity of the blood and juices.

The fymptoms peculiar to the firft fpecies, are, fpots, *exanthemata,* puftles, tubercles, and ulcerations, upon the external parts of the body; internally *cardialgia,* vomiting, *diarrhœa,* dyfentery, colics, together with frequent effervefcencies of the blood. When this fpecies of fcurvy is inveterate, the *genus nervofum* becomes affected. The fymptoms are then, a giddinefs; tenfive

headach,

headach; *fcotomia*; *coma fomnolentum*, or immoderate watchings; the night-mare, and fometimes madnefs.

Of the fecond fpecies, the fymptoms are, ftraitnefs of the breaft, palpitation of the heart, and faintings; numbnefs and laffitude of the body; convulfive motions, and erratic pains in the joints.

In the third, or acid fcurvy, there are continual irritations of the nerves; which are increafed by the flighteft paffion of the mind; frequent *rigors*, (a certain fign of acidity in the humours); a fenfe of cold in the back part of the head, and fpine of the back, fometimes running through the limbs; flatulent fpafms; convulfions, and what is commonly called the *hyfteric paffion*; fometimes coftivenefs; at other times the dyfentery; melancholy, with dread and defpair; atrophy; ulcerations; laftly, a gangrene, which generally clofes the fcene. From this acidity in the blood, proceed likewife, palpitations of the heart; a fudden ftoppage of the pulfe, attended with great anxiety, ending in a faint, with a cold fweat. When this fpecies of fcurvy has become inveterate and confirmed, it begets moft violent and dreadful fymptoms, *viz.* intolerable nocturnal pains, cancers, *&c.*

In the cure of the firft fpecies, we are to begin with gentle *cholagogue* purgatives prudently adminiftered and repeated, and venefection, if the difeafe is but commencing; proceeding to the digeftive or temperate alterative medicines, that may correct the hot *fulphureo-faline* ftate of the humours. If the patient be of a hot temperament, and lean, fcurvygrafs, and other hot antifcorbutics, are to be avoided. Affes milk with juice of dandelion, or a water diftilled from the milder antifcorbutics with cyder or cows whey, is then to be ufed. A pint of warm whey, with the addition of ten drops of *fp. cochlear.* or *fp. fal. d.* may be drank night and morning for fome weeks together. The mineral waters are likewife ferviceable; obferving at the fame

time proper rules with regard to diet and exercise. After those courses, (during which the patient must take a
purgative every week), the cure is to be completed
by restoratives and corroborants. The best is, a small
subacid wine, medicated with the temperate, but aromatic
and stomachic antiscorbutics, or confections of the subacid fruits, &c.

For cure of the second species, proceeding from a
fixed salt, the only proper medicines are those which a-
bound with a volatile salt, *viz.* the warm antiscorbutics.
Digestive and cathartic medicines must be interposed at
times, together with sudorifics and diuretics, according to
the tendency of the tartareous humour to the skin or kidneys. Steel mineral waters are to be used, if the patient is of a hot temperament. After those courses,
recovery is to be perfected by corroborants and analep-
tics. The best of these is fennel-wine.

The cure of the third species, or acid scurvy, is to
be begun with gentle *eccoprotics*, which make way for
bleeding; proceeding afterwards to deobstruents, (such
of this class as are mild), joined with temperate antiscorbutics, but especially such remedies as are proper in the
hypochondriac disease with obstructed *viscera*. Afterwards antacids are to be given, *viz.* volatile salts of any
kind, or the testaceous powders, lixivial salts, oily e-
mulsions, and chalybeate medicines. Milk almost of
any kind is proper; as likewise whey medicated with the
temperate antiscorbutics; broths of snails, cray-fish, &c.
The cure here, as in the before mentioned scurvies, is
to be concluded by corroborants; such particularly as
are recommended by authors at the close of the *melancholia hypochondriaca.*

He finishes his book with laying down the method of
removing several of the most urgent symptoms in this
disease. The principal of which are to be treated with
remedies appropriated to such diseases when *idiopathe-
tic*, joined with antiscorbutics.

Francisci

1674. *Francisci Deleboe Sylvii opera medica.*

This celebrated author has little upon this disease but theory. He only observes, (*prax. medic. append. tract.* 10. § 863. &c.*), that there is no distemper in which volatile salts are so efficacious and necessary as in the scurvy; herbs abounding with these salts, *viz. cochlear erysim. nasturt. raphan.* and mustard-seed, being its best remedies. In imitation of those, for many years past he had given, with great success in this distemper, volatile salts obtained from different parts of animals. Moreover, acids that are spirituous, either of the natural or chemical sort, are likewise serviceable in the scurvy, *viz.* juice of oranges, sorrel, &c. *sp. sal. nitr. dul.* For cure of the scorbutic spots observed after the epidemical constitution, of which he is there treating, he mixed these volatile salts and spirituous acids together; which proved very serviceable, and sudorific.

1675. *The disease of* London; *or, A new discovery of the scurvy.* By Gideon Harvey.

He divides the disease into two great branches, *viz.* a *mouth-scurvy*, and *leg-scurvy*. To which a third may be added, which he calls the *joint-scurvy*. They are thus denominated from the parts affected. The immediate cause of the first, is an acid lymph in the stomach; the occasional causes being the frequent use of mercury, a saline air, salt diet, brackish water used for brewing of ale, gluttony, debauchery, &c. The second, or leg-scurvy, he attributes to a cause opposite to that of an acid, *viz.* a lixivial alcalious salt. He terms it a *saponary state of blood.* The occasional causes of this are pretty much the same with the former, *viz.* salt air and food; the use of sea-salt, distilled spirits, and tobacco. An acid scurvy, upon its long continuance, changes into a saponary scurvy; or is followed with swelling and ulcers of the legs, &c. He afterwards makes many other distinctions in this disease, (see

part I.

part 1. chap. 2. p. 43.).   For a prefervative againft it,
he recommends change of air, and wholfome, nourifh-
ing, eafy-digefted food.   In the cure, bleeding is proper, and iffues both for that and its prevention.   In the
mouth-fcurvy, they are to be put in the left arm; in
fome cafes in the neck, or right arm; in the leg-fcurvy,
above the knee; in the joint-fcurvy, more than one are
to be made.   Aloetic pills are among the beft prefervatives againft this diftemper.   They are to be premifed
in the cure of a recent, or even inveterate fcurvy : but
at the fame time are proper only in the acid kind; as the
laxatives in the lixivial or faponary fcurvy muft be of the
mildeft fort.   The acid fcurvy requires warmer medicines; the lixivial the more temperate, cooling, mucilaginous, *&c.*   He concludes with the cure of a ftomachic fcurvy, hepatic, *&c.*

Abrahami Muntingii de vera antiquorum herba Bri-   1681.
tannica, ejufdemque efficacia contra ftomacacen feu fcelo-
tyrben, Frifiis et Batavis de Scheurbuyck, differtatio hi-
ftorico-medica.

He pretends, after much labour, to have difcovered
the true *herba Britannica* of the ancients, which had
been unknown to the world for many ages, *viz.* that
celebrated plant which, according to *Pliny's* account,
cured the *Roman* army, (fee p. 347.).   He would have
it to be *hydrolapathum nigrum,* the great water-dock;
and beftows the moft extraordinary encomiums upon it;
giving inftances of feveral remarkable cures performed
by its ufe, in the fcurvy.

Traité du fcorbut, par L. Chameau.   1683.

The fcurvy is in a particular manner endemic with
the *Englifh,* as the author had obferved during his refi-
dence for fome time among them, and for their fakes
chiefly he publifhed his book.   He makes it to be a contagious diffolution of the blood, by a very acrid fubtile

falt: confutes the diftinctions made of the difeafe by
Dr *Willis*, and extols milk as the moft excellent antifcorbutic; accounting all warm and acrid medicines for
the moft part pernicious.

1684.	*Nauwkeurige verhandelinge van de fcheurbuik en des
felfs toevallen:* or, A curious treatife on the fcurvy, and
its fymptoms. By *Stephen Blancard.* *Ejufdem praxeos
medicæ cap.* 15. *de fcorbuto.*

Though *Willis* and *Charleton* have written the beft
upon the fcurvy, they have not yet folved all the
difficulties that occur in it; which this author thinks he
does by his theory of fermentation, founded upon the
Cartefian principles. The malady proceeds from a thick-
nefs of blood. Of this there are two kinds, *viz.* a cold
and pituitous vifcidity; or there may be a heat and
an acidity in that fluid: hence the difeafe is properly divided into a *hot* and *cold fcurvy.* In the firft fpecies,
whatever incides and attenuates vifcid pituituous humours, fuch as the warm aromatics and fpices; in the
other (or acid fcurvy), the *teftaceous* powders, and all other
abforbents; fixed, volatile, and alcaline falts; chalybeates,
but particularly drinking of tea and coffee, are the proper remedies. Bleeding is of no ufe. Vomits and
purgatives are fometimes neceffary. All acids, vifcid
and falt foods, are pernicious.

1684.	*Jo. Dolæi medicinæ theoretico-practicæ encyclopædiæ
lib. 3. cap.* 12. *de fcorbuto.*

The fcurvy is a difeafe nearly allied to the hypochondriac affection, being an acid dyfcrafy of the blood.
He pretends to cure all fcurvies in twelve days, by
mercury dulcified in a particular manner.

1685.	*Michaelis Ettmulleri collegii practici de morbis humani
corporis part.* 2. *caput ultimum, exhibens duos affectus
complicatiffimos;*

complicatiſſimos; *nempe, malum hypochondriacum, et ſcor-*
butum.

He accounts the ſcurvy the higheſt degree of the hypochondriac diſeaſe. All the ſymptoms of this latter
occur in it, beſides many more. He has nothing new,
all he ſays being tranſcribed from other authors; but con-
founds the two diſeaſes together, ſo as to make ſteel, and
moſt other remedies proper in the hypochondriac diſeaſe,
uſeful in the ſcurvy. He obſerves, that mercury is extremely pernicious in the ſcurvy; and ſo much dreaded
in *Holland,* that even in venereal caſes, they were afraid
to uſe it, on account of their ſcorbutic conſtitutions.
Dutch ſeamen carry to ſea muſtard-ſeed, which both pre-
ſerves them from the diſeaſe, and cures it. In winter,
when the antiſcorbutic plants cannot be procured, a compoſition with muſtard-ſeed is to be preſcribed. *Phyto-*
log. p. 98. Vid. Sinap.

Thomæ Sydenham opera univerſa.   1685.
The author has no where treated expreſsly of this diſeaſe, but in a poſthumous work aſcribed to him, under
the title of *Proceſſus integri in morbis ferè omnibus cu-*
randis. There the ſcurvy is ſaid to be accompanied
with, 1. ſpontaneous laſſitude; 2. heavineſs; 3. difficulty of breathing, eſpecially after exerciſe; 4. rottenneſs
of the gums; 5. fœtid breath; 6. frequent bleeding at
the noſe; 7. difficulty of walking; 8. a ſwelling ſometimes, at other times a waſting of the legs; on which
ſpots always appear, that are either livid, or of a leaden,
yellow, or purple colour; 9. a ſallow complexion.
For cure, eight ounces of blood are to be taken from
the arm, provided there be no ſign of a dropſy; next
morning a purging potion given, and repeated twice,
at the interval of three days betwixt each doſe. On
the intermediate days the following medicines are to
be uſed, and continued for a month or two. ℞ *conſ.*
cochlear. hort. unc. ii. *conſ. lujulæ. unc.* i. *p. ari comp.*
                                         dr.

dr. vi. *ſyr. aurantior. q ſ. F. elect,* Of this the quantity of a large nutmeg is to be taken three times a-day,
with ſix ſpoonfuls of the *aq. raphan. comp.* or *aq. cochlear. recent* The patient is to have for common
drink, an infuſion of horſe-raddiſh, ſcurvygraſs, raiſins,
and oranges, in ſmall beer or in white wine. The a-
bove courſe is likewiſe beneficial in the ſcorbutic or hy-
ſteric rheumatiſm, bleeding and purging excepted. But
the more genuine ſentiments of this candid author are to
be found in his other works.

Cap. 4. *de febribus continuis, ann.* 1661, 62, 63, 64,
he obſerves, that the two great ſubterfuges of ignorant
phyſicians, were malignity and the ſcurvy; which they
blamed for diſorders and ſymptoms often owing to their
own ill management. Thus, whatever bad and irregular ſymptoms have been brought on in fevers, perhaps
by their unſeaſonable evacuations, theſe they aſcribe to
the malignity of the diſeaſe; but if the long continuance
of the diſtemper ſhould wipe off this aſperſion of malignity, whatever afterwards obſtructs the cure muſt be
the ſcurvy; both of which are blamed without reaſon.

Sect. 6. *cap.* 5. *de rheumatiſmo.* To deliver my
ſentiments freely, though I do not at all doubt that the
ſcurvy is to be met with in theſe northern countries,
yet I am perſuaded it is not ſo frequent as generally
ſuppoſed. For moſt of thoſe diſorders we term *ſcorbutic,*
are the effects of approaching ills not yet formed into
diſeaſes, or the relics of ſome diſeaſe imperfectly cured.
Thus, for inſtance, where a matter ſuited to produce
the gout is newly generated, there appear various ſymptoms, which occaſion us to ſuſpect the ſcurvy; till the
formation and actual appearance of the gout remove all
doubt concerning the diſtemper. And in the ſame manner, many ſymptoms aſcribed to the ſcurvy afflict gouty
people after the fit is over, eſpecially if it has been improperly treated. And this is to be underſtood, not only of the gout, but alſo of the dropſy. The proverb
is,

is, That where the fcurvy ends, there the dropfy begins; which is to be underftood in this fenfe, that, upon
the appearance of the dropfy, the preconceived opinion
of the fcurvy falls to the ground.   And the fame may
be faid of feveral other chronic difeafes that are but
forming, and others that are not totally cured.   He
however thinks, there is a fpecies of rheumatifm near a-
kin to the fcurvy in its capital fymptoms, and which requires the fame method of cure.   The pains fhift from
one place to another; rarely occafion a fwelling; there
is no fever; but it is attended with irregular fymptoms;
fuch efpecially as have taken much of the *cort. peruv.*
are fubject to it.   Though it is otherwife a very tedious
and chronic difeafe, yet it may be effectually cured by the
ufe of the antifcorbutic electuary before mentioned, and
a water diftilled from fcurvygrafs, brooklime, creffes,
&c.

Martini Lifter tractatus de quibufdam morbis chronicis 1694.
exercitatio 5. de fcorbuto.

He treats of the fcurvy next to the venereal difeafe,
becaufe they are nearly allied; having fo many fymptoms common to both, that they are not eafily diftinguifhed from each other, but by an experienced phyfician.   The fcurvy has not been exprefsly treated of by
the ancients, as being in their time endemic only in a
remote corner of the world little known to them.   *Eugalenus* was the firft who accurately defcribed this difeafe.   It was formerly confined to *Flanders* ; but has
acquired great ftrength fince our navigation to the *Indies,*
being now univerfal, and common to feamen of every nation.   He afcribes it to the ufe of falt food, old faltifh
cheefe, and the like; or it may be occafioned by ale
made of brackifh water.   He obferves the brewers have
a bad cuftom of adding falt and quick-lime to their
malt-liquors; which fines and preferves them without
hops.   He fancies the falt fea-air greatly productive of
this

this malady; as he had been informed, that even faltifh rains fell in hot countries. Notwithftanding the great virtues afcribed to fea-falt by *Diofcorides*; yet it is plain, that the ancients apprehended fome ill effects from it when crude, by their burning, wafhing, and drying of it. He afterwards very ingenioufly accounts for all the fymptoms of the fcurvy enumerated by *Eugalenus*; which he fuppofes to proceed from the ufe of this falt, occafioning a brinifh chyle, lymph, &c. and converting the whole humours of the body into a pickle. Juice of fcurvygrafs, lemons, and oranges, all forts of fruits, and pot-herbs, (the more acid the better), are excellent remedies; as alfo vinegar, and *fp. vitriol.* He pretends to be the firft who takes notice of fatal hæmorrhages fometimes occurring in this difeafe, and gives fome in- ftances of them from his *adverfaria*.

1696. *Sea-difeafes; or, A treatife of their nature, caufes, and cure.* *By* William Cockburn.

The fcurvy being generated by the falt provifions altogether unavoidable at fea, makes one of the conftant difeafes in navies. A fourth part of the feamen do not contract it directly, in declining from a ftate of health, but by being put too foon on the fea-provifions, after re- covering from fevers, and other diftempers. It attacks commonly the weak, lazy, and inactive. Refraining from the fea-diet, and living upon green *trade* (as it is called) on fhore, proves an abfolute cure. It is worthy obfervation, how fuddenly and how perfectly they recover of this diftemper by eating greens, *viz.* coleworts, carrots, cabbages, turnips, &c. Men put on fhore in the moft pitiful condition that can be imagi- ned, are able in three or four days, by means of this food only, to walk feveral miles into the country. When Lord *Berkeley* commanded the fleet at *Torbay* in 1695, the author prevailed with his Lordfhip to erect tents for the fick on fhore. Above a hundred of the

moft

moſt afflicted ſcorbutic patients, perfect moving ſkele-
tons, hardly able to get out of their ſhips, were landed.
They had freſh proviſions given them, with carrots,
turnips, and other greens.   In a week they were able
to crawl about; and before the fleet ſailed, they returned healthy to their ſhips.   He regrets, that this diſtemper had as yet been left without a remedy at ſea.   If
proper care was taken about their diet, ſeamen would
not be ſo liable to it.   He condemns the diviſion into
a hot and cold ſcurvy made by Dr *Willis.*   The firſt
alone is properly the true and real ſcurvy, and the latter nothing elſe but the *melancholia hypochondriaca.*   And
upon this occaſion he obſerves the neceſſity of having proper names and deſcriptions of diſeaſes; as the uſe of am-
biguous terms is apt to miſlead, and to have fatal conſequences in the cure of them.

*Archibaldi Pitcarnii element. medicinæ phyſico-mathe-
matic. lib. 2. cap. 23. de ſcorbuto.*

The reader muſt here be cautioned, that every thing
in this poſthumous work is not to be aſcribed to *Pitcairn.*
The ſymptoms of the ſcurvy are ſaid to be, a redneſs,
itching, putrefaction, and bleeding of the gums; looſe
teeth; ſpots on the legs, firſt red, then livid, and black-
iſh; an unuſual laſſitude; a red ſandy ſediment in the u-
rine, ſo that it appears lixivial; an unequal pulſe; wandering pains; toothachs; redneſs, or heat of the body;
fœtid breath; fluxes with or without blood.   The immediate cauſe is, a broken texture of the blood; and
this diſſolution of that fluid may be occaſioned even by
bleeding; which is by no means proper for ſcorbutic people.   But he talks only of the hot ſcurvy, or what *Willis* terms the *ſulphureo-ſaline*; this being properly the
diſeaſe, if we would diſtinguiſh it from the hypochondriac affection.   He recommends milk, or a milk-diet,
as the beſt cure.   But if it does not ſucceed, or any
thing forbids its uſe, then chalybeates are to be given,

3 E   with

with the addition of aftringents, and the fixed temperate antifcorbutics, efpecially if faintings, fluxes, or a
difficulty of breathing, afflict the patient. In the wandering gout, or fcorbutic pains, after gentle purging,
decoct. guajac. et farfaparill. is to be adminiftered; obferving, that if thefe pains are attended with few or
no other fcorbutic fymptoms, they are then to be deemed rheumatic. This may eafily be difcovered by their
admitting of repeated and plentiful bleedings; which
are fo very hurtful in the fcurvy. Next to a milk-diet,
chalybeates, decoction of the woods, and *fucc. antifcorbutic*; nothing will prove fo effectual as the transfufion
of the blood of a found animal into a fcorbutic patient.

1708.   *Hermanni Boerhaave aphorifmi de cognofcendis et cu-*
randis morbis. Aph. 1148. *&c. de fcorbuto.*
Befides the common caufes ufually affigned by authors
as productive of the fcurvy both at fea and land, he,
from *Sydenham*, adds that particular of having taken
too great a quantity of the *cort. peruv.*; then defcribes
the fymptoms peculiar to the malady in its beginning,
progrefs, and more advanced ftages, contained in the
four following fections.
Sect. 1. An unufual lazinefs; an inclination to reft; a
fpontaneous laffitude; a general heavinefs; pain of all
the mufcles as after too great a fatigue, particularly in
the legs and loins; an extreme difficulty in walking, e-
fpecially up or down a fteep place; in the morning, upon awaking, the limbs and mufcles feel as if wearied
and bruifed. *Sect.* 2. A difficulty of breathing, panting, and almoft fuffocation, upon every little motion; a
fwelling of the legs, often difappearing, and an inability
to move them, from their weight; red, yellow, or purple
fpots; a pale tawny colour in the face; a beginning
ftench of the mouth; a fwelling, pain, heat, and itching
of the gums, which bleed upon the leaft preffure; bare
and loofe teeth; pains of different forts, wandering, in
                                                          all

all parts of the body, external as well as internal, occafioning furprifing anguifh, refembling pleuritic, ftomachic, iliac, colic, nephritic, cyftic, hepatic, and
fplenetic pains. Hæmorrhages occur in this ftage, but
flight. *Sect. 3.* A deadly ftinking rottennefs, inflammation, bleeding, and gangrene of the gums; loofe,
yellow, black, and carious teeth; varicofe veins under
the tongue; hæmorrhages, frequently mortal, from
under the fkin, without any apparent wound; as alfo
from the lips, ftomach, liver, lungs, fpleen, *pancreas,*
nofe, *&c.*; ulcers of the worft kind upon every part
of the body, chiefly the legs, yielding to no remedies,
of a gangrenous difpofition, and moft fœtid fmell; *fcabies*; crufts; a dry and gentle leprofy; violent, piercing, univerfal nocturnal pains; livid fpots. *Sect. 4.*
Fevers of many forts, hot, malignant, intermitting all manner of ways, vague, periodical, continued, occafioning an
atrophy; vomitings; *diarrhœæ*; dyfenteries; fevere ftran-
guries; faintings; and an oppreffion upon the *præcordia,*
often fuddenly mortal; a dropfy; confumption; con-
vulfion; *tremor*; palfy; contraction of the finews;
black fpots; vomiting and purging of blood; putrefaction of the liver, fpleen, *pancreas,* and mefentery.

He fuppofes the immediate caufe of the diftemper to
be a fingular ftate of blood; in which part of that fluid
is too thick and vifcid; while, at the fame time, the other,
viz. the *ferum,* is too thin or diffolved, faltifh and a-
crid. Which latter, or its acrimony, is either of an a-
cid or alcaline quality: a diftinction here carefully to be
remarked. Upon this hypothefis he founds the following therapeutic rules, *viz.* That part of the humour which
is too thick, vifcid, and ftagnating, muft be attenuated,
rendered thinner, and put in motion; mean while, what
is already too thin, is to be infpiffated, and the predominating acrimony corrected according to its different
kind and fpecies. Now, as a fingular regard muft be had
at the fame time to thefe fo oppofite intentions of cure, he

thinks

thinks it the mafter-piece of art to cure the fcurvy. And after obferving that fmart evacuations always exafperate, and often render it incurable, he lays down the follow-ing procefs, adapted to the different ftages and fymp-toms, as diftributed in the four claffes or fections.

In the firft ftage (fee fect. 1.) we are to begin with a gentle, attenuating, deobftruent purgative, often repeated in a fmall dofe; next, to proceed in the ufe of attenu-ants, and what are called *digeftive medicines (a)*; con-cluding with a long continued courfe of the milder fpe-cifics, exhibited in almoft any form. In the fecond ftage, (fect. 2.), all that has been mentioned is neceffary, with the addition of the more acrid antifcorbutics. Baths for the body and feet, prepared with antifcorbutic ingre-dients; alfo hot, dry friction, and often blood-letting, for certain reafons he mentions, are proper. According to the acrid thinnefs of the fluids, heat, or danger of a hæmorrhage; or, on the contrary, the vifcidity and inaction of the humours, palenefs, coldnefs of the body, &c. the antifcorbutics given, are to be moderately a-ftringent, fomewhat cooling, or hot or acrid. In the third fpecies or ftage, (fect. 3.), all the already prefcri-bed meafures are to be ufed. The patient is alfo to take great quantities of foft antifeptic, antifcorbutic liquors, promoting for a confiderable time gentle evacuations, by fweat, urine, and ftool. In the fourth ftage or fpecies, (fect. 4.), the cafe is for the moft part incurable; medi-cines are to be varied according to the different fymp-toms; fometimes mercurials do fervice, as likewife what was ordered for the third fpecies.

He concludes the fubject with obferving, that, in or-der to a fuccefsful cure of this difeafe, it is princi-pally required to inveftigate the peculiar predominating acrimony in the humours: and as this acrimony may be

(a) Vid. *Willis.* It is needlefs to give *Boerhaave's* prefcriptions here, as almoft all of them in his *Materia medica* are taken out of *Willis*; as is indeed his procefs of cure.

either

either saline and muriatic, acid and austere, alcaline and foetid, or rancid and oily; so it requires different and opposite cures; what is serviceable to one scorbutic patient, proving poisonous to another. The name of the distemper is not so much to be studied, but each particular species of it, according to the different kinds of acrimony above specified, as if it was a distinct disease.

Jo. Henrici de Heucher cautiones in cognoscendo cu- 1712, *randoque scorbuto necessariæ.*

This pamphlet contains some of the most exceptionable doctrines of *Willis, Eugalenus, &c.* Of which the following may suffice as a specimen. Mercury is very justly sometimes recommended in the scurvy by *Boerhaave,* when it is accompanied with fevers of various kinds, vomiting, *diarrhœa,* dysentery, violent stranguries, faintings, and anxieties, often mortal; dropsy; consumption; convulsions; palsies; voiding of blood; putrefaction of the liver, spleen, *pancreas,* and mesentery.

An account of the scurvy at Wiburg. *Communicated by* 1732. *Dr* Abraham Nitzsch *to Dr* Schulze. Commerc. literar. 1734. Norimb. ann. 1734, *p.* 162.

It may be proper, first, to observe, that the scurvy is here an endemic *lues.* But what drew particular attention to it this year, 1732, was the uncommon number of the afflicted, and of those who died, together with its unusual duration. It persisted in its ravage from the beginning of the year until the month of *August,* with such remarkable violence, that I was sent thither by express orders in the month of *June.* I observed the appearances of the disease were not the same in all; but different in individuals, according to their constitution of body.

Those who were of a lax habit, laboured under an œdematous swelling of the legs, (rarely of the *abdomen*), yielding easily to the impression of the finger, but often becoming

becoming harder upon the continuance of the malady.
The *hypochondria* for the moſt part were tumid, the flexor
tendons of the *tibia* always contracted, with livid ſpots on
the legs, knees, thighs, and back.   Theſe in plethoric habits, particularly upon the *tibia*, became often inflamed,
attended with moſt acute pain, and quickneſs of the pulſe.
Now and then the white of the eye was altogether bloody;
and ſometimes the eye-lids were greatly ſwelled, being diftended with extravaſated, ſtagnating blood.   In ſome the
ſpots were pretty large, eſpecially upon the thighs and
back; in others they reſembled only flea-bites, and were
accompanied with ſwelling of the legs, univerſal laſſitude, ſwelled, bleeding, and putrid gums; as alſo a
pale wan countenance.   Several were diſtreſſed with a
great difficulty of breathing, moiſt cough, a *vertigo*,
and faintings, moſt commonly when in an erect poſture;
the latter often proved fatal to thoſe who had been
long afflicted.   The appetite from the beginning was
ſomewhat impaired, often leaving the patient upon his
being affected with *borborygmi* and *nauſea*, but returning
upon the acceſſion of a *diarrhœa*.   The feet, *ſcrotum*,
and *abdomen*, were ſometimes greatly diſtended with a
tranſparent watery ſwelling, and the ſkin inflamed.
The gums having become a maſs of ſpungy fleſh, difcharged, upon ſqueezing, a fœtid *ichor* ; and the ſali-
vary glands were ſometimes ſo ſtuffed, as to acquire the
hardneſs of a ſcirrhus, which could not be reſolved by
any other means than by a natural and ſpontaneous ſa-
livation.

Perſons of a dry habit were afflicted with ſymptoms
different from thoſe of repletion.   They were every day
more and more emaciated, and racked with violent ſhooting
pains on the *tibia*, accompanied with a fever.   The
anguiſh did not fix in one place, but by ſhifting produced arthritic pains, colics, the ſpaſmodic aſthma, headachs, toothachs, and contractions.   By the uſe of improper volatile medicines, the abdominal *viſcera*, the
liver

liver and spleen, became hard; upon which ensued either
an *ascites*, or an atrophy and *diarrhœa*, which constantly
proved fatal.   The gums were swelled and hard, painful to the touch, and often over-run with a cancerous
ulceration.

In order to put a stop to this dreadful calamity, it
was necessary that the treatment and remedies should be
suited to the habit and constitution of the patient.   I therefore prescribed for those who laboured under the slow
or cold scurvy, a decoction of *sum. pin. bacc. juniper.*
and *trifol. fibrin.*   Where there was reason to apprehend
a swelling of the abdominal *viscera*, I gave the neutral
salts, and alcaline tinctures: but where there was a fever, and inflammation on the *tibia,* the saline nitrous absorbents internally, and externally *sp. vin. camp.* with
saffron.   For the stiff tendons I used *ung. nervin. cum ol.*
philosop. &c. and baths; for the swelled, bleeding
gums, *ung. Ægyptiac. mel. ros.* and *spir. cochlear.* or
tinct. gum. lacc. and *sp. coch.* or common water acidulated with *sp. vitriol.* The air was corrected three times
a-day by a fume of juniper wood and berries.   The *pa-*
racentesis often succeeded with those who had the *ascites,*
when free from a fever, and an œdematous swelling of
the abdomen.   It restored them to perfect health; as
did also scarifications upon the calf of the leg and *scro-*
tum, when there appeared a tense watery swelling upon
these parts; provided proper internals were administered,
viz. aperient, diuretic, and strengthening medicines,
such as *tinct. tartar. mart. antimon.* neutral salts, *&c.*
If there was any danger of a gangrene from these scarifications, as often happened, it was stopped by nervous
and antiseptic applications.

In the painful scurvy, upon account of the dry habit
of body, medicines heating and exagitating the blood,
formerly given, were laid aside, and emollient remedies
were prescribed, *viz.* a decoction either of barley or
oats; or of *rasur. cornu cervi*, with *rad. scorzon. summit.*
millefol.

millefol. et flor. chamæmel. : as also oily medicines, *viz. ol. amygd. d. et sperm ceti*; which often miraculously al-layed arthritic pains, and the oppressive complaints in the breast. Antispasmodics were sometimes given, *viz. nitr depurat. cinnabar. antimonii*, epileptic powders, &c. and occasionally absorbents, and the *testaceous* powders. When the *hypochondriaca* were obstructed, *rad. cichor vel tarax.* was added to the decoction : and for the swelling, heat, and pain of the gums, the pulp of citron proved an excellent and agreeable remedy. By this treatment, and the blessing of Heaven, I put a stop to the cala-mity ; insomuch that the number of the diseased, and of those who died, diminished every day, and in the space of a month it quite disappeared.

This present year, the *Cuirassiers* lately come from the *Ukraine* to *Petersburg*, have furnished me with several farther observations upon this disease. The symptoms were as usual. It was always a salutary sign when the spots appearing continued out. In two cases their sudden disappearance proved fatal. Besides the use of the attenuating decoction before mentioned of *sum. pin.* I found it necessary, every second or third day, to give a half-spoonful of a mixture prepared of *gum. ammoniac. el. propriet ana p. æ.* diluted with *sp. vin. tartarisat.*; or *pulv. salin. dr. ss. cum diagrid. gran.* iv. *vel* v.: which had so remarkable good effects, that though many were ca-chectic, yet none became dropsical. Prudent blood-letting near the decline of the disease, when the pulse was strong, evidently assisted in the cure. I can solemnly affirm it was followed with an increase of strength, a perfect relaxation of the tendons, which had before been attempted to no purpose by warm steams and baths, and a more speedy recovery. The disease left us in *May*, having acquired its virulence in *February*.

1734. *Observationes circa scorbutum* ; *ejusque indolem, causas, signa, et curam. Auctore Joanne Fred. Bachstrom.*

From

From want of proper attention to the hiſtory of the ſcurvy, its cauſes have been generally, though wrongfully, ſuppoſed to be, cold in northern climates, ſea-air, the uſe of ſalt meats, &c.: whereas this evil is ſolely owing to a total abſtinence from freſh vegetable food, and greens; which is alone the true primary cauſe of the diſeaſe. And where perſons, either through neglect or neceſſity, do refrain for a conſiderable time from eating the freſh fruits of the earth, and greens, no age, no climate or ſoil, are exempted from its attack. Other ſecondary cauſes may likewiſe concur: but recent vegetables are found alone effectual to preſerve the body from this malady; and moſt ſpeedily to cure it, even in a few days, when the caſe is not rendered deſperate by the patient's being dropſical or conſumptive. All which is founded on the following obſervations.

He remarks, that the ſcurvy is moſt frequent among northern nations, and in the coldeſt countries. There it is not confined to the ſea alone, but rages with great violence at land, afflicting both natives and foreigners; of which the poor ſeamen left to winter in *Greenland,* who were all cut off by this diſtemper, afford a memorable inſtance. But the opinion of its being produced there by cold, he thinks irreconcileable with the daily experience of its attacking ſeamen in their voyages to the *Indies,* even when under the torrid zone.

That it is not peculiar to the ſea, the following hiſtories ſufficiently evince. During the late ſiege of *Thorn,* above 5 or 6000 of the garriſon, beſides a great number of the inhabitants, died of this diſtemper; the ſurrender of the town being more owing to the havock made by this dreadful calamity, than to the bravery of the beſiegers. Upon which he obſerves, that, allowing this diſeaſe to be moſt frequent among the northern nations in winter, yet the ſiege of that place was carried on in the heat of ſummer; and the *Swedes,* the beſiegers, a northern nation, kept altogether free from the ſcurvy.

3 F   The

The miſchief firſt attacked chiefly the blockaded *Saxon* garriſon. They being almoſt all cut off, the inhabitants were at laſt obliged to do duty upon the walls; of whom it alſo deſtroyed a great number. But no ſooner was the ſiege raiſed, and the gates of the town open for the admiſſion of vegetables and greens from the country, but the mortality quickly ceaſed, and the diſeaſe at once diſappeared.

In the end of the laſt war with the *Turks,* when the Imperial army wintered in *Hungary,* the country having been laid waſte about *Temeſwaer,* by the calamities of the preceding war, many thouſands of the common ſoldiers, (but not one officer, as having different diet), were cut off by the ſcurvy. The phyſician to that army employed his utmoſt ſkill, and the moſt approved antiſcorbutic remedies. Notwithſtanding which, the mortality went on increaſing during the winter. Unacquainted with the diſeaſe, or rather its remedy, he demanded a conſultation of the college of phyſicians at *Vienna*; whoſe preſcriptions and advice were of no ſervice. The diſeaſe ſtill perſiſted with increaſing virulence until the ſpring, that the earth was covered with greens and vegetables. And the phyſician now rejoiced as much in having found out the true cauſe of this evil, as before he had regretted his unhappy diſappointment in the removal of ſo general and dreadful a calamity.

As ſome are of opinion, that warm and inland countries are altogether free from this diſtemper, he gives an account from an officer of a *German* garriſon in *Italy,* many of whom were cut off by it at a great diſtance from the ſea. The officer himſelf, an *Italian,* was miſerably afflicted, and given over by his phyſicians, who were altogether ignorant of his caſe; when a *German* ſurgeon, by lucky accident paſſing that way, reſcued him from the jaws of death. He cured him in a few days, to the ſurpriſe of his phyſicians, by ordering his ſervant to the fields to ſupply him with green vegetables,

getables, eſpecially the *ſiſymbrium,* which grew there-abouts very plentifully.

The following relation is no leſs curious. A ſailor in the *Greenland* ſhips was ſo over-run and diſabled with the ſcurvy, that his companions put him into a boat, and ſent him on ſhore; leaving him there to periſh, without the leaſt expeƈtation of a recovery. The poor wretch had quite loſt the uſe of his limbs; he could only crawl about on the ground. This he found covered with a plant, which he, continually graſing like a beaſt of the field, plucked up with his teeth. In a ſhort time he was by this means perfeƈtly recovered; and, upon his return home, it was found to have been the herb ſcurvy-graſs.

From all which the author concludes, that as abſti-nence from recent vegetables is altogether and ſolely the cauſe of the diſtemper, ſo theſe alone are its effec-tual remedies. Accordingly he beſtows the epithet of *antiſcorbutic* on all of that claſs which are wholſome and eatable; obſerving Nature every where affords a ſupply of remedies, even in *Greenland,* and the moſt frozen countries. There no ſooner the ſnow melts from the rivers, but their borders are covered with brooklime, creſſes, and ſcurvygraſs, in ample prodigality. There Nature diƈtates to thoſe barbarous nations, that what ſhe thus bleſſes them with in ſuch bounteous profuſion, af-fords preſent health and relief in their malady. This all phyſicians acquainted with the nature of the ſcurvy, muſt be likewiſe ſenſible of. The moſt common herbs and freſh fruits excel the moſt pompous pharmaceutical preparations, eſpecially thoſe of the animal and mineral kinds. He divides antiſcorbutics into three claſſes. The firſt contains the common pot-herbs, and all plants of an inſipid, or rather ſweetiſh taſte, fruits of trees, &c. of this quality; and when in want of thoſe, even graſs it-ſelf may be eat. In the ſecond claſs, he ranks all ve-getables, roots, fruits, berries, &c. that are of a ſub-

acid or acid tafte : and thefe being of a middling quality
betwixt the infipid plants of the firft clafs, and the ftronger bitters he includes in the third, they will prove more
effectual than the firft, without being liable to fome inconveniencies which may attend thofe of the third clafs.
In this laft he comprehends all frefh herbs, roots, and
fruits, of a bitter and ftrong tafte, of the nature of fcurvygrafs, creffes, &c. Thefe laft are with caution to
be prefcribed at firft, or in great quantities. For prevention, he recommends living much upon green vegetables, when they can be got; otherwife, upon preferved fruits, herbs, roots, &c. He advifes feamen when
at land to be more careful of laying up a ftore of greens
than of flefh; and, in cafe of neceffity, would have
them when at fea to make trial of the fea-weeds that
grow upon the fhip's bottom ; being perfuaded, that the
great phyfician of nature had not left them without a
remedy, although he had never heard of its being
tried *(b)*. After a long abftinence from vegetables, the
difeafed are to begin with the milder antifcorbutics, proceeding by degrees to thofe of a ftronger nature. In
examining the mineral and foffil remedies, which have
been fo much recommended in the fcurvy, he obferves
of nitre, that as it is a copious ingredient in moft plants,
perhaps it may be ferviceable ; but, otherwife, all of
thofe claffes are to be avoided. He condemns the ufe
of fteel, mercury, and alum ; as likewife fulphureous
and vitriolic medicines, efpecially the ftrong acid of vitriol, which fome account a fpecific in the fcurvy; but
they will find themfelves difappointed.

1734.   *Parerga medica confcripta à Damiano Sinopeo.*
     In *Cronftadt*, which is a low marfhy ifland, and
where the weather for the moft part is cold, rainy, and
cloudy, the fcurvy is an endemic and common difeafe.
It is moft frequent and violent in the beginning of fpring;

(b) I am informed they were tried in Lord *Anfon*'s fhip.

but

but much rarer and milder during the rest of the seasons, unless the weather prove cold and wet: and for the same reason it is more frequent some years than others.

The symptoms are, a putrid swelling of the gums, lassitude, and a remarkable pain and weakness of the legs; swelling of the feet and knees; contraction of the tendons; a cachectic, and, as it were, anasarcous habit of body, with a dark yellowish hue; costiveness, and a thick lateritious urine. After those appearances, ensue pain, and even contractions of the upper extremities; livid spots of different sizes; pains in the shoulders, and small of the back. These latter prove very violent in such as are tainted with the venereal poison. Few die of this distemper; for the most part only those who have become consumptive or dropsical.

The learned author, in his very elegant and accurate account of the diseases which prevailed at *Cronstadt*, from the year 1730 to the end of 1733, observes, that when he first came there, *ann.* 1730, true pleurisies, peripneumonies, &c. reigned. Those acute fevers ceased with the spring; and an unusual dry and warm summer succeeding, there were few acute diseases, and even old chronical ailments became more tolerable. A dry and cold autumn, with a seasonable snowy winter, gave rise to but very few acute diseases; till about the beginning of *February*, when a catarrhal fever commenced. The weather proved then very unsettled; the spring was cold and moist; and the summer much the same, with little heat. This catarrhal fever raged about twenty days. Upon its remission, pleurisies, peripneumonies, rheumatisms, &c. took place; and an intermitting fever, which continued the whole spring; as also the scurvy. This last made its appearance in the month of *March* 1731, seizing at first only a few; but in a short time the number of scorbutic patients was equal to those in fevers; and afterwards exceeded them, the fevers then ceasing. It began with a bloated sallow complexion,

plexion, livid spots, &c. and was accompanied with
such symptoms as have been before mentioned.   In the
months of *April* and *May* it raged with uncommon violence, and continued almost till the middle of *July*;
when it was abated by the heat of the season.   Some
patients became anasarcous, or dropsical; others phthisical.
Some laboured under the most violent colics, with obstinate contraction of the belly; others were seized with
a *sphacelus* of the gums and *fauces*, scorbutic tumours,
&c.   Soft livid swellings arose upon the body : they
were judged to be full of matter; but, upon opening
them, nothing was discharged but a blackish dissolved
blood : the ulcer was surrounded by a fungous rotten
flesh, whose basis seemed very deep, and bled upon
the gentlest touch (c).

Although the scurvy was a distemper bad enough of
itself, it was, however, often rendered worse by being
complicated with other intercurrent diseases, *viz.* fevers,
and rheumatisms, but especially the intermitting fever.
All who recovered from this last, became scorbutic.
There was scarce any person, either in the hospital or
town, who laboured under even a chronic disease, who
was not more or less affected by the scurvy.   Hence
all diseases whatever became more troublesome and obstinate this spring.

The scurvy having entirely ceased in *July*, a few
mild fevers took place the rest of the summer, and autumn.

In the beginning of the year 1732 a gentle vernal
fever prevailed; soon after, the *pleuritis spuria* was more
frequent; and, lastly, the scurvy.   All those diseases entirely ceased upon the appearance of a warm and dry
summer.   This continued but for a month, when the
weather changed to rain and cold; which induced a u-

(c) A very accurate description of scorbutic tumours and ulcers.
Compare it with *Poupart*'s, p. 315. Dr *Huxham*'s, p. 92. and other
observations, p. 169. &c.

niverſal

niverfal diftemper, *viz.* a catarrh, with cough, *&c.* It fpread itfelf over all the countries about, raged much at *Peterfburg*, and affected even thofe who were at fea.

After many curious obfervations foreign to our purpofe, he remarks, that the vernal fcurvy, *ann.* 1733, was milder than any of the former; but, neverthelefs, contrary to cuftom, continued during the whole fummer and autumn, the feafons proving wet and uncomfortable. He has one fingular obfervation, That the *fcabies* and *purpura* prevailed at the fame time with the fcurvy. The remedies ufed, were, effences and conferves of the antifcorbutic plants, hot aromatics, bitters, *&c.* The author gave many medicines; but, unluckily, few or none that were truly antifcorbutic.

Jo. Geo. Henrici Krameri differtatio epiftolica de fcorbuto. 1737.

The cafe of the Imperial troops in Hungary; *tranfmitted* 1720. *to the college of phyficians at* Vienna, *by the author.*

The calamity which afflicts the Imperial troops, is not that fpecies of fcurvy defcribed by *Eugalenus* and others. It differs from it in three particulars.

1*ft*, It is not infectious. No officers are feized with it; and only the regiments of fuch nations as ufe too grofs a diet. 2*dly*, It is not a primary, but a fecondary difeafe. It attacks only thofe who have recovered from fevers, and efpecially fuch as have had frequent relapfes. 3*dly*, It is not attended with the many fymptoms defcribed by thofe authors. The appearances in all are conftantly uniform, and as follow.

In the firft ftage the gums are fwelled; they are apt to bleed, and ftained with livid fpots. Upon which enfue, great putrefaction, a moft offenfive ftench from the mouth, and a falling out of the teeth.

In the fecond ftage or degree of the malady, there is for the moft part a contraction of the joint of the knee, fo that the patient cannot extend his leg. Violent fhooting

ing pains are felt in this joint, as likewife often on the other joints of the body. The contracted knees are alfo fwelled, with incredible pain and *rigor* of the tendons; and the fkin is covered with bluifh extravafations, interfperfed with fmall miliary eruptions. In one night's time the eyes, and even other parts of the body, are covered with large livid fpots, as if the patient had received feveral bruifes. Thefe fpots are altogether without pain. The mufcles of the legs, thighs, and even cheeks, become greatly fwelled, and hard, nay, altogether indurated. But thofe fwellings, as alfo the large *ecchymofes*, never fuppurate. The pulfe is quick, fmall, and hard; the urine red, with a thick unequal fediment.

If the patient ftill continues the ufe of improper diet, as is the cafe of many of our common foldiers, from want of neceffaries and conveniencies in *Hungary*, the malady advances to its third ftage. The gums become prodigioufly fwelled, together with the cheeks. A gangrene, or *caries* of the jaw, enfues; both which prove incurable. The difficulty of breathing is fo great, that the patients not only faint away upon the flighteft motion of the body; but frequently, when walking about, drop down fuddenly dead. They generally complain exceffively of this *dyf-pnœa*, a few days before death, though they have neither cough nor fpitting. All the fpecies of dropfies, and œdematous fwellings on the body, accompany the advanced ftages of this calamity; in fo much that, by lying with the head in a declining pofture, the face in half an hour becomes fo fwelled, that the perfon cannot open his eyes. Such fwellings often difappear and return. They are fubject to profufe hæmorrhages from the nofe; and, in thefe deplorable circumftances, to a *diarrhœa* or dyfentery, which often clofes the fcene. In the beginning of the difeafe, the appetite and thirft are natural; but towards the clofe of the malady, the appetite fails, and the thirft is increafed. Of the many other fymptoms defcribed in this difeafe by authors, none

elfe

elfe occur but thofe alone which have been mentioned.

This is the fatal mifchief which deftroys many mifer-able wretches in *Hungary*, at fartheft in the fpace of two or three months, but for the moft part in three or four weeks. If the patient furvives till the fummer, he either perfectly recovers, or remains incurably con-tracted.

The remote caufes of this evil are, relapfes after tedi-ous fevers, which have been epidemic in the country; the moift and marfhy foil; but efpecially grofs and vi-fcid diet, *viz.* flefh, and the groffer farines, coarfe heavy bread, and pudding, (or a food called *rollatfchen*), eaten by the *Bohemians* more than by all others. They are al-moft the only nation affected. One thing remarkable is, that this difeafe does not appear in *Hungary* in fum-mer, autumn, nor in winter; but every year in the beginning of fpring.

I come now to what has been attempted, both by my-felf and others, towards the cure: And muft firft ob-ferve, that 400 of the troops near *Belgrade* having ta-ken mercury without my advice, the dreadful confe-quence was, they all died in a falivation! Shunning therefore that fatal drug, I generally premifed a vomit, on purpofe to clear the firft paffages, and fo to procure a more certain entrance of the fpecific antifcorbutics, with their full virtues, into the blood. I then admini-ftered, in every form that could be thought of, or that has been recommended by authors, the moft approved antifcorbutic remedies, *viz. Radices, raphan. taraxic. ari, afari, gentianæ, angelic. helen. acori, farfaparill. chinæ, &c. Folia, et herbæ aridæ*, (for here the green frefh plants cannot be procured), *becabung. nafturt. trifol. fib. cochlear. acetof. fcordii, rutæ murar. rofmar. falv. cent. min. fedi minim. &c. Ligna guajac. faffaphras, &c. Strobili pin. Cortices winteran. guajac. aurantior. Baccæ juniperi, lauri, &c.* I have alfo given falts of every kind, volatile and fixed, particularly *fal. vol. cornu cervi,*

arcan.

arcan. duplicat. sal. tartar. fix. sal: ammoniac. crud. cremor tartar. with chalybeates of all forts. *Spir. sal. ammon. sal. vol. ol. spir. et tinct. tartari, tinct. bezoard. spir. cochlear. &c.* In place of the juice of citrons and lemons, which cannot be got here, I gave *acet. theriac.* or vinegar, in which many of the before mentioned ingredients, particularly the celebrated *rad. armoraciæ,* were infused. I was not fparing of the moft coftly medicines, *tinct. mart. antimonii, lunæ helvet. &c.* But, alas, all was in vain!

In a word, there is nothing that has been recommended by the beft claffical and ftandard authors *(d)*, which I have not made trial of, except the juices of the frefh green plants, and their quinteffence recommended by *May (e).* It is not in my power to procure thofe herbs, or their juices; becaufe, as I obferved before, they do not grow in this country. We have nothing here but *eruca lutea* (wild rocket), and *rapiftrum arvorum* (wild muftard); but even of thefe, who can gather a fufficient quantity for fuch a number of the diftreffed? Milk, were it proper, cannot be purchafed for fo great a multitude of people: and the fame may be faid of whey.

After having met with fuch melancholy difappointments, in the trial of what has been recommended by others, and whatever I could think of myfelf; reflecting that tedious fevers had generally preceded, and that a flow fever ftill accompanied the difeafe, I fell upon the *cort. peruv.* given in the form either of electuary or infufion. By this, in a few days, I cured fixty foldiers in the regiment of *Bagnan,* who were in the fecond ftage of the difeafe. It is now two years ago; but at the fame time they had a proper diet, and fuch food as cannot at this time be procured. I have lately tried *fem.*

(d) Here he enumerates fixteen modern writers on the fcurvy, of the greateft repute, with an &c.

(e) A medicine of Dr *Michael's.* Vid. p. 183. The author afterwards obferves, that it was of no efficacy.

finap.

sinap. Muſtard-ſeed is ſaid to have ſaved the beſieged garriſon of *Rochelle,* when over-run with this diſeaſe; but here, like all other remedies, it is of no efficacy. I need not ſay any thing of topical applications: as ſuch powerful internal helps do not avail, little can be expected from them. I ſhall only obſerve, that different regiments have uſed the baths of the country; but all to no purpoſe.

I therefore humbly requeſt, that if any of you, gentlemen, are poſſeſſed of an *arcanum,* or a remedy able to overcome this *Herculean* diſeaſe, you would favour me with it; as alſo your beſt advice.   Perhaps ſome of you may have the knowledge of the fixed mercury boaſted of by *Dolæus* and *Helmont,* which will cure the ſcurvy without the aid of ſuch a proper diet as cannot at this time be procured for the wretched in *Hungary.*

A copy of this caſe of the troops was delivered to each member of the college at *Vienna*; and, by order of the Dean of Faculty, all were deſired in three days time to give in their opinion in writing.   Which produced the following anſwer.

We have received your very accurate account of the ſcurvy, which commits ſuch dreadful havock among the Imperial troops during the ſpring in *Hungary*; and it is ordered directly to be printed.   After having had all circumſtances duly weighed by the moſt experienced of our faculty, the firſt rule we preſcribe, is, great attention to the non-naturals.   Without this, the moſt heroic medicines may fail; but when a proper regard is had to theſe, ſimple remedies will do great things.   As the ſources of this calamity ſeem to be impure air   and an unwholſome marſhy ſoil, (evils not eaſily remedied); the troops muſt often ſhift their quarters, and be removed into better air.   When in unhealthful ſtations, they are, by way of prevention, to uſe the ſmoak of tobacco, juniper, &c.   They ſhould have always dry ſtraw to lay upon

the

the ground; and as wholfome food as can be provided
for them.

As to the cure, (after noting with infamy thofe who
have recommended a mercurial falivation in this difeafe,
as more properly deftroyers of the human race than
phyficians), we would advife a gentle vomit of *ipecacuan.* to be premifed; and afterwards the approved antifcorbutics of the vegetable kind to be given, *viz. cochlear. becabung. nafturt. fumar flor. hyperic. trifol. fibrin.
&c.* The juice, extract, tincture, decoction, &c. of
thefe, may be adminiftered either in whey or broth. As
you have none of thofe plants, we have fent you their
feeds to be fown in the country; and until fuch time as
they grow up, have fupplied you with a quantity of the
dried herbs, and of their infpiffated juice. Befides which,
we would recommend two remedies of great and experienced virtues *(f)*.

The author's farther explanations and experiences.

The fcurvy attacked only thofe who, after frequent
relapfes, and recovery from fevers, ufed a crude vifcid
diet. Hence not one officer was feized with it; nor even
any of the common men among the dragoons, as their
pay and living were better. It was always accompanied
with remains of the fever in the pulfe and urine. Both
in *Hungary*, and in *Piedmont*, where the troops were
lately afflicted with it, the natives were at the fame time
altogether free from it. The difeafe occurs oftentimes
in *Germany*, among fuch people as live altogether on the
boiled pulfes, without eating any green vegetables or
fummer-fruits. In the hofpital at *Drefden* there are
fcorbutic patients every year. It is a fatal mifchief often
in befieged towns, as alfo to feamen in long voyages. It
is, however, quickly cured in cold countries; as in *Green-*

(f) The one a pafte of *pulv. rad. chin. farfaparil. et hordei*,
from *Hoferus*; the other, a diftilled antifcorbutic water, from *Zwin-
gerus*. The author afterwards obferves they were of no efficacy.

land,

land, by fcurvygrafs; and in warmer countries, by the juice of oranges. *Dutch* failors effectually prevent this diftrefs, by eating once or twice a-week pickled cabbage. When blood was injudicioufly drawn for relief of the fcorbutic *dyfpnœa*, there was no feparation of the *ferum :* it was covered a-top with a white greafy film. The contraction occurs in no other joint but the knee. The difeafe conftantly begins, and regularly advances, in the manner as defcribed in the relation tranfmitted to the college. No perfon can be fuppofed to labour under the fcurvy, or any fymptom of it, unlefs the gums are affected. Putrefaction of the gums, is the primary and infeparable fymptom of the malady in its very firft ftage. *Orthopnœa*, dropfy, and dyfentery, attending the laft ftage, render the cafe often incurable. As to fcorbutic pains, it is remarkable they afflict equally both day and night, and are not increafed by heat, or by lying in bed. The knees, when fwelled, are generally covered with large *ecchymofes*. Thefe never come to fuppuration on any part of the body, except on the gums, where they often break and ulcerate. The flexor tendons of the *tibia* alone become rigid, *viz.* the tendons of the *feminervofus* and *femimembranofus* mufcles. Colics afflict in this difeafe when there is a *diarrhœa* or dyfentery, but never otherwife. In many thoufand fcorbutic patients, I never once faw the true pleurify, *nephritis*, ftrangury, nor hæmorrhages from the fkin, except where there was a wound; although fcorbutic people are fubject to hæmorrhages from the lungs, ftomach, inteftines, *&c.*; nor did I ever obferve any other ulcers than what have been defcribed, in the gums and cheeks, much lefs any fpecies whatever of a *fcabies*. Scorbutic people are never afflicted with epileptic fits, palfies, tremors, *&c.* Their death is for the moft part tranquil, if you except their laborious breathing.

    I can aver from experience in above a thoufand cafes, that this malady is moft effectually cured by the frefh
juice

juice of fcurvygrafs and creffes, either mixed, or feparately taken, to the quantity of three ounces twice or thrice
a-day in warm broth. Thefe juices occafion flight flufh-
ings of the face, are carminative, and promote urine and
perfpiration. As thofe herbs cannot be obtained frefh in
many parts of *Hungary,* nor in warm climates, the difeafe may be effectually cured by three or four ounces
of the juice of oranges or citrons, taken twice a-day in
a pint of water with fugar, or rather in whey. By
juice of citron in whey, twenty patients were lately cured in the hofpital of St *Mark* at *Vienna.* As to a prefervative medicine againft it, I know of none but the
effence (I fuppofe extract) of the *cort. peruv.* taken at
bedtime in the quantity of two drams, either by itfelf,
or mixed with other bitters. By this remedy the famous
Count *Bonneval* preferved himfelf and his domeftics,
many years in *Hungary,* free from the diftempers of the
country.

1739.   *Frederici Hoffmanni medicinæ rationalis fyftematicæ
tom 4. part, 5. cap. 1. de fcorbuto, ejufque vera indole.*
  In what he terms a compleat hiftory of this difeafe,
(in an enumeration of the fymptoms, claffed in *Willis*'s
manner, according to the different parts of the body affected), among other things he obferves, the fcorbutic
colic is diftinguifhed from all others, by the pain being
fo fhooting, acute, and intolerable. The belly is not,
as in other colics, diftended with a *flatus :* but the navel
is drawn inwards, fo as to form a cavity fufficient to
hold one's fift. It is very obftinate, yielding neither to
medicines nor fomentations ; and has often this peculiar
to it, that it terminates in a palfy. After a preceding
fcorbutic *dyfpnœa,* the patient is very apt to fall into a
dropfy, efpecially if draftic purgatives have been ufed.
The fcorbutic toothach is diftinguifhed from all others,
by its fuddenly attacking, and as fuddenly leaving the
patient. Headachs are moft troublefome in the evening ;

ing; but upon a fweat breaking out, they leave the patient.   Some in this difeafe keep awake for many weeks
without being fenfibly weakened by it.   Scorbutic ulcers appear in the following manner.   Firft, the part is
painful; then the *cuticula* feparates in like manner as
if boiling water had been poured upon the fkin; a ferous
humour oozes forth, and the part becomes extremely
painful; but true *pus* is fcarce ever obferved to flow
from the ulcer.   At other times, fcorbutic ulcers continue deep, and quite dry, without affording either *pus*
or *fanies*; and thefe are very apt to gangrene.

He thinks the beft cure for the fcurvy is the mineral
waters.   They are fufficient to effect it, as long experience had convinced him, together with a proper diet
and regimen.   For this purpofe, he recommends the
Carolinæ, Selteranæ, Egranæ, &c.   Where the convenience of mineral waters is wanting, he advifes drinking
fimple, pure, and light water, of any fort; which will
often remove the difeafe.   But it is ftill better if the
water partakes of fteel principles, fuch as the *Lauchftadt*
fpring, two miles from *Hall.*   It is to be both outwardly and inwardly ufed.   He likewife recommends a milk-
diet, efpecially affes milk.   When the fcorbutic *diathefis*
is complicated with obftructed *vifcera*, cachexies, the
hypochondriac difeafe, or the *purpura chronica*; then
the cure fucceeds better, if the milk be taken mixed with
the mineral water.   He obferves the great detriment of
mercury in this diftemper; and mentions various antifcorbutics, bitters, emollients, *&c.* that may be proper.

Siris: *A chain of philofophical reflections and inquiries* 1744
*concerning the virtues of tar-water.   By the Right Rev.
Dr* Geo. Berkeley *Lord Bifhop of* Cloyne.

The fcurvy may be cured (if the author may judge
by what he has experienced) by the fole, regular, conftant, and copious ufe of tar-water.

Theoretifch

1747. *Theoretijch praɛtiſche abhandlung des ſcharboɛtes, wie ſich derſelbige vornemlich bey denen kayſerlich Ruſziſchen armeen an verſchiedenen orten geauſſert und gezeiget hat, &c.:* or, A theoretical and practical treatiſe of the ſcurvy, as it has appeared chiefly in the Imperial *Ruſſian* armies, together with a circumſtantial deſcription of its cauſes, means of prevention, and cure. By *Abraham Nitzſch.*

Three different opinions of phyſicians concerning this diſeaſe deſerve cenſure. 1ſt, Some aſcribe many obſtinate ailments, eſpecially ſuch as have introduced any great impurity into the blood, *viz.* cutaneous diſeaſes, *purpura chronica, &c.* to the ſcorbutic taint. 2dly, Many who do not altogether deny the exiſtence of the ſcurvy, limit or circumſcribe it within too narrow bounds. 3dly, Others have deſcribed its cauſes, its different kinds, and cure, in too vague and looſe a manner.

The ſcurvy has been aſcribed to the uſe of ſalt, dried, and ſmoked fleſh-meats. But this opinion is confuted by daily experience. Others have blamed foggy moiſt air alone, and damp ſituations; or a mere want of a ſufficient quantity of vegetables: whereas it proceeds from no ſingle cauſe, but from a concurrence of cauſes, *viz.* improper, groſs, and corrupt aliment; moiſt air, accompanied either with cold, or with heat; and impure putrid water. Theſe acting in conjunction produce the ſcurvy, and are ſufficient to heighten the evil to an extreme degree of violence.

As thoſe cauſes operate but ſlowly in the body, the progreſs of the malady is very gradual. A change of colour is obſerved in the face. There is a general laſſitude. The thighs and legs feel heavy; and a remarkable weakneſs is perceived in the knees. At the ſame time the gums begin to ſwell and corrupt. The preternatural colour of the face afterwards increaſes, the legs begin to be painful, the cheeks and bones ſwell, the gums become monſtrouſly rotten, the body more feeble, and a difficulty of breathing enſues upon uſing of
exerciſe,

exercife. The knees and joints are alfo contracted. Finally, the appetite gradually decays, the body be- comes conftipated, the *abdomen* and *hypochondria* are af- fected. In fome kinds of this difeafe, feveral forts of blue fpots appear all at once. And this is *fcorbutus lentus feu frigidus*, the flow or cold fcurvy. But before we proceed to the hot fcurvy, of which there is but one fin- gle fpecies, it may be proper to diftinguifh the different kinds of cold fcurvies.

The firft is what occafions large, black, and blue *vibices*, or fpots, on the legs and joints; fometimes on the breaft and back, not unufually on one or both eye- lids, and on the white of the eye; which appears fwell- ed, and of a deep red colour; upon which enfues an *ophthalmia*, and afterwards the *chemofis lenta*. The gums are greatly fwelled, difcoloured, and very lax or fpungy; and when preffed, difcharge either a yellow ill- fcented blood, or matter. The parotid glands are alfo u- fually much enlarged. This fpecies, proceeding from a remarkable refolution of the red globules of the blood, is denominated *fcorbutus lividus vel livefcens*, a livid fcur- vy; being the only fpecies that is accompanied with partly dark, reddifh, and livid ftreaks, upon the fkin. The patient is feverifh, and the pains are very violent. It occurred moftly at *Wiburg, ann.* 1732; and again at *Peterfburg, ann.* 1733.

In the fecond fpecies, the red globules of the blood are not fo much refolved; it proceeding chiefly from a vifcidity of the lymphatic or ferous parts of the blood. The fpots appear of a deep red, turning afterwards to a darkifh yellow; being very fmall, fo as to refemble fmall peas, flea-bites, or *petechiæ*; and are difcovered no where elfe but on the fhins and ancles, attended with a forenefs in the fkin. Sometimes reddifh blue *vibices* appear upon the knee, and in the ham; the pain and fwelling there, as alfo the quicknefs of the pulfe, being always increa- fed, in proportion to the rednefs of thefe *fugillationes*.

The

The gums are not fo lax as in the former fpecies : the
upper part of them, however, is more excoriated.   On
the infide of the cheeks are obferved fwellings, fometimes hard, knotty, and wart-like, at other times fungous ;   and fometimes a uniform fungous fubftance extends itfelf even to the back part of the mouth.   This
fpecies, from the form of the fpots, is denominated a *len-*
ticular or *petechial fcurvy.*   The patient fpits more, and
the breath is more fœtid, than in any other fpecies.
Sometimes the temporal mufcle is fwelled and hardened
under the zigomatic procefs ; but the parotid glands never are.   It fhewed itfelf, *ann.* 1732, at *Wiburg,* only
here and there ; but afflicted much greater numbers, *ann.*
1737, in the intrenchments at *Uft-Samara.*

A third fpecies of this difeafe proceeds from a corruption of the fat or oily particles of the blood.   There
being no vifcidity either of its ferous or grumous parts,
there are confequently no fpots.   On the contrary, an u-
niverfal pale fwelling covers the body ;   which becomes
of a yellowifh colour, when thefe oily particles turn rancid.   When the fat affumes a hardnefs like tallow, the
thighs and arms are prodigioufly fwelled and indurated ;
and true *tophi* appear on the hands and fhins.   Now,
in this fpecies the ferous parts of the blood become much
more eafily and quickly vapid than in the others, and the
faline particles daily more and more acrimonious.   Hence
the cheeks are more fwelled, the knees more violently
contracted, the teeth loofer, and the gums much more
lax and rotten.   Sometimes a fungous flefh rifes at the
angle of the lower jaw, and the jaws are locked either
with or without an induration of the parotid gland, *cro-*
taphite or *maffeter* mufcles.   When this inert vapid *ferum*
is accumulated in the *tunica cellulofa,* an *anafarca* is induced ; when within the fubftance of the lungs, an afthma, upon which a true *hydrops pectoris* enfues ; when
in the lower belly, an *afcites per infiltrationem*; and when
in the glands of the guts, a *diarrhœa.*   When this vapid

ferum, by addition of oily and faline particles, has acquired an acrimony, it occafions the moft violent and gnawing pains in different parts of the body. Whereever it corrupts, the pains become there altogether intolerable, chiefly upon thofe parts where the ribs are articulated with the *fternum*; part of the bones of which may be taken out quite carious. It alfo produces a fpafmodic fuffocative afthma, a colliquative painful *diarrhœa,* and afterwards a gangrene of the cheeks, or an incurable *afcites.* This fpecies is of longer duration than any other, continuing often the whole fummer, until late in autumn. And as it is accompanied with no fpots, it may be denominated the *pale fcurvy*; but when the fat is thick. and vifcous, the *mucous pale fcurvy*; when it is become rancid, the *rancefcent fcurvy*; or when hard, and tallow-like, the *tophaceous fcurvy*; laftly, when the juices are very fharp, the *muriatic fcurvy.* In this fpecies the author faw great numbers of patients before *Afoph,* and in the general field-hofpital at St *Anne*; as alfo in the *Neifter* campaign: He obferved the tophaceous firft in *Finland,* at *Borgo, ann.* 1742; and the muriatic, where the cartilages of the ribs were really feparated from the *fternum (g),* as was plainly to be feen and felt, at the field-hofpital at *Abo, ann.* 1743.

These are the chief kinds of the flow fcurvy, which occurred in the *Ruffian* armies, and fell under the author's obfervation. There is indeed yet another fpecies of it, proceeding from a total refolution of the grumous parts of the blood; which occafions an extraordinary weaknefs and rednefs of the body, tumified pendulous cheeks, a deep cachexy, extremely ftinking, fungous, putrid, and purulent gums, contracted knees, &c. But this he never obferved, except in the intrenchments of *Uft-Samara.*

Thus much of the cold fcurvy. There remains the

(g) Cafes fimilar to thofe at *Paris.* Vid. diffections, part 2. cap. 7.

moft

moft oppofite branch of this difeafe, *viz.* the *hot* and *painful jcurvy.* It is diftinguifhed from the former, *1ft,* By there being no repletion or fwelling of the body; oir the contrary, there is rather a decay or wafting *(h).* 2*dly,* The gums are neither fo fungous nor fœtid; they are rather much fwelled, very hot, and fo painful, that the gentleft touch gives agony. 3*dly,* The pains are not fo fixed as in the cold fcurvy. The patient makes continual complaints, fighing and bemoaning his condition; and has a conftant, though irregular, fever. The pains fly from one member to another; fometimes from the back to the whole or half of the head, teeth, and neck; where, after occafioning the moft exquifite torture, they again inftantly attack the outfide or infide of the *thorax,* occafioning extreme oppreffion, ftitches, *&c.* : afterwards, feating themfelves in the *abdomen,* they produce colics, nephritic pains *(i),* and ftoppage of urine, and on the extremities all forts of convulfive contractions. 4*thly,* The knees are extremely rigid and contracted: but, unlefs it has been occafioned by fome outward accident, they are not fo much fwelled or inflamed as in the cold fcurvy. 5*thly,* No fpots are feen. 6*thly,* The principal difference lies in the urine: for in the livid and petechial fcurvies, though the urine is of a deep red, and undergoes little alteration by ftanding; yet this hot fpecies is diftinguifhed from them, by the fever which ac-

(*h*) Vid. part 2. p. 339.
(*i*) Vid. *Sinop.* part 3. p. 413. By the account of northern writers, it would feem, that venereal difeafes do not fo readily yield to mercurial medicines as they do in warmer climates. *Sinopeus* tells us, that he found great difficulty to cure even a common *gonorrhœa* at *Cronftadt.* And as for the pox, except it was very recent, the taint could not be fubdued by repeated falivations: for the difeafe generally broke out again, always in the fpring, together with the fcurvy; the latter feeming conftantly to awake any fparks of the venereal poifon lurking in the body. During a fcorbutic conftitution, thofe who, for venereal complaints, underwent a flight falivation, fell into a dreadful fcurvy; which being removed, left a worfe *lues* behind it.

companies

companies it; and the thick fandy fediment in the urine, which has a thin, white, greafy film a-top. This hot fcurvy he has remarked here and there; yet he no where faw more patients labouring under it than at *Wiburg*.

It may not be amifs to defcribe the various caufes which produced this calamity, in the order in which they occurred.

1*ft*, As to the fiege of *Afoph :* This place was attacked in the fpring *ann.* 1736, in very piercing cold weather, accompanied with frequent rain, fleet, and fometimes with fnow. And as there were no woods in the neighbourhood, the troops fuffered extremely, during this rigorous feafon, for want of firing. Nor did the regiments fare better who were ordered to join us; as moft of them were obliged to begin a long journey by land, upon a very fhort warning; or were tranfported in boats down the *Don*, together with the artillery, from the garrifon of *Nova Pawloffſky*, and the adjacent places. Now, as this fiege, by various accidents, was protracted three months, the inconveniencies and hardfhips which the troops fuffered, were extremely great. 1*ft*, The weather became exceffive hot; and was quite unfupportable during fun-fhine, and on ferene days. 2*dly*, We had a great deal of moift rainy weather; which greatly incommoded our army, which was incamped on flippery and hilly ground; as alfo the fick in their tents who were ill attended; their tents being alfo ill contrived. 3*dly*, Sicknefs was occafioned by the too frequent eating of fifh ill dreffed, with which the plentiful river *Don* abounds. 4*thly*, The bread was ill baked, for want of fewel. 5*thly*, The water was very impure, being taken up from the fordable parts of the *Don*, which became every day worfe and worfe. To which may be added, the preceding camp-diforders, *viz. diarrhœas*, and obftinate quartans; befides the paffions of the mind raging in the breafts of the foldiers, *viz.* difappointments, revenge,

revenge, anger, difcontent, *&c.* and the great fatigues they underwent.

As to what regards the fortrefs of *St Anne*; though the ground about it rifes pretty high, yet it lies fo low with refpect to *Great* and *Small Ruffia*, that it is from thence annually overflowed, generally in the month of *April*, for thirty verfts around, upon the break-ing loofe of the ice and fnow. The country about it appears like a great fea; and many parts within the for-trefs are funk feveral feet below water. This inunda-tion of the *Don* brings along with it an incredible num-ber of excellent and very fat fifh; which were fold ex-ceffively cheap, and eat in immoderate quantities, either frefh or dried. During the inundation, the air is very raw, cold, and windy. At the time of its drying up, the days are exceffively hot; and the fun is fcorching, when the weather is fair; but the nights, on the contra-ry, are intolerably cold, with a foggy moift air. As the moraffes dry up, and the remaining fifh (efpecially cray-fifh, of which there is an aftonifhing quantity left behind) begin to putrify, the air becomes more ftinking; and fo thick, that it is feveral hours every morning, before the fun has power to diffipate the noxious vapour. Upon the retiring of the flood, the ground fhews a fandy bot-tom, and is formed into little iflands and banks of fand, furrounded with fords filled with ftagnating water. What was drank, was often not taken where the ftream was quick and deep, but in fuch fords where it was muddy and greafy. The fifh remaining behind, were eat in im-moderate quantities ill dreffed. The barracks were built on morafs, damp ground, and too low. Laftly, The foldiers being the only inhabitants of the garrifon, were obliged to ftand every day up to their middle in water, in order to unload the neceffary wood; which is always fent them for fewel and building from the *Ukraine*.

The principal reafon why, of thofe regiments who marched to *Oczakow*, fuch a confiderable number were

attacked

attacked by the fcurvy, and brought into the hofpital at
Cobilack, was, the exceffive fatigues they underwent
through the whole winter, partly in cutting open the ice
of the *Neiper*, to prevent the incurfions of the *Tartars*;
and partly in performing other hard and fevere military
duties, either in ftormy fleety weather, or during exceffive froft and cold, without having proper conveniencies, lodgings, or diet. Even thofe who underwent
no fatigue, being afflicted with ailments of different forts,
for want of fufficient attendance, reft, and quiet, in the
army, became alfo fcorbutic.

As to what regards the great number of fcorbutic patients, which occurred not only during the march of the
army from *Oczakow*, but alfo during the *Neifter* campaign; the author treats only of the latter, as having
been there in perfon; and becaufe, according to his
beft information, the occafions and caufes of the malady
in both differed very little, or rather not at all.

The moft part of the recruits required to complete
the army, joined them feldom fooner than when either the
army was ready to march, or was actually in motion.
And though they were generally young raw fellows, exceffively fatigued after a long and tedious journey; yet
it was not poffible to grant them any reft or neceffary
refrefhment. They were directly incorporated into the
refpective regiments; and entered at once upon a new
way of life, *viz.* of conftant difquiet, military hardfhips and feverities, and of great fatigue. The marches
were begun early in the morning, often during thick
fogs and dews, heavy rains, or fevere cold. Towards
the middle of the day, they were oppreffed either with
intolerable fcorching heat, and clouds of duft, or with
much rain. The march was protracted for the moft
part till noon, and often beyond that time, according as
water, wood, and forage, were to be met with in thofe
defart places. Thus the poor foldier, after a fatiguing
journey, either quite enfeebled by the exceffive heat of
the

the fun, or drenched in rain, arrived at laft at the camp.
But often, even here, no reft could be permitted him. He
was obliged, according as it was his tour, to go upon the
piquets, *tabunen*, or the centinel's duty.   Another great
hardfhip was the want of good and clean water upon the
roads.   Overcome by the exceffive heat, fome threw
themfelves naked into every dirty muddy pond they met;
while others endeavoured to quench their violent drought,
occafioned by the duft and fun, by greedily drinking up
every drop of filthy ftagnating water they faw upon the
ground.   This bred many difeafes, efpecially continual
inflammatory fevers, &c.   Plethoric habits were attacked with apoplectic fits; which if not removed by immediate blood-letting, they quickly expired.   Their
blood was fo inflamed, that it came out as thick as pitch.
But the hardfhips which the fick underwent, were ftill
greater.   They were by moft regiments carried in open
carts, expofed to all the inclemencies of the climate and
weather, *viz.* to rain, duft, and wind, heat and cold.
In paffing the defiles, being generally the laft, it was always feveral hours before they arrived in camp after their
regiments; notwithftanding on the marching-days they
fet out early in the morning, long before the reft of the
army; and after having been quite foaked in rain in
their carts, were then taken out, and laid upon their bed
ftretched out under moift canvas, upon the cold wet ground.
Nor, in fuch afflicting circumftances for the fick, was it
a fmall addition to their mifery, that, in this defolate and
uninhabited country, proper food and drink could not be
procured, in order to reftore them to health and ftrength.
Hence it is not to be wondered at, that from fuch caufes, as alfo by reafon of the great preceding ficknefs
and fevers in the camp, (which, for want of conveniencies and proper treatment, were brought to no perfect
crifis), the fcurvy raged with fuch uncommon deftruction.

It is, however, remarkable, that this evil was greatly
prevented in the *Chocim* campaign, *ann.* 1739, by fending

ing the recruits much earlier; fo that they had fufficient time to be refrefhed after their journey, and were accuftomed a little to the military life and diet before they marched : as alfo by every regiment's being provided with four covered waggons for their fick; by which they were at all times fheltered from rain, duft, wind, and weather. The happy effect of thofe excellent regulations was, that in a whole divifion, confifting of ten or twelve regiments, we had fcarcely as many fcorbutic cafes as occurred in the former campaign in one regiment only; and then again an incredible lefs number died. For his method of cure, fee his account of the fcurvy at *Wiburg*, p. 407.

A voyage round the world, in the years 1740, 41, 42, 43, 44, *by* George Anfon, *Efq; now Lord* Anfon, *commander in chief of a fquadron of his Majefty's fhips, fent upon an expedition to the South feas.   Compiled from his papers and materials,* by Richard Walter, *M. A. &c.*   1748.

Soon after our paffing ftraits *Le Maire,* the fcurvy began to make its appearance amongft us : and our long continuance at fea, the fatigue we underwent, and the various difappointments we met with, had occafioned its fpreading to fuch a degree, that, at the latter end of *April,* there were but few on board who were not in fome degree afflicted with it; and in that month no lefs than forty-three died of it on board the *Centurion.*   But tho' we thought, that the diftemper had then rifen to an extraordinary height; and were willing to hope, that as we advanced to the northward, its malignity would abate : yet we found, on the contrary, that, in the month of *May*, we loft near double that number.   And as we did not get to land till the middle of *June,* the mortality went on increafing; fo that, after the lofs of above 200 men, we could not at laft mufter more than fix foremaft men in a watch, capable of duty.

This difeafe, fo frequently attending all long voyages,

3 I   and

and so particularly destructive to us, is surely the most singular and unaccountable of any that affects the human body. Its symptoms are unconstant and innumerable, and its progress and effects extremely irregular: for scarcely any two persons have the same complaints; and where there hath been found some conformity in the symptoms, the order of their appearance has been totally different. However, though it frequently puts on the form of many other diseases, and is therefore not to be described by any exclusive and infallible criterions; yet there are some symptoms which are more general than the rest, and occurring the oftenest, deserve a more particular enumeration. These common appearances are, large discoloured spots dispersed over the whole surface of the body; swelled legs; putrid gums; and, above all, an extraordinary lassitude of the whole body, especially after any exercise, however inconsiderable: and this lassitude at last degenerates into a proneness to swoon, on the least exertion of strength, or even on the least motion. This disease is likewise usually attended with a strange dejection of spirits; and with shiverings, tremblings, and a disposition to be seized with the most dreadful terrors, on the slightest accident. Indeed it was most remarkable, in all our reiterated experience of this malady, that whatever discouraged our people, or at any time damped their hopes, never failed to add new vigour to the distemper: for it usually killed those who were in the last stages of it, and confined those to their hammocks who were before capable of some kind of duty. So that it seemed, as if alacrity of mind, and sanguine thoughts, were no contemptible preservatives from its fatal malignity.

But it is not easy to complete the long roll of the various concomitants of this disease. For it often produced putrid fevers, pleurisies, the jaundice, and violent rheumatic pains. And sometimes it occasioned an obstinate costiveness; which was generally attended with a difficulty

of

of breathing; and this was efteemed the moft deadly of all the fcorbutic fymptoms. At other times the whole body, but more efpecially the legs, were fubject to ulcers of the worft kind, attended with rotten bones, and fuch a luxuriancy of fungous flefh as yielded to no remedy. But a moft extraordinary circumftance, and what would be fcarcely credible upon any fingle evidence, is, that the fcars of wounds which had been for many years healed, were forced open again by this virulent diftemper. Of this there was a remarkable inftance in one of the invalids on board the *Centurion,* who had been wounded above fifty years before at the battle of the *Boyne:* for though he was cured foon after, and had continued well for a great number of years paft; yet, on his being attacked by the fcurvy, his wounds, in the progrefs of his difeafe, broke out afrefh, and appeared as if they had never been healed. Nay, what is ftill more aftonifhing, the callous of a broken bone, which had been compleatly formed for a long time, was found to be hereby diffolved; and the fracture feemed as if it had never been confolidated. Indeed, the effects of this difeafe were in almoft every inftance wonderful. For many of our people, though confined to their hammocks, appeared to have no inconfiderable fhare of health; for they eat and drank heartily, were chearful, and talked with much feeming vigour, and with a loud ftrong tone of voice; and yet on their being the leaft moved, tho' it was only from one part of the fhip to the other, and that in their hammocks, they have immediately expired. And others, who have confided in their feeming ftrength, and have refolved to get out of their hammocks, have died before they could well reach the deck. And it was no uncommon thing for thofe who could do fome kind of duty, and walk the deck, to drop down dead in an inftant, on any endeavours to act with their utmoft vigour; many of our people having perifhed in this manner, during the courfe of this voyage.

Upon

Upon arriving at the ifland of *Juan Fernandes,* 167 fick perfons were put on fhore, befides at leaft a dozen who died in the boats, on their being expofed to the frefh air. The extreme weaknefs of the fick may be collected from the numbers who died after they got on fhore: for it had generally been found, that the land, and the refrefhments it produces, very foon recover moft ftages of the fea-fcurvy; yet it was near twenty days after their landing, before the mortality was tolerably ceafed: and for the firft ten or twelve days, they buried rarely lefs than fix each day; and many of thofe who furvived, recovered by very flow and infenfible degrees. Indeed thofe who were well enough, at their firft getting on fhore, to creep out of their tents, and crawl about, were foon relieved, and recovered their health and ftrength in a very fhort time; but in the reft, the difeafe feemed to have acquired a degree of inveteracy altogether without example.

It was very remarkable what happened to the *Gloucefter,* which, like the other fhips in that fquadron, had fuffered the moft unparallelled hardfhips, and buried three fourths of her crew in this difeafe; that, upon landing the remainder of her fick, lefs than eighty in number, very few of them died. Whether it was, (as the ingenious author obferves), that the fartheft advanced in the diftemper were already dead, or the greens and frefh provifions fent on board them when plying off that ifland, had prepared thofe who remained for a fpeedy recovery; their fick, however, in general, got much fooner well than the *Centurion*'s crew.

The havock which this dreadful calamity made in thofe fhips, was truly furprifing. The *Centurion,* from her leaving *England,* when at this ifland, had buried 292 men, and had but 214 remaining of her complement. The *Gloucefter,* out of a fmaller complement, buried the fame number, and had only 82 alive. This dreadful mortality had fallen feverer on the invalids

lids and marines than on the failors: for on board the
Centurion, out of fifty invalids, and feventy-nine marines, there remained only four invalids, including officers, and eleven marines; and on board the *Gloucefter*,
every invalid died, and only two marines efcaped out of
forty-eight.

In lefs, however, than feven weeks after leaving the
coaft of *Mexico*, having continued in perfect health for
a confiderable time before, this fatal difeafe broke out
again amongft them.   Upon which occafion, the ingenious author makes the following remarks.

Some amongft us were willing to believe, that in this
warm climate the violence of the difeafe, and its fatality,
might be in fome degree mitigated.   But the ravage of
the diftemper at that time convinced them of the falfity
of this fpeculation; as it likewife exploded other opinions about the caufe and nature of this difeafe.   For it
has been generally prefumed, that plenty of water,
and of frefh provifions, are effectual preventives of
this malady.   But it happened in the prefent cafe, we had
a confiderable ftock of frefh provifions on board, being
the hogs and fowls taken at *Paita*.   We befides, almoft
daily, caught great abundance of bonito's, dolphins,
and albicores: and the unfettled feafon having proved
extremely rainy, fupplied us with plenty of water; fo
that each man had five pints a-day during the paffage.
But notwithftanding this plenty of water, and frefh
provifions diftributed among the fick, and the whole
crew often fed upon fifh; yet neither were the fick
hereby relieved, nor the progrefs and advancement of
the difeafe retarded.   It has likewife been believed by
many, that keeping the fhip clean and airy betwixt decks,
might prevent, or at leaft mitigate the fcurvy: yet we
obferved, during the latter part of our run, that, though
we kept all our ports open, and took uncommon pains in
fweetening and cleanfing the fhips; yet neither the progrefs,

greſs, nor the virulence of the diſeaſe were thereby ſenſibly abated. The ſurgeon at this time having declared, that all his meaſures were totally ineffectual for the relief of his patients, it was reſolved to try the effects of *Ward*'s drop and pill; and one, or both of them, at different times, were given to perſons in every ſtage of the diſtemper. Out of the numbers who took them, one, ſoon after ſwallowing the pill, was ſeized with a violent bleeding at the noſe. He was before given over by the ſurgeon, and lay almoſt at the point of death; but he immediately found himſelf much better, and continued to recover, though ſlowly, till we arrived on ſhore near a fortnight after. A few others were relieved for ſome days. But the diſeaſe returned again with as much virulence as ever; though neither did theſe, nor the reſt who received no benefit, appear to be reduced to a worſe condition than they would have been if they had taken nothing. The moſt remarkable property of theſe medicines in almoſt every one that took them, was, that they operated in proportion to the vigour of the patient. So that thoſe who were within two or three days of dying, were ſcarcely affected; and as the patient was differently advanced in the diſeaſe, the operation was either a gentle perſpiration, an eaſy vomit, or a moderate purge. But if they were taken by one in full ſtrength, they then produced all the before mentioned effects with conſiderable violence; which ſometimes continued for ſix or eight hours together with little intermiſſion. Upon their arrival at *Tinian*, they ſoon began to feel the ſalutary influence of the land: for though they had buried in two days before twenty-one men, yet they did not loſe above ten more from the day after they were landed; and reaped ſo much benefit from the fruits of the iſland, particularly thoſe of the acid kind, that in a week's time there were but few of them who were not ſo far recovered as to be able to move about without help.

A

1748.

A voyage to Hudfon's-bay, *by the* Dobbs galley, *and* California, *in the years* 1746 *and* 1747, *for difcovering a north-weſt paſſage. By* Henry Ellis.

The bringing two caſks of brandy from *York*-fort for our *Chriſtmas* cheer, was attended with fatal confequences. The people had been healthy enough before this feafon of mirth came; but indulging themfelves too freely, they were foon invaded by the fcurvy, the conftant attendant on the ufe of fpirituous liquors. It is a melancholy, but withal a neceſſary taſk, to defcribe the progreſs of this foul and fatal diftemper. Our men, when firſt feized with it, began to droop, to grow heavy, liſtleſs, and at length indolent, to the laſt degree: a tightneſs in the cheſt, pains in the breaſt, and a great difficulty in breathing followed; then enfued livid fpots upon the thighs, fwelled legs, contraction of the limbs, putrid gums, teeth loofe, a coagulation of blood upon and near the back-bone, with countenances bloated and fallow; thefe fymptoms continually increafing, till at length death carried them off, either by a flux or a dropfy. Thofe medicines which in other countries are generally ufed with good effects, proved entirely ineffectual here. For unctions and fomentations, when applied to contracted limbs, afforded no relief: frefh provifions, indeed, when we could get them, did fomewhat. But the only powerful and prevailing medicine, was tar-water; and the fteady ufe of this faved many, even after the difeafe was far advanced, when all other medicines loft their efficacy, and were tried to no purpofe. As far as we could obferve, this falutary drink operated no other way than by urine *(k)*.

An

(k) Upon this relation, I muſt beg leave to obferve, that though the immoderate ufe of fpirits had certainly pernicious effects; yet the feverity of the winter, their being denied proper refrefhments from the *Engliſh* forts, and particularly, in fuch circumſtances, a want of greens and herbage, which do not feem to have appeared on the ground

1749. *An historical account of a new method for extracting the foul air out of ships, &c. with the description and draught of the machines by which it is performed; by Sa-muel Sutton, the inventor. To which are annexed, Two relations given thereof to the Royal society, by Dr Mead, and Mr* Watson; *and, A discourse on the scurvy, by Dr* Mead. Ejusdem monit. et præcept. medic. cap. 16. de scorbuto.

The learned author very justly describes the most es-sential symptoms of the scurvy. He imagines the air even more than any other agent concerned in bringing on this calamity. How the sea-air acquires such noxious qua-lities, he accounts for in the following manner. In the first place, moisture weakens its spring; next a combina-tion of foul particles, such as are contained in the breath of many persons crouded together, and some perhaps diseased; then the filthiness of water stagnating in the bottom of the ship; lastly, salts imbibed from the sea, some of which may probably have proceeded from pu-trified animals in that element, may insinuate them-selves into the blood, and, in the nature of a fer-ment, corrupt its whole mass. Other causes, as bad diet, *&c.* concur to breed the disease. For the preven-tion of it, he recommends the use of Mr *Lowndes's* salt

ground till towards the latter end of *March,* p. 204, were what principally occasioned the disease. As he very justly accounts for its return upon their passage home, p. 281. where he says, "The "uncomfortable weather we had, made so chiefly by the thick "and noisome fogs, proved the cause that many of our people be-"gan now to relapse into their old distemper, the scurvy." As to the good effects ascribed to the tar-water while at *Port-Nelson;* it were to be wished, both in this and many other relations of the effects of medicines in this disease, that we had always been inform-ed what other regimen the patients underwent, particularly as to their diet and lodgings. The mortality from this disease seems to have been increased in the latter end of *January;* and in the latter end of *March* several were in a bad way. Some likewise died of it on their passage home; which could not be for want of this me-dicine on board a ship, which has been often tried at sea.

made

made from brine, as preferable for falting provifions, both flefh and fifh, to that made from fea-water, even to the bay-falt; would have ftock-fifh ufed at fea, which is dried without any falt, inftead of falt fifh; and thinks, that the *Dutch gort*, which (as he had been informed) is a kind of barley ground, is not fo hot and drying as oat-meal. Wine-vinegar is likewife a proper prefervative. He obferves, that the difeafe is cured by vegetables, and land-air; and that hotter and colder vegetables, when mixed, qualify each other, efpecially as the acid fruits in Lord *Anfon*'s voyage were found of moft benefit. Milk of all forts, and its whey, when it can be had, are proper antifcorbutic food and phyfic. But as the defign of this difcourfe is principally to demonftrate the ufefulnefs of *Sutton*'s machine, he particularly infifts upon the advantage that might reafonably be expected from it. The book indeed contains feveral indifputable teftimonies of the ufefulnefs of thefe pipes; the operation of which is accounted for by the Doctor and Mr *Watfon.*

De tabe glandulari, five de ufu aquæ marinæ in morbis 1750. *glandularum, differtatio. Auctore Ricardo Ruffel, M. D.*

The ufe of fea-water would be very beneficial to failors in bilious colics, both to prevent the difeafe, and its return after the cure. This latter is to be effected by a *femicupium,* and purging falts, after the inflammation has been removed by plentiful bleeding. In his letter to Dr *Lee,* he obferves, that, after taking into ferious confideration the cafe of that fcorbutic putrefaction which afflicts feamen, he finds, that it is falfely afcribed to their falt provifions. Salt not only preferves meat from corruption, but mariners alfo from that corrupt ftate. This is confirmed, by remarking the ftrength and good ftate of health which poor country-people enjoy whilft living upon the fame food as feamen. Thus there are many in every country who have lived, perhaps

for

for thirty years, altogether upon falt beef, bacon, and coarfe puddings, unlefs upon a high holiday, when they are fometimes regaled with a bit of frefh meat; and yet continue perfectly healthy and ftrong. So that the difference between thofe people and feamen lies only in this, that the latter have not the benefit of fo much exercife, and live in a moift air, by which the tone of their fibres is relaxed, and perfpiration ftopt.

1750.   *An effay on fevers*, &c. *By Dr* John Huxham. *Appendix, A method for preferving the health of feamen in long cruifes and voyages.*

He thinks the fcurvy at fea owing to bad provifions, bad water, bad beer, &c. The pernicious effects of which will be confiderably augmented by living in a moift, falt atmofphere, and breathing the foul air betwixt decks. The moft effectual way of correcting this alcalefcent acrimony in the blood, is by vegetable and mineral acids: and for that purpofe he particularly recommends cyder; of which each failor fhould have at leaft a pint a-day.

1752.   *A differtation on quick-lime and lime-water. By Dr* Ch. Alfton.

The Doctor informs us, that he publifhed this paper chiefly for the ufe of mariners. He attributes the good effects of lime-water in putrid fcurvies, and fome other difeafes, not fo much to an antifeptic virtue, (which it is poffeffed of), as to its penetrating, detergent, and diuretic qualities. He has difcovered, that lime prevents the corruption of water, or infects breeding in it; and thinks this water will be ufeful in curing the difeafes to which fea-faring people are moft fubject. One pound of frefh well-burnt quick-lime of any kind, is enough to be put in a hogfhead of water; and this may be ufed, not only for common drink by the difeafed, or for prevention by the healthy; but alfo by boiling, and expofing it to the air for a fhort time, it will become, after long keeping,
fweet

fweet and wholfome water.   When lime-water, by
ftanding expofed for fome time to the air, has thrown up
all its crufts, none of the qualities of lime-water remain
in it.   From the notable quality he found in quick-lime
to prevent water from corrupting, he often thought,
that fome of it put in the fhip's well would effectually
prevent the corruption of the water there, and confequently the putrid fteams or foul air arifing from thence.
All thefe experiments are fafe, eafy, and attended with
no expence.

An effay on the fea-fcurvy: wherein is propofed an eafy 1753.
method of curing that diftemper at fea, and of preferving
water fweet for any cruife or voyage.   By Dr Anthony
Addington.

The defcription of the difeafe is borrowed from *Cock-*
burn, Boerhaave, Hoffman, Eugalenus, Lord *Anfon*'s voyage, *&c.* The cure propofed at fea, is to be begun, if there
be any marks of fulnefs, by blood-letting.   This is recommended upon the authority of *Hoffman, Boerhaave,*
Sennertus, and *Bruceus,* as alfo *Eugalenus.*   In order
to leffen the quantity of redundant blood ftill more, the
patient is afterwards to be put under a courfe of gentle
and daily purgation, with fea-water.   *Boerhaave,* without any reftriction to the habit of the patient, gives us
the greateft expectations from a moderate and protracted
courfe of purging in the fcurvy; and *Hoffman* fpeaks to
the fame purpofe.   But where there are marks of virulence in the fcurvy, it will be loft labour to rely on
fimple fea-water, unaffifted with any other antiputrid medicine.   So if, in conjunction with that water, we make
a prudent ufe of the fpirit of fea-falt, we fhall but feldom be difappointed in our hopes of a cure.   This is
that fafe and effectual corrector, which will counteract
the putrifying quality of rock and bay falt, when they
have been taken in fuch large quantities as to occafion
the fcurvy.   Twenty drops of this fpirit taken every day,

will probably fucceed with moſt patients. Five of them are to be given in the fea-water every morning, and the remainder at any other times in freſh water: to a pint of which, ten drops will impart an agreeable acidity. When the veſſels have been pretty well unloaded by the purgation with ſalt-water, and the bad ſymptoms begin to decline, the patient (with ſome exceptions) is to be bathed every morning in the fea juſt before he drinks his water. Sea-water is alſo to be uſed externally, where there are ulcers on the gums and legs, or rotten bones. To give the greateſt ſanction that can be given to the outward application of fea-water in ſcorbutic ulcers, it is adviſed for them by *Hippocrates*. In ſcorbutic fluxes, mortifications, and hæmorrhages, the ſalt water is to be omitted. The moſt probable way to remove the laſt ſymptom, is, to bleed the patient as often and as much as his ſtrength and age will permit; to open the belly, if coſtive, by glyſters; and to oblige him to live entirely on the unfermented farines, and to drink freely of water ſoftened with *gum. Arabic.* and ſtrongly acidulated with *ſp. ſalis.* About an ounce and a half of ſpirit of ſalt to a tun of water, will preſerve it from corrupting.

APPEN.

A P P E N D I X.

IT has been no eafy matter to obtain a knowledge of the many writings on this diftemper. There have been collections made from time to time, of the feveral authors on the plague, venereal difeafe, &c.; but no fuch have been compiled of writers on the fcurvy. *Sennertus, ann.* 1624, when he wrote his own treatife, reprinted the writings of *Solomon Albertus* and *Martini*, together with *Ronffeus,* and the authors which he had publifhed *ann.* 1583, *viz. Echthius, Wierus,* and *Langius* ; and this book, containing thofe feven authors, is the only collection ever publifhed of writers on the fcurvy. There was here as little affiftance to be obtained from medical *bibliothecæ. Lipenius,* in his *Bibliotheca realis medica,* publifhed *ann.* 1679, reckons up twenty-nine writings on this fubject, of which eight are academical difcourfes or difputations. *Mercklin,* in his *Cynofura meaica,* publifhed in the year 1686, enumerates twenty-four authors on the fcurvy. Of thefe, one, *viz. Henricus a Bra,* is claffed among them (though improperly) upon account of a letter written to *Foreftus,* upon a very different fubject (*a*). Another, *viz. Albertus,* he has by miftake inferted twice in his lift; and has given a place in it to *Jof. Stubendorfius* an editor of *Eugalenus, Simon Paulli, Joh. Langius, Arnold. Weickardus,* and *Ludov. Schmid* ; which three laft I have taken notice of in the *Bibliotheca,* though perhaps they are not deferving of it. He has befides included in it three academical difputations. The indefatigable Dr *Haller* publifhed *ann.* 1751, in his notes illuftrating *Boerhaave's Methodus ftudii medici,* the titles of almoft all medical

(*a*) *Vid. Forefti obferv. medicinal. lib.* 20. *obf.* 12.

writings

writings now extant, no lefs than 30,000 volumes. But it were to be wifhed, that fo good a judge had diftinguifhed fuch books as, not being able to maintain their character, are now out of print, or occafional pamphlets, and fome trifling academical orations and difputations, from writings of greater value.

The following lift contains the titles of fuch writings on the fcurvy, as have been omitted in the foregoing fheets, but are mentioned in thofe collections; and comprehends all that, after the moft diligent inquiry, have come to my knowledge; except a few academical difputations.

J. Roetenbeck und Cafp. Horns befchreibung des fcharboks. Nurnberg. 1633.

Chriftoph. Tinctorius de fcorbuto Pruffiæ jam frequenti. Regiom. 1639.

J. van Beverwyck van de Blaauw fchuyt. Dordrac 1642.

Henrici Botteri (b) tractatus de fcorbuto. Lubec 1646.

J. Schmids von der peft Frantzofen und fcharbock (c). Augfpurg. 1667.

Phil. Hæchftetteri (d) obfervationes medicinales raræ. Lip. 1674.

Hen. Cellarius bericht von fcharbock. Halberftatt 1675.

Jon. Zipfel vom fcharbock griesftein und podagra. Drefd. 1678.

Maitland on the fcurvy.

Melchioris Friccii differtatio de colica fcorbutica. Ulm 1696.

(b) Profeffor at *Cologne.* I have not feen his treatife; nor did *Haller.* I never found it fo much as quoted by any author, though it underwent two editions.

(c) I have feen the book; it contains nothing remarkable.

(d) A phyfician at *Augfburg. Decad.* 7. *caf.* 10. contains fome good obfervations on the fcurvy.

J. Humme!

J. Hummel de arthritide tam tartarea quàm scorbutica(e). Buding 1738.

Pierre Briscow traité du scorbut (f). Paris 1743.

Cadet dissertation sur le scorbut, avec des observations(f). Paris 1749.

Academical performances.

Jacob. Albini disputatio de scorbuto (g). Basil. 1620.

Abrahami Dreyeri disputatio de scorbuto (g). Basil. 1622.

Amb. Rhodii disputatio de scorbuto. Haffn. 1635.

Jac. Haberstro disp. inaug. de scorbuto. Jen. 1644.

Herm. Conringii disp. Resp. Behrens. Helmf. 1659.

Geo. Franci disp. Resp. Wyck. Heidelb. 1670.

And. Birch Angli disp. inaug. de scorbuto. Lugd. Bat. 1674.

Olai Borrichii disp. Resp. Joh. Melch. Sulzero. Haffn. 1675.

Caroli Patini (h) oratio de scorbuto. Patav. 1679.

Sam. Koeleser de Keresser de scorbuto Mediterraneo. Cibinii 1707.

G. Thiesen de morbo marino. Lugd. Bat. 1727.

Michaelis Alberti (i) disp. de scorbuto Daniæ non endemio. Hall. 1731.

Christoph. Mart. Burchard disp. de scorbuto maris Balthici accolis non endemio. Rostoch. 1735.

Sim. Pauli Hilscher (k) programma de scelotyrbe memorabili casu illustrata. Jen. 1747.

Mich. Law dissert. medic. inaug. de scorbuto. Edin. 1748.

(e) An indifferent character of it is given by *Haller.*

(f) These two *French* authors are now out of print, as would seem at *Paris.* I imagine the latter to have been an academical performance.

(g) Both are preserved in a collection of academical disputations, published by the bookseller *Genathius.*

(h) Professor at *Padua;* more celebrated for his other writings than this.

(i) Present professor of medicine at *Hall* in *Saxony.*

(k) Present professor at *Jena.*

A

A CHRONOLOGICAL INDEX

of medical authors who have written particular books on the scurvy; as also the principal systematic, and other medical writers, whose sentiments are delivered in this treatise.

1534. *Euritius Cordus*, a celebrated Botaniſt. He died ann. 1538.

1539. *Jo. Agricola (Ammon.)*, Profeſſor of Medicine, &c. at Ingolſtadt.

1541. *Jo. Echthius*, a phyſician at Cologn, by birth a Dutchman. He died *ann* 1554.

1560. *Jo Langius*, chief phyſician to the Elector Palatine.

1564. *Balduin. Ronſſeus*, ordinary phyſician to the city of Goude in Holland.

1567. *Jo. Wierus*, chief phyſician to the Duke of Cleves and Juliers.

    Adrian. Junius, an eminent phyſician and hiſtorian. He died *ann.* 1575.

1581. *Rembert. Dodonæus*, chief phyſician to the Emperor of Germany.

1589. *Hen Brucæus*, Profeſſor at Roſtock.

    Balthaſ Brunerus, chief phyſician to the Prince of Anhalt.

1593. *Solomon Albertus*, Profeſſor of Medicine at Wittenburg.

1595. *Petrus Foreſtus*, phyſician at Alcmaer, Profeſſor at Leyden, &c. (a).

1600.

(a) Beſides the above authors, it is taken notice of by ſeveral other medical writers in the ſixteenth century, viz. *Cornelius Gemma* (*Coſmocritic. lib.* 2. *cap.* 2.), *Petrus Pena* (*adverſar. ſtirpium, p.* 121. & 122.), *Schenckius* (*obſervat. medicinal.*), *Carrichterus* (*prax. Germanic. lib.* 1. *cap.* 41.), *Mithobius de peſte*, *Tabernæmon de thermis,*
Peucerus

Peucerus de morbis contagiofis, &c. There were likewife two *thefes*, or difputations, publifhed upon it; one by *Tweftrengk*, at *Bafil*, in the year 1581, and another by *Hambergerus*, at *Tubingen*, in the year 1586. One *Gul. Lemnius*, a *Zealander*, is faid to have wrote upon the fcurvy. He feems to have been a very trifling author, believing it to be the fame difeafe in man that the meafly diftemper is in hogs. It would appear from *Solomon Albertus*, that his performance was out of print in the year 1593.

(b) It was one of the moft celebrated faculties of medicine at that time in *Europe*; of which *Olaus Wormius*, two of the *Bartholines*, and *Simon Paulli*, were then members. The latter, who was phyfician to the King of *Denmark*, has ufually been ranked among the writers on the fcurvy, upon account of an appendix which he added, *ann.* 1660, to his *Digreffio de vera caufa febrium, &c.*

1662. *Balth Timæus*, chief phyſician to the Electon of Brandenburg

1663. *Valent. Andreas Moellenbrochius*, a phyſician of Erfurt.

1667. *Thomas Willis*, an Engliſh phyſician, Seidleian Profeſſor at Oxford.

1668. *Everard Maynwaringe*, a phyſician at London.

1669. *Paul. Barbette*, a Dutch phyſician.

1669. *Frederic. Deckers*, Profeſſor at Leyden.

1672. *Gualterus Charleton*, phyſician in ordinary to his Majeſty King Charles II.

1672. *Herman. Nicolai*, a Dane.

1674. *Franciſcus Deleboe Sylvius*, Profeſſor at Leyden.

1675. *Gideon Harvey*, phyſician in ordinary to his Majeſty King Charles II.

1676. *Bernard. Below*, phyſician to the King of Sweden.

1681. *Abraham. Muntingius*, Profeſſor of Botany in Groningen.

1683. *L. Chameau*, a French phyſician.

1684. *Stephanus Blancardus*, a Dutch phyſician.

1684. *Jo. Dolæus*, chief phyſician, &c. to the Landgrave of Heſſe-Caſſel.

1685. *Michael Ettmullerus*, public Profeſſor in the univerſity of Leipſic.

Thomas Sydenham, the Engliſh Hippocrates.

1694. *Martin. Liſter*, an Engliſh phyſician.

1696. *William Cockburn*, phyſician to the Royal navy of G. Britain.

1699. *Franc. Poupart*, phyſician at Paris.

Arch Pitcairn, an eminent Scots phyſician.

1708. *Herman. Boerhaave*, the celebrated Leyden Profeſſor.

1712. *Jo Hen. de Heucher*, Profeſſor at Wittenburg.

1720. College of phyſicians at Vienna.

1734. *Jo. Freder. Bachſtrom*, a Dutch phyſician.

1734. *Damianus Sinopæus*, chief phyſician to the marine hoſpital at Cronſtadt.

1737

1737. *J. G. H. Kramer*, phyſician to the Imperial army in Hungary.
1739. *Frederic. Hoffmannus*, a celebrated author, Firſt
Profeſſor of Medicine at Hall in Saxony, &c.
1747. *Abraham Nitzſch*, phyſician to the Ruſſian army.
1749. The learned Dr *Richard Mead*, phyſician to his
preſent Britannic Majeſty, &c
1750. Dr *Richard Ruſſel*, phyſician at Lewes in Suſſex.
1750. Dr *John Huxham*, a celebrated phyſician at Plymouth.
1752. Dr *John Pringle*, Phyſician-General to the Bri-
tiſh army.
1752. Dr *Charles Alſton*, learned Profeſſor of Botany
and Medicine at Edinburgh.
1753. Dr *Anthony Addington*, phyſician at Reading.

An

An *Alphabetical Index of Authors*, &c.

Those who do not treat of the scurvy, are marked in Italic *characters.*

Authors are sometimes quoted in this treatise, without inserting the title of the book. In such cases, the pages in which the titles are mentioned, are here distinguished by being put within crotchets.

F I N I S.

Printed in the United States
By Bookmasters